Leadership and Change in Human Services

D0102982

For over forty years Wolf Wolfensberger has been a significant figure in the world of human services, especially in the field of learning disability. His work on normalization and Citizen Advocacy in the late 1960s and early 1970s has been acknowledged by supporters and critics alike to have been fundamental to developments in a number of countries, most notably his adopted country, the USA, Canada, Australasia and the UK. His further work in developing the theory of Social Role Valorization, the successor to normalization, and as a commentator on broader trends in society and their effects on vulnerable people and services for them has ensured his place as a major voice for values and the human worth of all people. Never afraid of controversy, his views have brought him into conflict with institutional vested interests and radical groups alike.

In *Leadership and Change in Human Services* David Race introduces the reader to Wolfensberger's key ideas through a series of extracts from his published work. Throughout the edited selection, the emphasis is on placing Wolfensberger's work in a contemporary context and examining its continuing relevance today. Including a comprehensive bibliography of Wolfensberger's written output, this Reader offers an invaluable source of reference to all those concerned with the recent history of human services.

David Race is a Lecturer in the School of Community, Health Sciences and Social Care, University of Salford.

Leadership and Change in Human Services

Selected readings from
Wolf Wolfensberger

Compiled and edited by
David G. Race

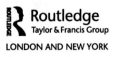
Routledge
Taylor & Francis Group

LONDON AND NEW YORK

First published 2003
by Routledge
2 Park Square, Milton Park, Abingdon, Oxon, OX14 4RN

Simultaneously published in the USA and Canada
by Routledge
270 Madison Ave, New York NY 10016

Routledge is an imprint of the Taylor & Francis Group

Transferred to Digital Printing 2010

Typeset in Times and Humanist by
HWA Text and Data Management Ltd, Tunbridge Wells

British Library Cataloguing in Publication Data
A catalogue record for this book is available from the British
Library

Library of Congress Cataloging in Publication Data
Wolfensberger, Wolf.
   Leadership and change in human services : selected readings
from Wolf Wolfensberger ; compiled and edited by
David G. Race
      p. cm.
   Selections from about 335 of Wolfensberger's publications
published over a span of 45 years, with comments and summary
statements by the editor.
   "Full bibliography of Wolf Wolfensberger": P. .
   Includes bibliographical references and index.
   1. Human services–Philosophy. 2. Social advocacy. 3. Social
role. 4. Marginality, Social. 5. People with mental disabilities–
Social conditions. 6. People with mental disabilities–Services
for–Moral and ethical aspects. I. Title.

HV40.W65 2003
364–dc21
                                                  2002037133

ISBN 0–415–30562–4 (hbk)
ISBN 0–415–30563–2 (pbk)

Contents

Foreword

Writers find it difficult to keep their writings in a proper and objective perspective. This is why I am greatly indebted to David Race for the enormous amount of work he did of looking at about 335 of my publications printed over a span of 45 years. I am very pleased with the way he has exercised his judgment on how to stay within the publisher's stipulation to keep the text to about 100,000 words, and yet include publications – or parts thereof – that might either still be of interest or relevance today, or that at least shed light upon the era in which they were produced.

Looking at the book overall it is clear that one could have read all the selections included in it, and more, over the years as separate items, either when they first came out or even later. But by having them organized in this way, by theme rather than chronologically, one can begin to see the body of work as a coherent whole rather than as its segmented parts.

Wolf Wolfensberger
Syracuse University
October 2002

Preface

The origins of this book came in an informal lunchtime meeting in the middle of a workshop given by Wolf Wolfensberger and his associates at Andover, Massachusetts, in March of 2001. That meeting contained the core of what became the planning group for the third international conference on Social Role Valorization, to be held in June 2003 at the University of Calgary in Canada. As someone who just happened to be at the lunch table, but who also had written some things in regard to Wolfensberger's work, my interest was aroused when the suggestion was made that a collection of his writings be prepared for the conference. Such a collection had been something I had hoped to become involved with prior to this meeting, and I was only too pleased to offer to take on the project.

After some exploratory work with potential publishers, I was sufficiently encouraged to visit Professor Wolfensberger at his Training Institute in Syracuse to draw up a 'long shortlist' of his writings for inclusion in the book. In discussion with Wolf Wolfensberger and Susan Thomas, key decisions regarding the shape of the book began to emerge. The first decision was between a collection of complete articles, or an edited selection, which would enable more to be included. Given the likely size of the book, the latter course was pursued.

The second, related, decision was whether the book should seek to be primarily for scholars, and aim at a chronological retrospective on Wolfensberger's work, with detail of sources, academic critiques, and considerable editorial comment on these; or whether it should be aimed at a wider audience, with a theme-based approach, leaving the ideas in the various extracts to 'speak for themselves.' Again, the likely size came into the picture, but also the fact that, as we shall see in the body of the book, Wolfensberger's influence has reached far beyond academia, and into the whole gamut of those influenced by, and involved with, human services. People who use services, their families, front-line service workers, advocates, service managers and planners, leaders and 'change agents' (to use Wolfensberger's own term); all have been affected in some way by one or more of the ideas that he has set in train in the course of 45 years.

The book is therefore an attempt to reach all of that audience – including the academics – with a clear laying out of the range of ideas and issues that have figured in Wolfensberger's writings. A number of themes emerged from the time at Syracuse, under which an initial selection could be made, and these were used to approach a publisher. The outline was sent to the publisher's referees, and some helpful suggestions as to the ordering of themes emerged. Work then commenced on a firmer outline, and my role of editor came into full force. The result was a smaller number of items than the original outline, but one which it is felt fulfils the aims of the book set out above. Throughout this process, the comments and suggestions from Wolf Wolfensberger and Susan Thomas have been both encouraging and invaluable, though naturally I take responsibility for the end product.

To enable the reader to be clear about the way the book is laid out, a brief note on format may be necessary. The book begins with a general Introduction, followed by seven chapters arranged around the themes found in the list of Contents. Each chapter has a brief editorial introduction, followed by comments and summary statements by the editor before and during each extract. All editorial comments and writing is in a sans serif font (as here), with Wolfensberger's writing in a serif font. Where editing has been carried out on any passages, the use of ellipses (...) indicates this. Titles and dates of extracts only are listed below the chapter headings in the list of Contents, with full reference details given before each extract in the body of the text, in the Acknowledgements and in the References. Because the extracts were originally published in a variety of countries, there will be some variation in the spelling and format conventions.

As well as those already mentioned, my thanks go to the various authors and publishers, listed separately, for their co-operation to enable me to use the extracts selected for the final version. In addition, I would like to thank Edwina Welham at Routledge, for her flexibility and willingness to back her judgement regarding this book.

Finally, I dedicate this book to my son Jonathan, for many hours spent scanning articles into our computer, despite the competing pressures of exams, courting, football and the pub. The world he and his three brothers now face, as vividly expounded in many parts of this book, is not a particularly pleasant one, and I hope they may come in time to reflect on some of the challenges that Wolfensberger's analysis raises. Whether they do so or not, I believe that their experiences of personal involvement with at least two vulnerable people will, as the last chapter hopes, better equip them to rise to those challenges.

David Race
October 2002

Acknowledgements

The editor and the publisher gratefully acknowledge the following bodies for their co-operation in the preparation of this book. The order of these acknowledgements and the lists within them is, except for the first, the same as the order in which the extracts appear in the book

Wolf Wolfensberger, and the Training Institute for Human Service Planning, Leadership and Change Agentry at Syracuse University

For general permission to select and edit all his publications, and for extracts from the following items published by the Training Institute, and/or in non-commercial publications or those with Dr Wolfensberger's individual copyright:

'The bad things that typically get done to devalued people, 1998, *A Brief Introduction to Social Role Valorization: A High-order Concept for Addressing the Plight of Societally Devalued People and for Structuring Human Services*, 12–24, Training Institute for Human Service Planning, Leadership and Change Agentry, Syracuse University, NY.

'The definition of normalization: update, problems, disagreements and misunderstandings', 1980, in R.J. Flynn and K.E. Nitsch (eds) *Normalization, Social Integration and Community Services*, 71–115, Baltimore: University Park Press.

A Balanced Multi-Component Advocacy/Protection Schema, 1977 (Law and Mental Retardation monograph series), Toronto: Canadian Association for the Mentally Retarded. (Republished in 1999 by the Training Institute for Human Service Planning, Leadership and Change Agentry, Syracuse University, NY.)

'What advocates said', 2001, *Citizen Advocacy Forum*, 11(2), 4–17.

'A brief reflection on where we stand and where we are going in human services', 1983, *Institutions, Etc.*, 6(3), 20–3.

'Extermination: disabled people in Nazi Germany', 1980, *Disabled USA*, 4(2), 23–4.

'Of human courage and dignity', 1970, *Mental Retardation News* (newsletter of the National Association for Retarded Children, TX), 19(9), 6.

'The prophetic voice and presence of mentally retarded people in the world today', 2001 (edited presentation to Religion Subdivision of the AAMD, May 1976), published as part of the collection in W.C. Gaventa and D.L. Coulter (eds) 2001, *The Theological Voice of Wolf Wolfensberger*, Binghamton, NY: The Haworth Pastoral Press.

The Roeher Institute, Toronto, formerly National Institute on Mental Retardation, Canada

For extracts from the following:

'The role of ideology in shaping human management models', 1972, Chapter 1 of *Normalization: The Principle of Normalization in Human Services*, 6–10, Toronto: National Institute on Mental Retardation.

'The concept of deviancy in human management', 1972, Chapter 2 of *Normalization: The Principle of Normalization in Human Services*, 13–25, Toronto: National Institute on Mental Retardation.

'Typical programmatic and architectural implications of the normalization principle', 1972, Chapter 4 of *Normalization: The Principle of Normalization in Human Services*, 31–42, Toronto, National Institute on Mental Retardation.

'Societal integration as a corollary of normalization', 1972, Chapter 5 of *Normalization: The Principle of Normalization in Human Services*, 44–54, Toronto, National Institute on Mental Retardation.

The Third Stage in the Evolution of Voluntary Associations for the Mentally Retarded, 1973, Toronto: International League of Societies for the Mentally Handicapped, and National Institute on Mental Retardation.

The American Association on Mental Retardation and their journal Mental Retardation

For extracts from the following:

'General observations on European programs',1965, *Mental Retardation*, 3(1), 8–11.

'A brief overview of Social Role Valorization', 2000, *Mental Retardation*, 38(2), 105–23.

'An "if this, then that" formulation of decisions related to Social Role Valorization as a better way of interpreting it to people', 1995, *Mental Retardation*, 33(3), 163–9.

'Social Role Valorization and, or versus, "Empowerment"', 2002, *Mental Retardation*, (40)3, 252–8.

'Embarrassments in the diagnostic process', 1965, *Mental Retardation*, 3(3), 29–31.

'How to exclude mentally retarded children from school', 1975, Guest Editorial, *Mental Retardation*, 13(6), 30–1.

'Bill F.: signs of the times read from the life of one mentally retarded man', 1989, *Mental Retardation*, 27(6), 369–73.

'Eulogy for a mentally retarded jester', 1982, *Mental Retardation*, 20(6), 269–70.

'Common assets of mentally retarded people that are commonly not acknowledged', 1988, *Mental Retardation*, 26(2), 63–70.

New Statesman Ltd, and Spencer Neal, publisher

For the extracts from the following (copyright New Statesman Ltd, all rights reserved):

'Models of mental retardation', 1970, *New Society*, 15(380), 51–3.

Raymond Lemay and Robert Flynn, and the University of Ottawa Press

For extracts from the following:

'A contribution to the history of normalization, with primary emphasis on the establishment of normalization in North America between 1967–1975', 1999, Chapter 3 of R.J. Flynn and R.A. Lemay (eds) *A Quarter-century of Normalization and Social Role Valorization: Evolution and Impact*, 51–116, Ottawa, University of Ottawa Press.

The Taylor and Francis group, and their individual companies

For extracts from the following:

'Social Role Valorization: a new insight, and a new term, for normalization', 1985, *Australian Association for the Mentally Retarded Journal*, 9(1), 4–11.

'Social Role Valorization is too conservative. No, it is too radical', 1995, *Disability and Society*, 10(3), 245–7.

'Human service policies – the rhetoric versus the reality', 1989, in L. Barton (ed.) *Disability and Dependency*, 23–41, London: Falmer Press.

Raymond Lemay (Editor) and SRV/VRS: The International Social Role Valorization Journal/La Revue Internationale de la Valorisation des Rôles Sociaux

For extracts from the following:

'Some of the universal "good things of life" which the implementation of Social Role Valorization can be expected to make more accessible to devalued people', 1996, *SRV/VRS: The International Social Role Valorization Journal/La Revue Internationale de la Valorisation des Rôles Sociaux*, 2(2), 12–14.

The University of Lincolnshire and Humberside

For extracts from the following:

'Major obstacles to rationality and quality of human services in contemporary society', 1997, in R. Adams (ed.) *Crisis in the Human Services: National and International Issues – Selected Papers from a Conference held at the University of Cambridge, September 1996*, 133–5, Kingston upon Hull: University of Lincoln-shire and Humberside.

The Division on Developmental Disabilities (formerly the Division on Mentally Retardation) of the Council for Exceptional Children, USA

For extracts from the following:

'Normalization of services for the mentally retarded: a conversation with Wolf Wolfensberger', 1974, interview in the 'Now way to know' series, *Education and Training of the Mentally Retarded*, 9, 202–8.

'A call to wake up to the beginning of a new wave of "euthanasia" of severely impaired people, 1980, Guest Editorial, *Education and Training of the Mentally Retarded*, 15, 171–3.

Brookline Books

For extracts from the following:

'Let's hang up "quality of life" as a hopeless term', 1994, in D. Goode (ed.), *Quality of Life for Persons with Disabilities: International Perspectives and Issues*, 285–321, Cambridge, MA: Brookline Books.

The Canadian Council on Social Development, and their journal Canadian Welfare

For extracts from the following:

Review of *Enough Room for Joy: Jean Vanier's L'Arche: A Message for our Time*, 1974, *Canadian Welfare*, 50(6), 14–17.

Introduction

Wolf Wolfensberger – changing leadership and leading change

It has become fashionable in biographies and retrospectives for authors to indulge in what some have called 'historical revisionism' – or more crudely, to speculate on what an author or public figure 'must have thought' on this or that topic, regardless of the evidence of what they actually said or did. Equally prevalent, and rather more sinister, is the seeking out of a person's flaws. These can be either characteristics that most people would regard as such, or those that offend against current political orthodoxies. In either case such revelations then taint the ensuing analysis with the notion that the views of 'such a person' are not worth considering. The actual content of those views, or any real observable influence they may have had on an aspect of human activity can thus be conveniently ignored.

This book will follow neither of those fashions, for two reasons. First, as stated in the Editor's Foreword, the book's purpose is to bring together, for as wide a range of readership as possible, a selection of the writings of Wolf Wolfensberger. Readers can therefore make their judgement on the *ideas* in those writings, not on the man himself. The second reason is to avoid the tendency to oversimplified generalizations about cause and effect in a person's actions and writings that can be amplified by the abbreviation that inevitably arises in a book of this size.

What this introduction will confine itself to, therefore, is an attempt to give the reader a context for the chapters which follow. This will be achieved through a brief outline biography of Wolfensberger, derived from his own published accounts of his time in human services and his intellectual development. Key influences on the ideas expressed in his writings can thus be highlighted. Though there are naturally many connections between all of these, we are not asking the reader to take Wolfensberger 'all or nothing'. Indeed, except for a brief reference in this Introduction and at the end of the book, Wolfensberger's specifically theological writings and thoughts, which have undoubtedly had a strong influence on his secular work, are not dealt with. That task has been addressed to a large extent in the 2001 publication *The Theological Voice of Wolf Wolfensberger* (Gaventa & Coulter (eds)).

Further, though reference to it will be made fairly frequently, we will not attempt to discuss in detail what Wolfensberger has called the 'teaching culture', through which many of his ideas have been put forward and discussed. Since at least the early 1970s, in many countries, this has taken the form of teaching events, or 'workshops' in which the ideas are put forward in a sequential series of presentations, often over many days. This form of teaching has attracted controversy, which has often failed to distinguish debate over the *process* of delivering the ideas from debate on the ideas themselves. This book will not enter that debate, though reference to the teaching culture as a source of certain articles will be made. Given the immense amount of material contained in, and time invested in, the teaching events, much abbreviation is necessary for written accounts of them, even in Wolfensberger's original articles, let alone edited versions of them for this book. That being said, the written word has a key part to play in the wider dissemination of ideas, especially if, as is our aim here, the themes of a person's work can be presented in one volume. The teaching culture then becomes part of the context for this collection, with the potential for readers whose interest is aroused on some or many of the issues, not only to explore the original articles, but also to seek out a teaching event for even greater depth.

A full list of current events is normally available from the Training Institute for Human Service Planning, Leadership and Change Agentry, Syracuse University, 800 South Wilbur Avenue, Suite 3B1, Syracuse, NY 13204, USA.

A note on terminology

One of the subsets of the tendency to judge people's ideas on the basis of their personal attributes, especially in certain academic circles, and especially in England, concerns the use of language. Wolfensberger was, ironically, one of the first people to teach and write about the place of terminology in the devaluation process (e.g. Wolfensberger, 1972 – see Chapters 1 and 2). Yet he has been subject more than most to this form of pre-judgement. This may be partly because, as I have discussed elsewhere (Race, 1999, 2002a), a helplessness to do something about the plight of certain groups of people has often resulted in a diversion of energy into arguing about what they are called. Such arguments have then resulted in polarity of opinion, or even outright hostility, between groups who should be in alliance in combating oppression. It may also be, as we shall see on other controversial issues throughout this book, that people hearing ideas that ring true but are unpleasant to face seek diversion from facing them by finding ways not to hear them.

The Editor comes from a country that seems to be afflicted more than most by this tendency, in that the condition that Wolfensberger (and most official bodies in his country and a number of others) call mental retardation, is currently referred to in the UK by at least two terms – namely learning difficulty and learning disability – that are used nowhere else in the world. The exercise of some humility therefore seems appropriate. In selecting and editing works spanning over 40 years, and aimed at a worldwide readership, an attempt at some sort of politically correct Bowdlerization of Wolfensberger's writing would strike one as intensely arrogant. This is apart from the sheer impossibility of selecting one out of the vast number of possible terms to replace those used by Wolfensberger. The extracts in this book are therefore reproduced as written, with whatever language was used at the time of their original publication. My own commentary will reflect this, at the risk of academic opprobrium, but in the hope – stated once again and not for the last time in this book – that the ideas, rather than the descriptive language, will be what readers will consider.

A brief biography of Wolf Wolfensberger

Wolf Wolfensberger was born in Mannheim, Germany in July 1934, to what he describes as a 'family of Catholics, Protestants and Jews'. That make-up, as for many families in Germany at the time, led to considerable dangers as the country, and the world, moved into war. Like many young children in the war, Wolfensberger experienced many horrors, and was sent to the countryside for two years in order to escape some of the bombing of the cities. He credits his months alone then, on the pastures herding cattle, for forming his capacity to be alone, and think independently. Of further relevance to our concerns was the emigration to the USA, together with his mother, of the young Wolfensberger in 1950.

From the age of 17 to 21, whilst attending Siena College in Memphis, Tennessee, Wolfensberger worked as a laboratory technician for a chemical company. He gained his BA in philosophy in 1955. Graduate study followed, at St. Louis University, Missouri, with a part-time job as a research clerk-statistician. He then served a year in a clinical psychology internship at Norfolk (Nebraska) State Hospital, a mental institution, during which time he completed his MA in Psychology and Education in 1957.

Wolfensberger then moved on to doctoral studies at George Peabody College for Teachers (now part of Vanderbilt University) in Nashville, Tennessee, intermittently working as a staff psychologist at Muscatatuck State School (for the retarded) in Butlerville, Indiana, and serving another year's internship, this time of a research nature, at E.R. Johnstone Training and Research Center, Bordentown, New Jersey, 1959–60, under Dr. Leonard Blackman. He finished his dissertation and graduated with a PhD in Psychology and Special Education in 1962, while working as Chief Psychologist and Director of Human Development at Greene Valley Hospital and School (for the retarded), Greeneville, Tennessee, 1960–62. At that time, he successfully applied for a one-year National Institute of Health post-doctoral research fellowship in mental retardation at Maudsley Hospital, London, England, 1962–63, under Drs Jack Tizard and Neil O'Connor. These two were the leaders of what has been called the 'psychologists group' in the UK, standing somewhat against the large 'subnormality hospitals' and advocating, through their own and others' studies, a developmental approach to working with their occupants (Race, 2002a). Wolfensberger credits both Tizard and O'Connor with having contributed enormously to his professional growth, and believes that Tizard specifically gave him an orientation to think systemically about mental retardation and services, which at that time was a rather rare perspective.

Travelling to the UK for a year was rather more arduous than nowadays. On an outward journey by train and aeroplane, and a sea voyage to return, Wolfensberger was accompanied by his wife Nancy, whom he had met in Indiana and married in 1960, and their two daughters Margaret, not yet two, and Joan, a babe in arms (Paul, the youngest of their three children, arrived in the December of 1966). The 1962–63 visit also included trips to other European countries, and formed the beginning of what was to become a small group of highly influential, but also highly radical and controversial, people in the mental retardation field, who were to have a significant impact on services in the late 1960s and early 1970s.

On returning to the US, the next year (1963–64) was spent in a very instructive but rather unhappy position as Director of Research and Training at Plymouth State Home and Training School, Northville, Michigan. Wolfensberger began to publish on his European trip, perhaps the earliest of his writing on broader aspects of services, and certainly one of the earliest of his critical accounts of services in the US (see extract 2).

The next move, to Nebraska, could be described as providing the channel by which Wolfensberger, and his ideas, rose to more than local prominence. Initially employed as a Mental Retardation Research Scientist at the Nebraska Psychiatric Institute, University of Nebraska Medical Center, Omaha, Nebraska, he rose from assistant to associate professor of Medical Psychology in the Departments of Psychiatry and Pediatrics in a joint appointment. Influenced, by his own account, by continuing contact with Europe, and by wider attention being given to Goffman's writings (e.g. 1961) in the mental retardation field, especially in the work of Vail (1967), Wolfensberger not only became part of a growing anti-institutional movement in the USA, but was also able to put some of the burgeoning ideas into practice, via a project called Eastern Nebraska Community Office of Retardation (ENCOR). This has been well documented (e.g. Menolascino, 1974; Schalock, 2002) but its significance for the field as a whole is relevant to note here. This was, in particular, that it was possible to provide a comprehensive service system for mentally retarded people in a given region, with minimal recourse to institutions, based on developmental assumptions about such people. Findings from Europe, especially the work of Tizard and his colleagues, and increased contact with Scandinavia, including visits in 1967 by Bengt Nirje from Sweden, gave credibility to the scheme. But it was also as board member of the Greater Omaha Association for Retarded Citizens, the parents' organization, that Wolfensberger was able to influence the ideas in practice. The ENCOR project itself then became a place of pilgrimage for the radical end of the mental retardation field.

At the same time, the putting together of a report for the President's Commission on Mental Retardation (described in detail in extract 6) brought together many of the radical groups worldwide, with Wolfensberger as the driving force. It was also, as we shall see, the first written account, in the chapter by Bengt Nirje, of the 'normalization principle'. Following that report, produced and distributed in book form (Kugel and Wolfensberger, 1969) an immensely productive period, both in terms of direct involvement with services, as well as writing and teaching, took place in Wolfensberger's life. In a number of mostly voluntary offices and roles, he was able to refine and develop the notion of comprehensive services, and was influential in the development of a number of alternatives to institutions. The notion of citizen advocacy, an equally radical idea to normalization, and one which has had possibly an even greater worldwide effect (see extract 17) emerged from Wolfensberger's dealings with the parents' group in Nebraska. Also, the first edition of the evaluation tool based on normalization, Program Analysis of Service Systems, was devised with Linda Glenn. The criticisms and pressure for reform of the existing system contained in all of these efforts, especially since the Kugel and Wolfensberger book, was well received among parents' groups and the small radical movement. It also, however, brought an equally vituperative response from the establishment in the mental retardation field, and eventually led to Wolfensberger's position at the Nebraska Psychiatric Institute becoming untenable. As he put it much later 'Unlike other professors who perished when they did not publish, I perished in good part because of what I published.' (Wolfensberger, 1999, p.88).

It could be said that Nebraska's loss was Canada's, and the wider world's, gain. Wolfensberger's recruitment by G. Allan Roeher to the Canadian National Institute on Mental Retardation (part of the overall body of Canada's national parents' group) set in train another key aspect of this highly influential period in Wolfensberger's life. With the official position of Visiting Scholar to the NIMR, with joint appointment as special lecturer, Psychology Department, York University, the time from September 1971 to August 1973 firstly saw the publication of the Normalization text and the second edition of PASS by the NIMR (after the former had been rejected by a number of major publishers). Secondly, through the use of PASS in teaching and evaluation, and the general focusing of activity of radicalized people on Toronto, there began the development of a cadre of leaders, who were to have an influence on services well beyond Canada, in many cases lasting to the present time.

The Normalization text was to have an immense effect, a fact that has been recognized over the ensuing decades. In 1991, in a review of 11,300 articles and books published in the field of mental retardation over a 50-year period, a panel of 178 experts identified the 1972 text as the most important 'classic' work in the field. (In the same survey the 1983 article 'Social Role Valorization: a proposed new term for the principle of normalization' – see Chapter 3 – was named the seventeenth most important 'classic' work. Only 25 works in total were identified as 'classics', and only one other person had two publications cited among these 25.)

The use of PASS, as an evaluation instrument but especially as a tool to teach about normalization, was also to have effects lasting well into the ensuing decades, and with its successor PASSING (Wolfensberger and Thomas, 1983 – see Chapter 3) has acted as a focal point for leadership recruitment and development. It is therefore no surprise that when Wolfensberger moved to Syracuse University, New York State, in 1973, in addition to his role as Professor in what was then called the Division of Special Education and Rehabilitation, he also established and directed his own Training Institute for Human Service Planning, Leadership and Change Agentry. The focus of that Institute was, and is, implied by the name. Continuing as an associate consultant (on planning, training, and research) to the NIMR, from 1973 to 1986, the Canadian links were not forgotten, and contact with groups in England, Australia and New Zealand developed as the 1970s progressed.

In his address to the 1994 International SRV conference (Flynn and Lemay, 1999), Wolfensberger makes humorous reference to the suggestion that 'If I had done normalization the favor of dying when I was at the peak of my reputation and effectiveness, it probably would have been embraced and more systematically studied'. He was referring to events after the heyday of the late 1960s and early 1970s that, in his view, contributed to his marginalization, not only in terms of normalization, but also in terms of his influence on leadership and change in human services. The fact of this book, and the conference at which it is expected to be launched, puts those remarks somewhat in doubt. It is certainly true, however, that developments in his thinking and teaching made Wolfensberger even more of a figure attracting either strong adherents or strong opponents. This was, interestingly, a description that he was to apply to Jean Vanier and the L'Arche movement (see extract 29), and one of the developments has a considerable connection with that movement.

Wolfensberger lists the following:

a) his articulation of what he describes as the 'dynamics of social decadence' (see Chapters 5, 6 and 7)
b) his warning of the dangers of 'deathmaking' of vulnerable and devalued people (see Chapters 6 and 7)
c) his analysis of the stages of change of voluntary associations, particularly parents' groups such as those by whom he had been lauded in the USA and Canada. This posited that they had become stuck as service-providing agencies, thus diminishing their campaigning zeal, along with their voluntary membership (see extract 18)
d) his increasing statements criticizing as bankrupt the human service system, which were contrasted with earlier attempts at values-led comprehensive services (see Chapter 5)
e) his criticism, after being a powerful voice against segregated education, of the over-simplified and arbitrarily applied 'mainstreaming' of the 1970s, often with adherents citing normalization as their watchword.
f) in response to his contact with L'Arche, the attempt to bring his religious faith and work into greater harmony. This was also strongly influenced by contact with the writings, and the teachings, of a theologian called William Stringfellow, in particular his 1973 book subtitled *An Ethic for Christians and Other Aliens in a Strange Land.*

As we have noted, this last aspect of Wolfensberger's writings is not fully covered in this collection, but the combination and interaction of these ideas with the other ones listed did begin a process by which Wolfensberger became increasingly isolated in certain circles. This did not, however, stop the continuation of leadership development, or the spread of the core ideas of normalization and citizen advocacy, but it could be said to have been influential in a great deal of confusion and misrepresentation around those ideas, resulting amongst other reasons in a reformulation of normalization as Social Role Valorization (see extract 10).

The 'teaching culture' continued, with Wolfensberger himself tending to focus for the period of the late 1970s and 1980s more on the issues under a) to d) above, though his Training Institute, and the leaders developed from it, continued to teach about normalization, to become involved in changing the service world, especially in the field of mental retardation. Certain countries began this teaching later than it had started in North America – in England for example, the first PASS workshop was not until 1980, and Australia seems to have developed a broader and stronger movement around SRV and PASSING, though normalization had had its effects. This is not to suggest that Wolfensberger was ignoring normalization – the development of SRV, and the creation of PASSING as essentially the successor to PASS as SRV succeeded normalization shows his continued involvement in this area (see Chapter 3).

In terms of publication, however, after the early 1980s papers on the change to SRV, there are more articles on the bigger issues of 'deathmaking' and the 'disfunctionality' of human services, and on his return to the UK after a 22-year absence, Wolfensberger began a series of visits presenting workshops on those issues. It was not until the prospect of the 1994 international conference celebrating 25 years since the publication of the Kugel and Wolfensberger book that attention, at least as far as publication is concerned, returned to SRV. Subsequent publications are dealt with in Chapter 3, but despite this, and the formation in 1992 of the North American SRV Development, Training & Safeguarding Council, Wolfensberger's main output has been on these larger issues, covered in Chapters 5 to 7.

Ultimately, the threads of the 40 or more years of Wolfensberger's working life are, in the view of this editor, coming together, and, typically, fitting uneasily into a postmodern world, especially in academia. The lessons of history do not always sit well with this group, and it is ironic that many of the articles appearing in this book raise issues that have a compellingly contemporary ring. One of them closes this introduction. It is placed here because, in this editor's view, it has remained as a key to practically all the selection of writings in this book, and certainly at the root of the development of leadership and influence on change of Wolf Wolfensberger. This is his analysis of the crucial part played by values and ideologies in the behaviour of societies, their human services, and the place of vulnerable people.

In the first chapter of the 1972 Normalization text, Wolfensberger provides an overview of that analysis. It would, as noted, seem to be just as apposite 30 years later, with only some of the descriptive labels changing in that time.

1   From: "The role of ideology in shaping human management models," 1972, Chapter 1 of *Normalization: The Principle of Normalization in Human Services*, 6–10, Toronto, National Institute on Mental Retardation.

Man's behavior is in good part determined by what I want to call his ideologies. By ideology, I mean a combination of beliefs, attitudes, and interpretations of reality that are derived from … experiences, … knowledge of what are presumed to be facts, and above all, … values.

Ideologies can be thought of as being "big" or "little". Religions, political systems, philosophies of life, etc., these are all big ideologies, or conglomerates of ideologies. Little or at least medium-sized ideologies deal with a wide range of our functioning in our private and professional lives. For instance, … while the number of human management professionals and agencies is large, the services they render are profoundly affected and often even governed by a relatively small number of fundamental assumptions or concepts. Thus, in the field of mental retardation, services were for years dominated by the idea that the retarded were a menace to society. …

We not only need to recognize relatively broad human management ideologies, but also those that may be strongly held by specific professions or schools of thought, or even by specific agencies. Unfortunately, such … ideologies are often merely agency myths or dogmas, and there is a point where an ideology, a myth, and a dogma merge into one. For instance, today, we recognize that the prevalent ideology of welfare agencies in regard to foster and adoptive placement of retarded infants (e.g. "everybody knows you can't place mongoloids") was a dogma, and being false, was also a myth. But this ideology was powerful, and determined what was done for many decades.

Ideologies are extremely powerful forces that rule and determine a host of behaviors. … Even scientists who pride themselves on being purely empirical in their scientific work are ruled by ideologies. … Kuhn (1962) has rendered a widely acclaimed analysis which appears to have demonstrated that science progresses in discontinuous steps which are attained by rather radical reconceptualizations, many of which are ideological rather than merely empirical in nature. Thus, scientific theories come and go, although they are never provable, and only occasionally disprovable.

They come and go because of the prevailing scientific as well as social and even political ideologies. The history of science is replete with examples where even a formidable body of evidence was ignored or denied because the prevailing ideology could not tolerate or account for such evidence. In medicine, the evidence against bloodletting was overpowering – yet it was practiced for hundreds of years. Today, one of the most widely practiced psychiatric techniques, namely psycho-therapy, is supported by only scant good experimental evidence, despite more than 50 years of practice. I, too, have my transempirical scientific ideologies. For instance, I am most skeptical about extrasensory perception, even though the evidence for it is very strong. My scientific ideologies find it difficult to account for such evidence. Therefore, I dismiss the evidence.

If a human management assumption, concept, or ideology has rather global implication and is consistently expressed, we often refer to it as a human management "model," in the sense of the word "paradigm." It is not necessarily something that others should model themselves after, but an example – a typical expression – of a concept or pattern.

Another way of conceptualizing a human management model is as a consistent pattern in which the behavior of persons is structured by other persons who exercise authority over them. Human management models affect and often even dictate the location, design, and operation of human management facilities... .

Not only daily management practices, but also the social organization of service systems and manpower structures are usually consistent with and related to the prevailing human management concepts and models (e.g. Gruenberg, 1966). ...

From the above, one might almost infer that ideologies, and human management models based upon them, are bad. This is not necessarily so. There are good and bad ideologies, and good and bad models. Some good models become bad only when they are inappropriately applied. For instance, the medical model is superb – in appropriate contexts; it has been destructive in others, as when it has been applied to certain problems which are primarily of a socio-pedagogic nature.

Perhaps it is in the sciences where the power of ideologies is to be regretted, because in contrast to human services, science is much more based in empiricism than values, and because ideologies can override facts and empiricism rather easily. However, in human management, I hope that values shall forever reign supreme, at least to a degree. Values are valuable, and our lives should be ruled by them. But at the same time, we must strive for three goals: good ideologies rather than bad ones; ideologies which either transcend empiricism or at least are not inconsistent with it; and conscious ideologies rather than unconscious ones. Below, I will elaborate upon each of these.

Good ideologies rather than bad ones

Some ideologies are obviously more adaptive than others; and ideologies differ from each other in regard to the degree to which they are consistent with the holder's other and higher-order ideologies. Yet, obviously, it is only by wisdom or hindsight that we can differentiate good ideologies from bad ones. Otherwise, there would be no bad ideologies, because everybody would embrace only the good ones.

Unfortunately, there are probably only two ways to improve the quality of our ideologies. One way is to strive with sincerity to root out all of one's unconscious ideologies which usually are unconscious only because they are "bad." If they were good, we would be less apt to tuck them away. Secondly, there are times when we can apply a bit of decision theory. For instance, some ideologies may be redundant but at least they will not do any harm, while others can do a lot of harm; or some may increase our options, while others reduce them. A belief in the theory that mental retardation is primarily hereditary logically leads to treatment nihilism, while an environmental theory impels toward treatment activism. If the hereditary theory is wrong but we adopt it, we lose all human values, by doing nothing where much could be done, and that is what we did for many decades. On the other hand, if we adopt the environmental theory, and it is wrong, we lose little in human values, only in money. If retarded infants can be fostered, but we do not try because we do not believe it can be done, we will have thrown away a valuable option and harmed a lot of children. If it cannot be done, but we try and fail, we have only wasted a little effort and money, and the children fare no worse off than they were before. ...

Ideologies transcending empiricism but not inconsistent with it

Let us compare the following two ideologies: as many of the retarded as possible should engage in work that is as culturally normative as possible; or homeless retarded children should be institutionalized because no one will foster or adopt them. The first ideology transcends empiricism. It states a principle and leaves it up to the future and empiricism to determine what "as many as possible" or "as culturally normative as possible" may mean. On the other hand, the second ideology is so phrased as to be directly empirically testable. There is nothing wrong with an empirically-based ideology, but it must not be inconsistent with empiricism, and the second ideology is. An example of an empirically-based ideology that is consistent with empiricism is: because most of the severely retarded, and some profoundly retarded, can perform work which, though probably sheltered, is culturally normative in quality if not always in quantity, they should perform such work rather than work which is culturally deviant.

Conscious rather than unconscious ideology

One thing that can be very bad about our ideologies is that more often than not, we are not aware of them. Sometimes we take them so for granted that we lose sight of their existence. ... At other times, we simply are not equipped intellectually to formulate our ideologies in words. At yet other times, our ideologies are so bad that we cannot consciously face up to them.

For example, we all claim to believe in equality – and then we practice gross discrimination, but deny it because we cannot admit it and therefore do not realize that we discriminate. In our human management services, we claim to render treatment – and then we dehumanize, and yet deny that we dehumanize. Our educators call for segregated special education of the mildly retarded – and then the evidence shows that with specially trained teachers, small special classes, and special materials, the special children learn less than they would if left integrated in large classes with regular teachers and classmates years ahead of them. But first we deny the evidence, and when we can no longer deny it, we ignore and usually repress it, and we keep doing that which makes us feel comfortable with our ideology.

There are few things more vicious, more maladaptive, more inimical to individual and collective well-being than unconscious ideologies. The fact that for 200 years, we have adhered, largely unconsciously, to racial discrimination while claiming to adhere to equality is an extreme example. It is a phenomenon that might destroy us. ...

Chapter 1

The analysis of devaluation and wounding

Introduction

In the hundreds of publications that Wolf Wolfensberger has produced over the years, one theme recurs, sometimes in a small portion of the paper concerned, sometimes dominating it, but always around in one form or another. Whether in the early days as a psychologist, in the height of his influence in the early 1970s, in his controversial later works and workshops – whether on the subject of service organization, planning, advocacy, normalization, social role valorization, relationships between people or lessons from history – the way we as humans think about certain groups of people and what we then, as collections of humans, do about that is the basis of this recurring theme. As the extract in the Introduction above reveals, the basis for our thoughts and actions are, Wolfensberger believes, grounded in values. As the years have passed, his views on the content and/or relative weight of those values may have changed, as we shall see in later chapters. Overall, however, the result of our values and subsequent actions, in terms of the creation and perpetuation of devalued groups, has not changed. The groups themselves may also have changed, though Wolfensberger's origins in the mental retardation field have kept that group as a constant in his work (just as they remain the most consistently devalued group, at least in so-called developed countries). The *process*, however, does not change.

As we shall see, greater refinement of analysis has added some new words to describe this process, from 'treatment of deviancy' to devaluation, with the incorporation, via contact with Vanier and L'Arche, of the descriptive term 'wounding'. Other authors and groups (e.g. Oliver, 1990; Morris, 1993) have described the process in different terms, and with different emphases on causes and responses, but appear to be talking about much the same thing (much though some of them would not be prepared to acknowledge such a view). At its root, however, the process would seem to this editor to be so clearly set out in so much of Wolfensberger's work, and to produce in those who read and hear his account of the process such strong reactions, emotional as well as intellectual, that it represents what he would call a 'true universal'.

All of us can recognize, at the level of our most basic instincts (some would say deep in our soul), and identify with, this process of devaluation and wounding. We may then deny it, try to pick small or large holes in it, try to attack the man proposing it, or close our ears because of the language in which it expressed, but the underlying truth remains.

This opening chapter, therefore, goes straight to the heart of the matter; in fact, subsequent chapters can be said to summarize the many aspects of Wolfensberger's response to, or refinement of, the central theme of devaluation and wounding that these opening extracts present.

2   From: 'General observations on European Programs', 1965, *Mental Retardation*, 3(1), 8–11.

One of Wolfensberger's earliest published thoughts on the issue was encountered in the third of three articles, written for the journal *Mental Retardation*, on his 1962 European trip discussed in the Introduction. It represents, for its time, very radical thoughts about the link between the way services are carried out, and the view of the service system, and society, about the people for whom they are provided. The articles make a number of comparisons favourable to the European services, especially in terms of their developmental and community orientation, and in his conclusion, Wolfensberger first of all dismisses the simplistic belief of services that more money could make US services better, then points to the lack of a community base for those services. Finally, and in terms of the theme of this chapter, Wolfensberger speculates on the 'complex and profound' questions of why different societies treat similar groups of people in significantly different ways.

...

Conclusion

Since my return to the United States, I have spoken to a number of parent and professional groups, frequently showing slides and pictures I brought back. One point often made from the audience is that if we only had more money we would be able to provide more or better services, too. This is a fallacious and even dangerous argument. First of all, money alone cannot assure quality of service. Over and over, I observed that the better endowed programs were not always the best, or, to the contrary, that they were often very ineffective. Secondly, many states provide considerable financing for institutions but little in terms of community services. For the same amount of money it takes to provide one place in an institution, one could maintain from three to five retardates in the community by means of day care services, home visitors, parent counseling, mother's helpers and sheltered workshops. Yet even though this is now known, several states are presently in the process of enlarging, building, or planning traditional, large, uneconomical omnibus type institutions, often far removed from the area of greatest need. It would appear that there is a lot of money available even now, but that it is being spent uneconomically and not in the best interest of the retarded. ...

In this series of articles a number of programs and issues have been discussed which are not likely to leave us feeling content and happy with what we have been doing. Our programs and attitudes have come a long way in the last decade, but many of us, while verbalizing the fashionable watchwords, do not appreciate how much could actually be done. ... there are enough publications in our literature which glorify the achievements of this or that program, and too few which point to conditions which are unsatisfactory or which, in some institutions or states, are outright scandalous.

Particularly, I see one almost inexplicable paradox in the contrast of care and training the retardate receives here and in Europe. Ours is a society based on democratic and idealistic principles. We voice beliefs in self-sufficiency, hard work, human dignity, freedom of movement, minimal controls and equality of opportunity. Furthermore, we are affluent while European countries either are not or much less so. Also, they have been traditionally restrictive of human rights and opportunities, and more class conscious. For example, Germany, even today, is a country where the police has vast power, where the state keeps up with the whereabouts of every individual; where every resident age 14 and over must have his passport if he goes out upon the street; where you must give your wife's maiden name, place of birth, and your own passport number, place, and date of issuance if you wish to register in a hotel; and where a man can be held in prison for months without a public charge. Yet, when it comes to providing programs for the retarded, the Europeans are both wise and generous where we have been careless and stingy; they grant rights which we so often take away; they provide opportunities we deny; they educate for independence where we prefer to give meager charity; they permit open movement of retardates where we yet have innumerable locks and fences; they tackle problems we prefer to repress.

Why this reversal of traditional modes of behavior when it comes to mental retardation? Is it because our Protestant ethic rejects individuals we believe to be idle, unproductive and unfavored by God? Is it that in our striving for ascendancy, independence and strength, the retardate reminds us of what we might be, and we thus proceed to repress his needs or even his existence? Or, in our affluence, are we gratified to have an object of charity, and to maintain the retardate in a state of well-fed dependency? The answer is probably complex and profound, and the questions keep nagging. But regardless of past and present paradoxes, the time has come to demand that the best of ideas from everywhere be combined with the material resources of our society in order to produce better solutions to the problem.

---

3   From: 'Models of Mental Retardation', 1970, *New Society*, 15(380), 51–3.

In the period between the series of articles mentioned earlier and the next article in this chapter, a considerable amount of activity took place in the mental retardation field in the USA and certain European countries. In relation to the development of normalization, this is outlined in Wolfensberger's own account at the start of Chapter 2. In terms of the analysis of devaluation and the experiences of vulnerable individuals and groups in Wolfensberger's writings, however, the early reflections above now go on to consideration of the 'models' of service that characterized the field at the time. The next extract is from an English journal, *New Society*, which was not an academic journal, but more a journal for the intelligent lay reader (mainly of a 'soft left' persuasion – it has subsequently merged with the more famous journal of the left, the *New Statesman*). It was adapted from a key chapter in the famous report for the President's Commission on Mental Retardation, published as *Changing Patterns of Residential Services for the Mentally Retarded* (Kugel and Wolfensberger 1969 – see extract 6 for greater detail). The chapter, entitled 'The origins and nature of our institutional models', was also summarized in the journal *Mental Retardation* (White and Wolfensberger, 1969) and later edited to form a best-selling monograph with photographic illustrations (Wolfensberger, 1975). It also sees one of the earliest references to the 'historic roles' of devalued (especially impaired) people, the link between those perceptions, and the reinforcement of such perceptions in the 'settings' of human services, by the physical environment, the social environment, and the language used about people. The article itself, of course, uses then contemporary sociological and social psychological language, that of 'deviancy theory' which, as we have discussed and shall see below, also informed elements of normalization ideas and has had its critics, both from within sociology and outside. As with much of Wolfensberger's writing, however, the article has a broader historical referential sweep, and in addition acknowledges some of the key influences and contemporaries on his thinking. (N.B. As an article in a non-academic journal, referencing was not made in the ordinary way, but with a list being given in the margins, rather than references in the text. To aid readers of this book, the basic citations are given after the extract, with the full references in the main list at the back of the book.)

Man's attempts to deal with deviance can be classified into three categories: destroying the deviant, making him undeviant, or segregating him. Segregation can take two forms: protecting the deviant from society, or protecting society from the deviant. Apparently, it is difficult to the point of impossibility for society at the same time to view people as deviants and interact normally with them. A good example of the three main reactions to deviancy is the treatment of the Jews in Europe. During early Christianity, efforts aimed at converting them; in the Middle Ages, they were segregated by banishment or ghettoes; in the recent past, they were first segregated in concentration camps and then destroyed.

Another important fact about deviancy is that although it can take many forms, these tend to be treated in very similar ways at a given time. When Hitler destroyed the Jews, he also destroyed the mentally disordered and the retarded, the aged, habitual criminals, gypsies and vagabonds. The history of the treatment of the mentally retarded over the past 100 years illustrates very well the changing ways in which society can "manage" deviancy. Here, too, there were remarkable parallels in the handling of the retarded, the disordered, the epileptic, the blind and deaf and even criminal offenders. ...

There is, obviously, a clear link between the way a deviant is perceived, and the way he is treated. On studying the history of mental retardation, you find seven chief social roles in which people have been cast at different times and places. The retardate has been seen as subhuman (an animal or vegetable), as a sick person, as a menace, as an object of pity, as a burden of charity, as a holy innocent, and as a developing person. By their very nature, it appears that all but the last of these seven perceptions leads directly or indirectly to treatment which "dehumanises".

In a research programme I have confirmed – by the factor analysis of attitude statements put to various groups of people – that several of these "role perceptions" of the retarded are still identifiable in American society. When we create a human management "setting" (agencies, institutions, …) for the handicapped, the dominant perceptions – in society as well as among specialists – will result in a building, a staffing hierarchy, and rules and procedures which add up to a consistent model.

An institution based on the view that a retardate is "sick" – the "medical" model – will have certain characteristics. It will be called a hospital, and its director will be a physician. The hierarchy and daily schedule resemble those of a hospital. Non-medical staff sport white coats. Resident care is called nursing care; residents are called patients, and their retardation is referred to as an illness or disease. Assessment of their problems is called diagnosis, and all "management procedures" are called therapy or treatment, even to the point where education, work and recreation become educational, industrial and recreational therapy. Those who "administer" such therapy (perhaps in "doses" rather than lessons) may be called therapists. Finally, there may be a preoccupation with the issue of the curability versus incurability of retardation, and a decided pessimism – despite occasional "convalescent leaves" for patients – because of the "chronicity" of the condition.

Some institutions combine perceptions. The subhuman and the menace model are often mixed. Usually, such institutions have features like these: strong fences and windowguards; locked doors, rigid segregation of the sexes; little or no use of knives and forks; unbreakable windows, dishware and furniture; staff looking at residents from protected stations rather than interacting in their midst; an open view of residents' beds, toilets, lavatories and bathrooms; prohibition of the carrying of matches, lighters and pocket knives; and rigid control and censorship over incoming and outgoing mail, parcels and telephone calls.

It was in the middle of the 19th century that enthusiastic educational pioneers launched on concerted efforts to reverse the deviancy of the retarded. They intended to make the deviant undeviant, but their goal was not so much to make the retarded person "normal" as to make him productive, adjusted and independent. It was during this period of optimism that institutions for the retarded were founded throughout the western world. The "perception" was the humane one – of the retarded as developing persons.

In America and other countries, these early institutions based on the development model were defined as residential schools. It was believed to be very important for the residents to have many contacts in the outside community and to have other experiences which today would be called "normalising". One of the first

American institutions was, we are told, "organised on the family plan; the pupils all sat at the same table with the principal … It was the belief of the managers that only a relatively small number of inmates could be successfully cared for in our institutions." To be in the public eye, these early institutions were, in America, sited in the principal or capital cities of their states. A large family residence in a crowded neighbourhood of Boston was the first public institution for the retarded in the United States. …

One of the early pioneers in the United States, Samuel Howe, was an internationally renowned social and political activist. In 1866 he said: "All great establishments in the nature of boarding schools, where the sexes must be separated; where there must be boarding in common and sleeping in congregate dormitories; where there must be routine, formality, restraint and repression of individuality; where the charms and refining influences of the true family relation cannot be had – all such institutions are unnatural, undesirable and very liable to abuse. We should have as few of them as is possible … Witness the old nunneries and monasteries, darkened and saddened by lack of the sunlight of affection and love … soured by crushed hopes and yearnings … Witness soldiers in detached garrisons; sailors on long voyages; prisoners under long sentences. Wherever there must be separation of the sexes, isolation from society, absence of true family relation, and monotony of life, there must come evils of various kinds which no watchfulness can prevent nor physician cure."

In his book, *Asylums*, published in 1961, Erving Goffman also pointed out the similarity between mental hospitals, prisons, monasteries, boarding schools and army camps, calling them "total institutions". Under the direction of Professor Jack Tizard of the University of London Institute of Education, researchers have used Goffman's work to devise a scale for measuring the quality of residential service given to children. Interestingly, this scale includes such items as whether the staff and children eat together.

The reason why Goffman and Tizard can still be concerned about this problem is because, unfortunately, what intervened between Samuel Howe and the other pioneers, and the present day, makes ghastly reading. If more people knew this tragic history, it might prevent a recurrence of the kind of dehumanisation of the deviant which was at its most common and most extreme between about 1910 and 1960.

First by about 1870, the "developmental" attitude changed, and a "pity" model took its place. This occurred because the early institutions, although remarkably successful, were not as successful as many people expected them to be. One expression of the pity model was the view that the deviant should be segregated from society in order to protect and shelter him. So institutions were moved into the purportedly bucolic and Eden-like setting of the countryside, with fences around them to keep out the predations of a cold and vicious world.

But a successful human management model must be based on respect, not pity. Pity may be benevolent, but it contains an element of regarding those who are pitied as not so fully human as he who is doing the pitying. This pity model was only transitional (perhaps this is always the function of pity). It only lasted for 20 or 30 years, reaching a peak in the United States in the mid-1880s.

By about 1890, theories like Morel's gained ascendancy. Morel and his followers held that physical, mental and social handicaps tend to have a common genetic base. These "degeneracies" would get worse from one generation to the next until they resulted in widespread severe retardation. Soon the new intelligence tests appeared to show that retardation was much commoner than people had suspected. Other evidence suggested that the retarded reproduced much faster than the rest of the population. As biased and poorly conducted family studies – like that of the Kallikak family by Goddard – appeared to verify these thoughts, the conviction grew that society was doomed unless degeneracy was axed at the roots – to use the language of the period.

Early attempts at prevention included persuasion, restrictive marriage laws, and "a-sexualisation" (meaning castration or sterilisation). For various and readily understood reasons, these measures were either ineffective or too controversial. Euthanasia, though suggested, was never accepted except in Nazi Germany. In desperation, the workers in the field turned to segregation. On this, there was no controversy. One of the most influential documents in this alarmist "indictment" period was the 1908 report of the Royal Commission on the Care and Control of the Feebleminded: "If the constantly recurring fatuous and irresponsible crimes and offences of mentally defective persons are to be prevented, long and continuous detention is necessary." As this type of segregation was seen as protecting society from deviancy, it took on aspects of sanctioned mass dehumanisation perhaps unrivalled in western countries outside Hitler's concentration camps. Institutions were shaped according to the "menace" and/or "subhuman" model.

Some writers emphasised the menace more. They use terms like "the menace of the feebleminded", "inherent social menace", ... "rapacious social ills", ..." parasitic, predatory", ... "almost invariably immoral", ... "evil of the greatest magnitude".

Other writers built up the general perception of the retarded as being subhuman. Thus, Kerlin wrote of a retardate: "With his great luminous, soft, jet eyes, he reminds one of a seal." And Fernald, after whom we in the United States named buildings and institutions, said: "We now have state commissions for controlling the gypsy moth, the boll weevil, foot-and-mouth disease ... but we have no commission which even attempts to modify or control the vast social, moral and economic forces represented by the feebleminded persons at large in the community." Sometimes the retarded were even referred to as the "waste products" and "by-products" of society. In 1924, F. G. Crookshank wrote a book with an almost atavistic theory of mongolism, ominously entitled *The Mongol in our Midst*. It would have been more appropriate if the hapless mongols had been able to cry out: "Help! A Crookshank in our midst".

In order to segregate vast numbers of menacing deviants, institutions had to enlarge and be operated economically. Buildings were packed like herring cans, and some institutions housed over 5,000 residents; expenditure was cut and economic productivity maximised. Institutions had to be built where land was the cheapest – i.e. far from centres of population. Maximised productivity specifically implied the ruthless exploitation of the labour of the resident retardate to the point of working him literally to death. Death rates in institutions were catastrophic.

But the very largeness of these institutions, apart from other reasons, dehumanised residents. They lost their identity and their individuality. The institutions became a Procrustean bed that never exactly fitted any newcomer. He had to be either stretched out or cut down to size. When I was working in such an institution, and before I realised what I was doing, I too, did my share of stretching and cutting.

It is interesting that when the scientific rationale on which the large, dehumanising, segregated institutions were based was rejected – between 1918 and 1925 – no new rationale emerged. It seemed as if the frenzy of the alarmist period had drained the vitality out of the professionals in the field. Indeed, the pessimism of the period – mistakenly still lingering to this day – had driven many workers who might have enlivened the field into areas they thought would be more rewarding, and it still keeps many young people from choosing a career concerned with mental retardation.

When you look at the anachronistic social systems that are our older institutions today, you can only understand them if you see them as living relics coasting on the momentum of the fire of another age – like the astronomer's "white dwarfs" (spent stars), except that they are large.

Today we are beginning to realise the power that different perceptions of social roles exercise, not merely in shaping behaviour toward deviancy, but also in shaping the behaviour of the deviant himself. Today we know, from an increasing number of studies, that when positive demands and challenges are made to a person, he will almost always respond positively, provided he gets support and help. When a person is called stupid and expected to act stupid, he eventually falls into the stupid role, and acts and even becomes stupid. When we define a person as an animal and structure his environment accordingly, he will begin to act like an animal. By confirming the original perceptions and predictions, this sort of thing sets in motion a cycle that can be either vicious or beneficial.

This phenomenon will impress itself strongly on an observer who visits both Scandinavian and American institutions for the retarded. He will probably see less animal-like behaviour in the more severely retarded in all of Denmark or Sweden than he will in a single one of our typical American institutions (documented so movingly by Blatt and Kaplan in a photographic essay entitled *Christmas in Purgatory*).

The task ahead in treating retardation is to recognise dehumanisation where it exists, label it as such once it is recognised, and then replace it with enlightened forms of management. Community services, and family guidance and assistance, can help cut the total of residential places needed, as the 1959 Mental Health Act hoped in Britain. What residential places are needed could be provided primarily by means of numerous small special-purpose residences dispersed throughout the community which would let us phase out the large, traditional, often isolated or at least insulated, institutions over the next twenty or thirty years.

The "menace", "subhuman" or even "medical" models on which these institutions were based should be replaced again by the "developmental" model which, despite its benefits, has been only sporadically implemented so far. Leadership has been provided by organisations of parents of the retarded and by a few professionals like Jack Tizard, who long were voices crying in the wilderness.

We shall then have come full circle, back to the words of Samuel Howe spoken a hundred years ago:

"Any class of young persons marked by an infirmity ... depend more than ordinary persons do for their happiness and for their support upon the ties of kindred, of friendship, and of neighbourhood. All these, therefore, ought to be nourished and strengthened during childhood and youth – for it is then, and then only, that they take such deep root as to become strong, and life-lasting. ... Beware how you needlessly sever any of those ties. ... lest you make a homeless man, a wanderer and a stranger. ... If the field were all clear, and no buildings provided, there should be built only a building for schoolrooms, recreation rooms, music rooms and workshops; and these should be in or near the centre of a dense population. For other purposes, ordinary houses would suffice."

[References used in the article: Blatt and Kaplan, 1966; Crookshank, 1924; Goffman, 1961; Howe, 1866; King and Raynes, 1968; Nirje, 1969; Report of the Royal Commission on the Care and Control of the Feebleminded, 1908; Wolfensberger, 1969; Vail, 1967.]

---

4   From: 'The concept of deviancy in human management', 1972, Chapter 2 of *Normalization: The Principle of Normalization in Human Services*, 13–25, Toronto: National Institute on Mental Retardation.

The notion of deviancy, the historic social roles, and the effect of perceptions on how people are treated, were to be elaborated at full length in Chapter 2 of the 1972 *Normalization* publication. The connection between these ideas and the fully formulated exposition of the 'wounds' of devaluation described in the last extract in this Chapter, written nearly thirty years later, should be clear from the next piece. Even at this early stage, though mental retardation is at the fore, the examples from other devalued groups serve to reinforce the wide applicability of the observations. It also addresses some of the later critics, in dealing with the issue of intent, and the key concept of deviancy, and later devaluation, being in the eye of the beholder, or perhaps, to use a later term, 'socially constructed'. The reader of this extract is invited, some thirty or more years later, to reflect on the applicability of the 'historical roles' to their own contemporary society, and to vulnerable groups therein.

...

The social definition of deviancy

...

(I acknowledge the strong influence which the sociologist Richard Kurtz has exerted upon the formulation of this chapter which has drawn partly upon an earlier publication (Wolfensberger, 1969).

The concept of deviancy has been elaborated in the recent past by social scientists, and it is a very useful one. A person can be said to be deviant if he is perceived as being significantly different from others in some aspect that is considered of relative importance, and if this difference is negatively valued. An overt and negatively valued characteristic that is associated with the deviancy is called a 'stigma'.

Some sociologists (e.g. Farber, 1968) do not consider the terms 'deviant' and 'deviancy' as appropriate for some groups, such as the retarded, because to these sociologists, the definition of deviancy implies an intent to be deviant. I find this definition to be very weak, since it would necessitate the determination of the presence or absence of intent in each individual instance, and in practice, this would imply reliance on a mentalistic and intangible construct that is rarely ascertainable in a convincing manner.

It clearly must be kept in mind that deviancy is of our own making; it is in the eyes of the beholder. An observed quality only becomes a deviancy when it is viewed as negatively value-charged. And the same quality that may be negatively valued in one culture may be positively valued in another. Obesity in women is a good example, being valued in some mid-eastern cultures. As a German proverb proclaims: what is an owl to one person is a nightingale to another.

Handicapped individuals are frequently perceived as deviant. One only needs to consider the history of attitudes toward and the management of the mentally retarded and disordered; the visually, aurally, physically, or speech handicapped; the cosmetically disfigured; the aged and epileptic; and the delinquent and legal offenders. Even those whose differentness may not constitute a disability may be perceived as deviant, for instance those who are unusually tall, short, thick, or thin; members of ethnic, racial, or non-conformist minorities; and even those who stand out because of special talents, high intelligence, or virtue.

The generality of attitudes toward deviancy

Too often, we are only concerned about attitudes toward one type of deviancy, perhaps the type that is of primary concern in our own work. Yet frequently, the attitude that we may see expressed toward a person with a certain deviancy may not really be specific to that deviancy at all; such an attitude is very apt to be part of a more generalized attitude complex about a group of deviancies, or perhaps about deviancy in the broadest sense.

We should keep in mind that such assertions have considerable empirical and historical evidence behind them. Persons rarely appear to be prejudiced against only one type of deviancy. For instance, English (1971) showed that negative attitudes toward blindness were related to similar attitudes toward racial and ethnic minorities. Adorno *et al.* (1950) identified an 'authoritarian personality' type that is particularly apt to be prejudiced. Also, history shows that different types of deviancies were often managed in very similar ways, and that a wide range of deviancies may elicit similar responses or expectancy patterns from people.

To explain such generalization of response, Wilkins (1965) suggests that our attitudes toward deviance derive from the platonic notion that goodness, truth, and beauty are related to each other, and that any deviations from norms, i.e. truth, are 'errors' which, by analogy, must be related to evil and ugliness. For instance, a person may react with similar emotions toward retardation as he does toward blindness, delinquency, and senility. ...

The tenth (1880) United States census first combined 'defectives, dependents, and delinquents' for reporting purposes. In its reports, the Public Health Service combined criminals, defectives, and delinquents as late as the 1920s. Between about 1875 and 1920, one of the most important organizations of human service workers in the United States was the National Conference on Charities and Correction, and in its proceedings during this time span, it often grouped the idiotic, imbecilic and feeble-minded with the deaf, dumb, blind, epileptic, insane, delinquent and offenders into one general class of 'defectives'. Few of us today are aware of the fact that the more contemporary term 'mental defective' was coined to distinguish the retarded from these other 'defectives', and it is no coincidence that there were many public institutions serving both the retarded as well as epileptic nonretarded. During the eugenic alarm period (circa 1890–1925), an incredible variety of deviancies were believed to be associated with retardation; indeed, they were seen to be caused by it: illness, physical impediments; poverty; vagrancy; unemployment; alcoholism; sex offenses of various types, including prostitution and illegitimacy; crime; mental illness; and epilepsy. All these were called the 'degeneracies'. ...

During the early part of the century – a very chauvinistic period – numerous writers claimed that a large proportion of the retarded and otherwise degenerate came from foreign-born stock, contributing to the call for more restrictive immigration laws (Wolfensberger, 1969). This is perhaps an extreme example of how retardation was linked in the minds of many to other types of deviance. One could go on endlessly demonstrating the point that societal responses toward one type of deviancy were not specific, but were part of a more generalized pattern of response toward deviance.

Major historic roles of deviant persons

When a person is perceived as deviant, he is cast into a role that carries with it powerful expectancies. Strangely enough, these expectancies not only take hold of the mind of the perceiver, but of the perceived person as well. It is a well-established fact that a person's behavior tends to be profoundly affected by the role expectations that are placed upon him. ... This permits those who define social roles to make self-fulfilling prophecies by predicting that someone cast into a certain role will emit behavior consistent with that role. Unfortunately, role-appropriate behavior will then often be interpreted to be a person's 'natural' mode of acting, rather than a mode elicited by environmental events and circumstances. ...

When we review history and literature, it becomes apparent that regardless of time or place, certain roles are particularly apt to be thrust upon deviant persons. The way in which these roles transcend time, distance, and culture is remarkable. Most of these socio-historical role perceptions reflect fairly clear-cut prejudices which have little relationship to reality. However, as with many prejudices, the lack of objective verification is not a crucial element in the shaping of a social judgment or social policy. ...

The deviant individual as a subhuman organism

Historians and sociologists have long recognized that deviant subgroups within a culture may be perceived as not fully human. To this day, for example, there are large segments of our population, which deny full human status to members of certain minority groups, such as Negroes and Indians. Even ordinary army recruits may be said to need 'being broken' or tamed, like wild beasts or horses. But the retarded are particularly apt to be unconsciously perceived or even consciously labeled as subhuman, as animal-like, even as 'vegetables' or 'vegetative'. The literature of retardation is richly endowed with allusions to the alleged subhuman nature of retarded individuals and with labels that suggest subhuman status. The term 'garden-variety retardation', widely used by professionals in the past to refer to so-called cultural-familial retardation, has definite vegetative connotations.

It is interesting to note that the vegetable concept may, in part, have been derived from an appropriate transfer of the medical concept of 'vegetative functions'. In medicine, the 'vital functions' controlled by the autonomic nervous system and/or the hypothalamus may be referred to as 'vegetative'. These functions, which include temperature, heart rate, blood pressure, respiration rate, etc. are possessed by all humans and most animal species, and yet the concept of vegetative functions is sometimes translated into the social context in such a way as to abrogate even animal, not to mention human, qualities. ...

Deutsch (1949) pointed out that the mentally disordered were often apt to be stripped of their human attributes, together with their rights and privileges as human beings. Logically, if one dehumanizes a person who once had reason but lost it, then it is even easier to dehumanize a person who never possessed much reason in the first place, such as a retarded individual. For instance, a comment in the *Atlantic Monthly* (October, 1967, p. 49) called for '... sacrifice of mentally defective humans, or human vegetables' to provide organ transplants and '... increase the intellectual betterment of mankind. ...'

...

Dehumanization of the retarded is so accepted, even in this day, and even by workers in the field, that we can witness a public statement by a contemporary superintendent of a state institution referring to some of his retarded residents as '... so-called human beings ...' '... below what we might call an animal level of functioning ...' (*Frontiers of Hospital Psychiatry*, 1968, 5(1), 5–6).

Some of the implications of the subhuman role perception to human management are obvious. Aside from these obvious points, the following corollaries of the subhuman perception are of note: attribution of animal-like qualities or even skills; belittling of the learning capacity; abrogation of a sense of aesthetics; need for extraordinary control, restriction, or supervision; denial of citizenship rights and privileges, which may partially explain why, since about 1900, retarded residents in public institutions have been treated in a fashion that today is being (or will probably soon be) ruled illegal or unconstitutional; abrogation of human emotions, sensibilities, shame, and even sensation and perception.

In regard to the last point, the idea that the mentally afflicted lack sensory acuity, e.g. that they are insensitive to heat and cold, was popular into the mid-1800s (Deutsch, 1949). This myth resulted in their often being denied heat during the winter for their cold institution cells, and may well have contributed to the image of the retarded as insensate vegetables. Indeed, even new buildings designed specifically for the disordered did not provide for heating of the residents' cells, nor were their windows glazed (Tiffany, 1891). Parallels to this interpretation of a devalued group as being insensate non-humans can be found even in contemporary society. As recently as 1972, the South African government was planning to build high-rise housing for non-white laborers, in which these laborers would be 'kept' segregated by sex, four persons to a room, and without any heating (*Time*, May 15, 1972).

Devaluation of a human being into a subhuman role is so contrary to other ideals and values which a perceiver may hold as to prohibit the conscious recognition and labeling of the dehumanization. Therefore, it is important to be aware that while many persons hold subhuman perceptions, they cannot admit these perceptions to their own awareness because the implied interpretation of a human being would clash with other, concurrently held, perceptions and values. Thus, it is very common to encounter a person who dehumanizes a group of devalued individuals without being conscious of the meaning of his overt behavior and the reality of his attitudes. Only by understanding this process of repression of an unacceptable impulse can we also understand certain dehumanizing behaviors, or why some dehumanizers are remarkably unaware that their behaviors and attitudes are dehumanizing and are perceived to be so by others.

Vail (1967) has probed this problem with considerable sophistication. For instance, how can the fact be explained that individuals who, by all ordinary criteria, can be described as model citizens, suddenly become the cold-blooded killers of millions. This can only be understood if one understands the reality and process of the dehumanization of devalued individuals. The explanation is that if an organism is perceived as being not fully human, then it does not matter whether this organism is destroyed, dislocated, disowned, or otherwise used at the convenience of those perceived to be human. Animals are thus used all the time.

What is remarkable is that individuals who are relatively moral in every other sphere of their lives are capable of imposing nonhuman role perceptions upon certain groups, and are then very readily capable of treating such groups no better than animals. Only this reality can explain how otherwise moral and loving individuals can be unfeeling and dehumanizing human managers in certain spheres of their functioning. … It explains a phenomenon such as the senior personnel of an institution with about 75 years of experience in work with retarded children designing a new building for severely handicapped children which has toilets that are too large and high to be usable by such children, and soap dishes and towel racks attached so high on the wall as to be unreachable by the children. Had the designers been charged with planning a building for human children, they would have anticipated such problems; designing for entities perceived to be nonhuman, it was impossible for the designers to muster the empathy necessary to anticipate this problem, even with generations of experience behind them.

Only by fully understanding the dynamics and the accompanying unconsciousness of dehumanization will one be able to fully perceive and relate to the symbolic ways in which dehumanization often manifests itself. For example, there are many documented instances in which a parent has destroyed his handicapped child. The motives have been varied, and have included disappointment, frustration, hostility, pity, etc. However, it is not often that a middle-class parent not merely destroys his own child, but also commits the highly symbolic act of discarding the child literally in the garbage, as has happened recently in a large North American city.

As Buddenhagen (1971) points out, there may be similar symbolism in the fact that severe aversive punishment is particularly apt to be used with the retarded, and perhaps for reasons which are not quite conscious. With less impaired individuals, we are much more apt to use rewards, and while it might take some ingenuity to devise an appropriate reward system for the profoundly retarded, such ingenuity is probably quite within the scope of ability and grasp of most experimenters. … Similarly, the use of the electric cattle prod to administer aversive stimuli in the shaping of the behavior of the profoundly retarded may carry with it profound symbolic meaning. …

Finally, Rowland and Patterson (1971) suggest that past and recent efforts of prominent scientists to explain the social problems associated with certain minority groups as being due to genetic intellectual inferiority is merely a sophisticated way of interpreting such minority groups as subhuman.

The deviant individual as a menace

Unknown events or objects, if alien enough, tend to arouse negative feelings in both man and beast. Man's history is filled with incidents of man's persecution of fellow men of different features, skin pigmentation, size, shape, language, custom, dress, etc., and it is apparent that man has been very apt to see evil in deviance. Therefore, it is not surprising that one role perception prominent in history is that of the deviant person as a menace. He might be perceived as being a menace individually, because of alleged propensities toward various crimes against persons and property; or he might be perceived as a social menace because of alleged contribution to social disorganization and genetic decline. This role perception has been a very prominent one during the so-called genetic scare or alarmist period. ... when most of society's problems were attributed to inherited defect.

The deviant individual as an unspeakable object of dread

Somewhat related to other role perceptions of the deviant person as subhuman or a menace is the perception of him as a dreadful entity or event. In some respects, this role perception is similar to the one of 'Man as other' defined by Vail (1967). Man as changeling, discussed earlier, may fit here, as may perceptions of a deviant person as sent by God as a punishment for the sins of his parents, discussed further below.

The deviant individual as an object of pity

Frequently, a deviant individual is viewed as a person who is handicapped because of a misfortune for which he bears no responsibility, and who therefore should receive special attention, services, etc. The deviant person may even be seen as 'suffering' from his condition ... . While there may be made efforts to relieve this alleged suffering, the person may also be seen as possibly unaware of his deviance. Much as in the sick role perception, the pitied person is likely to be held blameless for his condition, and perhaps unaccountable for his behavior. He is very apt to be viewed with a 'there but for the grace of God go I' attitude.

Usually, this form of the pity perception is benevolent and is accompanied by compassion and acceptance, although it may be devoid of respect for the deviant person. However, there also exists another variant of the pity perception, upheld more by a sense of duty than compassion. Particularly persons possessing a strongly moralistic conscience but not much genuine humanism are apt to perceive deviant persons as objects of sour charity. ... While the affected person was usually (but not necessarily) viewed as innocent, his parents often were not. Thus the advent of a handicapped child was sometimes interpreted as a punishment for parental sins, and occasionally, the handicap was even attributed to a sin committed by the handicapped person himself prior to the presumed onset of his impaired condition. ...

Thus, the sour humanist may look upon a deviant recipient of services as a 'kept' object of charity, and while such charity clients may be seen as entitled to basic assistance and sustenance, they are not seen as entitled to anything interpretable as luxuries, frills, or extras. The object of such charity is expected to be grateful, and to work as hard as possible for his 'keep'.

As Coll (1969) pointed out, the Puritan Ethic had a strong influence in the formulation of the 'less eligibility' doctrine in the history of welfare services and charitable agencies. The doctrine states that no matter what the need of a person may be who is supported by public funds, assistance to him must be below the level of the lowest prevailing wage.

The deviant individual as a holy innocent

In a number of cultures and eras, deviant individuals, particularly the mentally afflicted, have been accorded a religious role interpretation as the special children of God, as saints, or as holy or eternal innocents. Those incompetent to perform everyday tasks might be perceived as having religious thoughts on their minds, or as being endowed with saintly powers. It may also be believed that such persons have been sent by God for some special purpose. Perceived in a religious light, the afflicted are usually seen as incapable of consciously or voluntarily committing evil, and consequently they may be considered to be living saints. Religious role perceptions of some kind were reportedly prevalent among the Eskimos, North American Indians, and Arabs; and in Russia, Central Asia, and medieval Europe. ...

At times, deviant persons have been perceived as not merely incapable of sin, but as actually being representative of, or possessed by, a sacred spirit. In such cases, a certain awe or even cult may surround such persons, as was reportedly the case among some North American Indian tribes. A person perceived in such a way may be quite valued, and he or his family may be perceived as specially favored by the Lord. To this day, certain Central American Indian cultures perceive their albino members as being on special terms with the sun god, and as being less inclined to commit evils (Shatto and Keeler, 1971).

Vanier (1971) relates the story of an Algerian who said to the parents of a retarded child 'How lucky you are to have a child like that. We believe that a family that has a child like that is blessed by Allah.' In the Arab world, the word 'saint' may actually be used for persons of altered mind, including the retarded, disturbed, epileptic, and religious ascetic. The term 'marabut' might be applied equally to the lowly retarded servant girl or to a respected saintly figure (Edgerton, 1970).

Jewish tradition, like many, is divided as to attitudes toward handicap. While one current of attitudes is very devaluing, another provides a positive and religious interpretation. Thus, the following ancient Hebrew prayer, over 3000 years old, is intended to be said upon encountering a deformed person : 'Praise to you, Lord God, king of the universe, who varies the forms of thy creatures.' A Jewish proverb states that 'the power of prophecy is given to children and fools'.

In Western culture, the holy innocent perception is still particularly prevalent in Catholicism. There is a 'Prayer for Holy Innocents' in the Roman ritual, and one encounters many poems on the theme, such as the much-publicized 'Heaven's Very Special Child'. ...

The holy innocent perception is one of the most benign role perceptions in human management. However, it has one element that is objectionable. It implies a reverse form of dehumanization, by elevating a human being almost above the human level, and by suggesting a 'little angel' status.

However, the perception of the holy innocent must be differentiated from the interpretation of the impaired person as innocent but not necessarily holy. This is a perception forcefully synthesized by Vanier (1971), and if applied with discretion to some impaired persons (such as to some of the retarded), it may be quite accurate for them. This interpretation is based upon certain child-like traits which may be found especially in retarded persons, without implying that such persons are either holy or eternal children. In other words, selectively applied, this perception can be a highly realistic one which, in a sensitive and properly motivated person, can elicit a rich and enriching response style toward the perceived person.

The deviant individual as a diseased organism

An additional historically prominent role perception is that of the deviant individual as sick, i.e. as an incumbent of what sociologists refer to as the 'sick role'. ... Conditions which have been widely subsumed under such a model include homosexuality, mental disorder, mental retardation, stuttering, alcoholism, and drug addictions. ... Perceived as sick, the deviant person may be seen as entitled to the privileges, as well as subjected to the demands, that have been proposed by Parsons (1951; Parsons and Fox, 1958) as characteristic of the sick role generally, and as partially verified empirically by Gordon (1966).The privileges include exemption from normal social responsibilities, and recognition that the condition is not the individual's fault; the demands are that the individual must want to get well or at least better, and must seek suitable and appropriate remedy for his condition.

It should be noted that the disease model can be expressed in two variants, one of these embodying the best tradition of medical service to fellow humans, and the other one being concerned with health but not with human values. The latter model can be likened to veterinary medicine, and is particularly apt to be encountered in residential institutions.

The deviant individual as an object of ridicule

This role perception is closely associated with another one in which men are perceived as 'trivium' (Vail, 1967), i.e. as unimportant or not to be taken seriously. Thus, for many years, the Negro was virtually always depicted by the mass media, such as movies, in the role of a servant; a comic figure. ... or, at best, a light entertainer. Similarly, the retarded have frequently been cast into the role of village idiots, and in folk humor they are almost without exception depicted as an object of ridicule. A relatively recent manifestation of this role perception is the so-called moron joke of a few years ago, and an outstanding depiction of the retarded person as an object of ridicule was contained in the award-winning film *Charly*, based on Keyes' (1966) book *Flowers for Algernon*. ...

The deviant individual as an eternal child

A very strong role perception of some deviant individuals is that of persons who are and perhaps always will be much younger than their age. For instance, the book *The Child Who Never Grew* by Pearl Buck (1950) and a Canadian film entitled *Eternal Children* render such a depiction of the retarded person. ...

Generally, those who hold the eternal child role perception do not place strong or even reasonable developmental and adaptational demands upon the person so perceived. Instead of expecting the person to adapt to the environment, those who see him as a child would adapt the environment to him. For example, Eaton and Weil (1955) report that when a child is recognized as retarded among the Hutterites, extensive adjustments are made in his social environment. His baptism may even be 'cancelled', so that he can do no wrong as an adult. In no case is the retarded person institutionalized, as happens in the mainstream North American culture when the social systems surrounding a retarded person cannot or will not adapt to his limitations. ...

---

5 From: 'The bad things that typically get done to devalued people', 1998, *A Brief Introduction to Social Role Valorization: A High Order Concept for Addressing the Plight of Societally Devalued People and for Structuring Human Services*, 12–24, Syracuse, NY: Training Institute for Human Service Planning, Leadership and Change Agentry.

As discussed in the Introduction, a 'teaching culture' has paralleled Wolfensberger's writing, since at least the early 1970s. Some might claim that the development of the core ideas of this chapter owed more to that culture than the writing itself, at least until much later in the 1990s and after. Their origins in what has gone before in this chapter should, however, be clear. Indeed, the use of the 'historic roles', supported by contemporary examples, became a key element in the teaching of normalization, and then Social Role Valorization (SRV). As the introduction to this chapter discusses, however, there has also developed a formulation of the experiences of devalued people that informs a great many more teaching events than simply those about SRV. Many of the broader ideas dealt with later in this book are presaged, in teaching events, by the exposition of what has become known as the 'wounds' of devalued people.

As the years have proceeded, however, perhaps because of the attempts of those responding to the devaluation process in human services to devise 'solutions', the focus for some people has shifted to devising such solutions in the first instance, without looking at the problems they were intended to tackle. Thus, in many places where normalization and SRV were taught, the 'wounds' were not addressed at length, or sometimes at all. There may have been other reasons for this, such as an understandable desire to tell 'good news' to support the fledgling pockets of services that attempted to provide a more valued life for people, often very much against the mainstream. Whatever the reason, and even if it represents a common understanding, almost a 'taking for granted' of the devaluation process, failure to present the devaluation process can also result in the repression into unconsciousness, talked about by Wolfensberger in the previous extract, of the reality of that devaluation and its continuing effect. Hence, in at least the training events that claim to be following the leadership of Wolfensberger's Training Institute, the 'wounds' presentation continues to be made.

Those who have moved from this approach, but are nevertheless sympathetic to the overall thrust of Wolfensberger's work, have then been joined by a number of critics who label the public description (i.e. in training events or publications) of such societal devaluation as 'collusion' in the very process itself (e.g. Ramcharan et al., 1997). In certain circles, particularly in the UK, this has resulted in the removal, or at least a drastic diminution, of discussion or presentation of the 'wounds'. Over the twenty or more years since they were first formulated as such, therefore, though there have been many presentations of the 'wounds' all over the world, there has equally been a significant group of people, aware and even supportive of normalization and SRV, who have nevertheless no awareness of the depth and breadth of applicability of the 'wounds' description.

The following extract is therefore the fullest and latest available written description by Wolfensberger. Though it is taken from his 1998 monograph on SRV, the extract should again be read in terms of the wider applicability of the devaluation process and its relevance to modern society, whenever the timeline of 'modern' is defined. It should also be read with the proviso that it summarizes material that can take anything up to a whole day of presentation, with many examples of the points raised from many different spheres of human services being used to illustrate their empirical validity.

The bad things that typically get done to devalued people

People who are the objects of devaluation, and especially of devaluation by their society, typically have all sorts of hurtful things done to them. Sometimes, these things are done with conscious and explicit intent; sometimes, these things are done unconsciously; and sometimes, these things are simply the result of life conditions and circumstances which are the way they are for the devalued party because of that party's devalued status and life conditions.

Very briefly, the following are the hurtful things that on a probabilistic basis are very apt to befall societally devalued people, and even characterize their lives. ...

1   Many devalued people are, or become, impaired in body, including in brain or sense organs. Some get devalued because they have impairments of body that were either evident at birth or acquired afterwards. However, so often, the opposite also happens, in that people who were devalued for other reasons become impaired in body as a result of that devaluation, and this usually

makes them even more devalued. For instance, people may become impaired as a result of poverty, poor nutrition, unsafe living conditions, poor health care, or being assaulted – all things that are very likely to happen to them as a result of being devalued.

2   Many devalued people are impaired in functioning. Examples include deficiencies in seeing, hearing, speaking, mobility, or self-care. Because of their devalued state and bad living conditions, children from devalued classes may grow up less intelligent, and/or mentally conflicted, even if they are physically whole. Many devalued people are or end up impaired in some area of functioning that most valued people possess and take for granted, such as basic literacy, getting along adaptively with other people, running and maintaining a household, attending to one's personal appearance, etc. Functional impairments may have been the reason some people got devalued in the first place, or the functional impairment may be a result of a person having been devalued for some other reason. In either case, the functional impairment may be a result of an earlier physical impairment, though functional impairments can also exist in the absence of physical impairment.

3   Devalued people get relegated to low social status in society, and are looked down upon. They are considered second-class citizens – or even worse – and treated accordingly.

4   As a result of being relegated to low social status, or being devalued even if not status-reduced, people also get systematically rejected, not only by society as a whole but quite often even by their own family, neighbors, community, and even by the workers in services that are supposed to assist them. Rejection means that other people really do not want that person around. Several of the subsequent forms of wounding can be understood to be the overt behavioural expressions of people's internal feeling of rejection.

5   One consequence of wounds 3 and 4 that is of special relevance to SRV is that devalued people get cast into roles that are devalued in society, and their access to valued roles is severely diminished, or even eliminated. Typically, there is some kind of link between the reason why a person is devalued, and the specific devalued role that gets imposed on the devalued person, or the valued roles that get withheld from such a person. In other words, the devalued person is given a role identity that confirms and justifies society's ascription of low value or worth to the person. Some of the major common negative social roles into which members of societally devalued groups are apt to be cast are given in Wolfensberger (1972). ... [See previous extracts – Ed.]

6   Another wounding expression of rejection is that devalued people get systematically and relentlessly juxtaposed to images that carry very negative messages in the eyes of society. Services to them get put in locations where valued people do not want to be; devalued people get placed with other people whom society also does not want; image-degrading language is used with or about them, and image-degrading names get given to their services;

elements of their personal appearance that attract negative attention are not addressed, or their deviant appearance may even be enlarged by people in charge of their lives; services to them are funded by appeals that are image-tainting. All these (and other) sorts of negative images convey messages such as that these people are worthless, subhuman, menaces, dangerous and despicable – and this negative imaging perpetuates the social devaluation and de facto invites other people to do bad things to the devalued people.

7   Rejected and negatively-imaged devalued people are at extreme risk of being made society's scapegoats. Whatever the problem is, devalued people are apt to be suspected of causing or exacerbating it, and punishing them in some way is widely promoted as the solution to a societal problem. For instance, devalued people are more likely than valued people to be suspected of an offense that has been committed, accused of it, arrested, prosecuted, convicted, and given a harsh sentence. Entire devalued classes may be accused as guilty when a society experiences a natural disaster or social or economic problem. ...

8   Another behavioral expression of rejection (No. 4) is to push a devalued rejected person away, i.e., people put distance between themselves and those they devalue and reject. The valued people may do this by removing themselves – i.e., by withdrawing as far as possible from those they devalue – or by moving the devalued people away. For instance, they may segregate devalued people into separate settings, perhaps even ghettoes and reserv-ations, or send them into a form of exile. Thus, the distance may be physical, as in segregation; and when people are segregated because they are deval-ued, they usually also get congregated with other devalued people, often in huge groups. But the distance may also be social, as in various forms of degradation that make it clear how lowly the devalued party is seen to be even when no physical distance is put between the two parties. ...

9   People who are devalued also experience loss of control over their lives. It is other people who gain power over them and make decisions for them, in both overt and subtle ways, some of them already mentioned above.

10   Furthermore, devalued people experience a very wounding discontinuity with places and physical objects, including possessions. At least in part, this kind of discontinuity is the result of being distantiated, of having little control over one's life, and of being moved about a lot. Often, physical moves are interpreted to be for the devalued person's own good, or as progress and growth in independence. There can be scores of these kinds of discontinuities in a person's lifetime, and many can be quite dramatic.

11   Commonly, the devalued person also suffers a great many social and relationship discontinuities, meaning that people come and go in that person's life, endlessly. Often, relationship discontinuity accompanies, or is the result of, physical discontinuity (No.10), but even when a person is stable in one place, there may still be many, many people who walk in and out of that person's life. What makes this even more hurtful is that many of these very

people (especially paid ones) make either explicit or implicit promises that they want to be friends, that they are going to help, that they are "not like the others" – and yet all of them may end up leaving, perhaps after only a brief presence. When such an explicit or implicit promise has been made and then gets broken, the wound of discontinuity is compounded by the wound of betrayal.

12   Quite naturally, when a party is devalued and rejected, when other people withdraw from contact with that devalued party, and when what relationships there are do not last, this also means that natural relationships – such as those with family and friends – either never develop in the first place, or get withdrawn or severed. When natural relationships are no longer freely and voluntarily given to devalued people, other people have to be recruited to do what is needed for them. These other people almost always have to be paid, because that is the only reason they would be involved with the devalued person, and when such payment ceases, so does their presence. So the lives of devalued persons often begin to be filled with artificial and "boughten" relationships that are really substitutes for the "real thing" that valued people enjoy, such as the voluntary and willing relationships of family, friends, loved ones, and acquaintances. Some devalued people do not have even one single enduring unpaid relationship. Thus, the essence of this wound is the absence of natural relationships.

13   Devalued people also tend to get deindividualized. They are subjected to regimentation and mass management, and they so often have to accommodate themselves to whatever is available, rather than getting what they need or want when they need or want it, and the way that they need or want it – at least the way that valued people often do.

14   People who are devalued commonly end up poor. In both overt and subtle ways – some so subtle that they may not be recognized for what they are – devalued people end up with very little in the way of material possessions. If they need services, they may have to impoverish themselves in order to receive them, or they may end up poor as a result of receiving services. Some devalued people come from families and classes that have been poor for generations.

15   Devalued people also suffer impoverishment in the world of experience, which is often very narrow for them. They are denied participation in valued society and its activities, and there may even be places to which they are forbidden – or otherwise unable – to go. Many experiences that valued people take for granted may be withheld from, and be strange to, devalued people.

16   One particular experience from which devalued people may get cut off is knowledge of, and participation in, the religious or spiritual life of society. There are handicapped people who have never really been given instruction in the religion they may have been born into, nor been permitted to participate in the religious community life of their fellow believers.

17   One of the major results of several of the above wounds is that devalued people's lives so often get wasted. Days, weeks, months, years, a lifetime goes by while they are denied opportunities, challenges, experiences, and their earlier potential is wasted or destroyed. When they do receive service, it is often the wrong kind, or at any rate, of less intensity or quality than they could benefit from, or than valued people would get. Many devalued people spend much of their time just sitting and waiting, wasting away, often even in the service programs in which they are enrolled. We call this the wound of life-wasting.

18   Devalued people are very much at risk of being so badly treated as to be outright brutalized and violated, even to the point of being made dead. They may get assaulted on the streets, in their families, or by their service workers. Other people will think they are justified in getting rid of them permanently, i.e., ending their lives.

All of the above wounds deal with bad things that rather normatively happen to, or get done to, devalued people. These things can badly wound a person's psyche, spirit or soul, and result in a very distorted or disturbed relationship of the wounded person to the world, and especially to other people. Some of the most common expressions of such deep woundedness along this line are the following.

1   The wounded person may be, act, and feel like, an alien in the world, particularly the world of valued society. Devalued people can become very much aware that they do not fit in, that they are not welcome. If deeply wounded, people may become alienated not only from the valued world and its privileges, responsibilities, patterns, and opportunities, but even from humanity generally.

2   Wounded people may begin to dislike themselves and think that they really are despicable, unlovable, worthless; that everything bad that happens to them is their own fault, and that they deserve bad fortune. In that case, they may succumb to despair, perhaps become self-destructive.

3   Many of the wounds tend to make the wounded person very insecure. This sense of insecurity may be profound and pervasive, as it may concern a person's stability of place; of relationships, acceptance and belonging; of role, function and contribution in society; and of sense of ability and accomplishment.

4   These wounds can also generate an expectancy in the wounded person to fail at everything, or what psychologists have called a "failure set," which then tends to actually lead to avoidance of challenges, and to failure after failure, in a vicious circle.

5   People who are the objects of devaluation may be very aware that they are a source of anguish to whatever people may still be around who love them, especially their family members. Many realize that they are not what others wish they were, and that others − especially their loved ones − are inconvenienced or even suffering because of who and what they are.

6 Some people who have been deeply wounded by rejection and/or real or perceived abandonment – especially early in life – will embark on a real or symbolic quest for the abandoner. Often, this is an idealized mother (e.g., one who gave up her baby for adoption), or parents (e.g., who had institutionalized a child at birth or in childhood, and then drifted out of that child's life). This quest may be life-long, and even if it is successful, it may be bitterly disappointing.

7 Relatedly, people who have been deeply wounded in their relationships may develop fantasies about having once had positive relationships, and they may even invent new relationships that do not exist. Such fantasies express a deep, unfulfilled longing.

8 Relationship-wounded people may also seek a great deal of physical contact with others, perhaps going as far as becoming sexually promiscuous or prostituting themselves, out of a desperate desire for the things they have been deprived of, and that the physical contact represents: affection, and being loved.

9 Deeply wounded people can become very distrustful of relationships, and are apt to put them all to the test – sometimes tests that are so hard that no-one could pass them, e.g. "will you still accept me and not send me away even if I assault you, or set fire to your house, or choke your baby?"

10 Many devalued people become embittered, and perhaps even full of resentment and hatred towards the privileged world for having done, and continuing to do, such hurtful things to them.

11 Some people have been so badly wounded that they withdraw from all contact with other human beings, and perhaps even from reality altogether.

12 Of course, many deeply wounded people are so enraged about what has been, and perhaps continues to be, done to them that they become overtly violent towards other people and the world.

13 And coping with one's wounds can take so much energy that a deeply wounded person actually ends up reduced in intelligent, rational and adaptive functioning, reduced in mental and emotional competence, and perhaps even reduced in intelligence itself.

Obviously, the bad things that happen to devalued people are not only hurtful but can also become life-defining. Examples are having to live in poverty, being perceived for much of one's life as a social menace or as subhuman, being systematically segregated, being excluded from major opportunities in life, having one's life wasted, etc.

What I have just sketched is the real way that people who get devalued tend to experience the world. Versions of this story keep happening over and over, and could be retold – at least in part – about the life of almost everybody who has been in a devalued state for a significant period of time. And yet, training programs for human service workers hardly ever convey this phenomenology to their students.

Chapter 2

Normalization

Introduction

Though the theme of devaluation and wounding is present in one way or another in most of Wolfensberger's work, it was, at least initially, for the ideas that have been associated with the word 'normalization' that he became internationally known. As discussed later in this chapter, many of the ideas attributed to this word were not those of Wolfensberger, and many of the actions taken by services in the name of normalization have moved a long way from the origins of the ideas, or even Wolfensberger's specific formulation of it. Because of this, and also perhaps for reasons discussed in later Chapters, especially Chapters 5 and 6, a great deal of the clarity that came with the early formulations, especially in the late 1960s and early 1970s, has been lost in a mass of controversies, personalized attacks, and even outright banning of discussion of anything coming from Wolfensberger.

This chapter therefore aims to remind readers of some of that early depth and clarity, and also to put into context, via later recollections of Wolfensberger, just how fragile were the chances of the ideas achieving the sort of worldwide effects and acclaim that were outlined in the Introduction. The first extract traces some of the ideas and early history of how Wolfensberger's formulation of normalization was developed, and the influences on that.

---

6 **From: 'A contribution to the history of normalization, with primary emphasis on the establishment of normalization in North America between 1967–1975', 1999, Chapter 3 of *A Quarter-Century of Normalization and Social Role Valorization: Evolution and Impact*, 51–116, Ottawa: University of Ottawa Press. (Revised and edited version of paper originally presented at the conference "Twenty-Five Years of Normalization, Social Role Valorization and Social Integration: A Retrospective and Prospective View" held in Ottawa, May 1994.)**

The picture presented in this keynote address at the 1994 Ottawa conference, though it is obviously from Wolfensberger's perspective and based on his diaries and recollections, presents the modern reader with a sense of wonder at a) the fragility of the initial movement, with many events being subject to chance circumstances and the coming together of relatively few people, and b) how much of what is now taken for granted was totally radical, even unthinkable, in the late 1960s and early 1970s. In addition, the extract puts the intellectual antecedents of normalization, some of which have been already mentioned, into some context, at least as far as Wolfensberger's thinking is concerned. His gentle chiding, in the introduction, of scholars not going to original sources would appear to this editor to be just as relevant nearly ten years later as it was in 1994.

Introduction

In recent years, there have been many references in the literature to the early days of Normalization where the authors cited references that were not from the founding period, but secondary or retrospective ones from the 1980s. Among the reasons people cite post-1980 literature when discussing events that occurred up to 20 years earlier appear to be four: (a) they were not on the scene at the time; (b) they do not know the primary literature (perhaps the computer bases that were consulted did not go back far enough); (c) if they do know it, they do not have ready access to it; and (d) they prefer recent revisionist ideas to the historical truth, and therefore avoid the original literature.

So I went to my extensive personal archives and drew on these for this presentation. In fact, this was the first time that I methodically mined my relevant archives from the 1960s and 1970s for Normalization material. Historical revisionists may commence quaking in their boots because I can now cite genuine original sources and prove many of the points I will make. ...

Ideas and schemes that were widely promoted as major answers in human services, and/or for the conditions addressed by these, prior to the advent of Normalization and/or shortly after it, and some in competition with it

In this section, I want to take a look at what the conceptual landscape in human services was like in the years or decades prior to the advent of Normalization. ...

Of course, literally billions of people during the last century thought that Marxist arrangements would bring about something close to a paradise on earth, since a huge number of problems were seen to be no more than the fruits of economic and power inequalities, capitalism, and other ills for which Marxism claimed to have remedies. ...

For several decades, eugenic measures were seen as the most overarching package of solutions to social problems, and to many clinical and personal ones. This included a massive program of institutionalization, with specialized institutions erected for a large variety of afflicted people. ... The poverty of service conceptualization was such that even when the social alarm associated with eugenics had been heavily discredited by about 1930, institutionalism barreled right on for another 30 years. ... [See Chapter I – Ed.] As I will emphasize repeatedly, there was also very little critique of institutionalism prior to about 1965. Almost everybody was willing to say that this or that could be better about institutions, but one will not be likely to find much in the *professional* literature – at least not from the human service sector – that said (a) that institutions were awful places, or even (b) that there was anything intrinsically defective about the very idea of large institutions. If there were people who believed these things, they were not afforded a forum to voice such thoughts. What published critique there was of institutions came mostly from a few exposés, and mostly from outside the service system.

In response to both the terrible conditions in institutions of all sorts and to the fact that, nevertheless, waiting lists for them were normatively very large and long, a major reform concept for about 100 years was "more institutions" and "better institutions." After circa 1930, the cry for more institutional space was not so much motivated by eugenic reasons as it had been before, but simply to reduce overcrowding in existing institutions and to service the huge institutional waiting lists. ...

What did people mean by "better institutions"? Above all, they meant less crowding, and reducing it was widely considered to be the single biggest key to improving institutional conditions. They also meant things such as smaller dormitories, smaller wards, more cleanliness, less ugliness in the environment, less stench, a better toilet-to-resident ratio, better educated attendants and a few more of them, a few more professional staff members, and fewer who were very deviant themselves, and for most residents, a small cabinet for keeping some personal clothes and perhaps a few other items. An institution that had even some of these was considered a model institution to which observers streamed in envious admiration.

By the 1950s, 1960s, and 1970s, "better institutions" also began to mean two more things: (a) smaller institutions with only a few hundred to a low thousand or so residents; and (b) more equitable distribution of institutions across a state or province, both for humane reasons and reasons of local economy.

One of the "better institution" concepts that captivated many minds and was seen as a major reform idea was the "therapeutic community" concept originated by Maxwell Jones after World War II (e.g., Jones, 1953). This concept spread to many other kinds of institutions and seemed to experience occasional reincarnations through similar schemes, such as so-called "remotivation" schemes in the 1960s and 1970s. Many people looked to therapeutic community schemes as at least a major foundation of "good institutions." In one of my first published articles on Normalization, namely, the one for a psychiatric audience in 1970 (Wolfensberger, 1970a), I had to explain why and how Normalization was not the same as the "therapeutic community," and that we should quit invoking images of the medical model with "therapy" language and instead think in terms of a "normalizing community" (p. 296). The article was promptly reprinted by the Pennsylvania Association for Retarded Children, together with a statement that "we must begin to practice the *Normalization PRINCIPLE*," and widely disseminated over the state. ...

During the 1940s and 1950s, many people looked on psychotherapy and personal counseling – and some on psychoanalysis specifically – as a major answer to problems of living. Many people really thought that individual problems of a psychic nature would yield to this service modality if only (a) enough therapists or counselors could be trained, and (b) the people with the problems would come to them. Obviously, some still cling to this notion, as is evident from the extremely widely syndicated advice column of Ann Landers during recent decades, and to this day. The advent, and relatively sudden dissemination, of Rogerian counseling had much to do with this, because it was widely seen as both more readily learnable by more people than other forms of psychotherapy and as applicable to more situations and needs than the "heavy" psychotherapies, such as psychoanalytic ones.

A strategy that was perhaps the most broadly promoted one since World War II was a very vague construct of "attitude change.". ... Out of this reasoning must have come the intense efforts to educate the public about mental disorder and mental retardation by means of tours of institutions, and such tours became very common in the 1950s and 1960s. Apparently totally unrecognized at that time was the fact that education by itself does not combat prejudice, and that contact with devalued persons or classes that is experienced as unpleasant is even apt to have an effect opposite to the desired one. ...

Before the advent of Normalization, and during its early days, behavior modification (which then was usually still known as operant conditioning) presented itself as a quasi-savior for certain groups, including the mentally retarded. Many films were made that tried to show what behavior modification could do, and some of the accomplishments in individual instances were impressive – even amazing. However, so many of these films were made in institutions, and displayed little sense of awareness – or none whatever – either of the badness of the institutional arrangements or that the clinical methods of behavior modification were a very displaced response to institutionalism. ... Also, almost all these films displayed an appalling unconsciousness of image issues and quite unnecessarily interpreted retarded people in all sorts of negative ways.

One of the most threatening major potential competitors of comprehensive normalized community services was the idea of ... the "comprehensive community services facility" into which many people in the 1950s and 1960s put much hope. In essence, this was a single building in which, and to a lesser degree from which, it was believed all or most needed services could be rendered to a service region. Such a facility would have components such as a children's day service center, a sheltered workshop, some residential units, soft services (such as assessment and guidance) rendered to people coming in on an "ambulatory" basis, some specialized "ambulatory" medical services, and offices for people who might go out and render limited services in the community, probably mostly consulting other services, plus a very modest amount of home visiting. Obviously, this idea was rooted in the then-prevailing medical model, and the idea of Louis XIV's *hôpital général* and its later offspring, the *Allgemeine Krankenhaus* (Foucault, 1973; Thompson & Goldin, 1975). ...

Many people had the idea that with many services co-located in neighborhood centers, citizens would rarely have to go outside their neighborhoods to be served. This just underlines how naive people were as to what constitutes comprehensiveness.

Unfortunately, it is this idea that ensouled the ill-fated community mental health centers, and the so-called "university-affiliated facilities" in mental retardation all over the US that became (a) financial milch cows for universities, and especially medical schools, (b) major consumers of mental retardation funds, and (c) only relatively minor contributors to the welfare of retarded people. That this idea would win out over community services that were normalized, diversified, dispersed, and citizen-controlled was for years a distinct possibility and a major fear among people like myself.

The single biggest service related to mental retardation that such centers, and other center-based units, rendered was the hugely expensive and stereotyped multi-disciplinary assessment of retarded people – mostly children. These assessments tended to have a strong neuropsychiatric slant, and to be rather meaningless dead ends. I wrote an exposé of this scandal (Wolfensberger, 1965a, 1965b) and had the hardest time getting a brief version of it published in the US, and only in something like an opinion column. [See extract 22 – Ed.] ...

During the 1960s, one step ahead of Normalization, a movement gathered a great deal of momentum that was high-level and only medium naive, namely, a "rights" orientation. But there was always some fuzziness about whether people intended to invoke legal or transcendent rights, the latter often called "human rights" or "moral rights," and how the two should be linked. I remember promoting the idea in those days that human rights should be pursued, as being of a higher order and greater universality than legal rights. The rights movement reflected at least some European influences, because the idea that certain services were a right rather than a privilege had long been established in the laws of several European countries, with additional such rights being defined in the mid-1960s ... . In the US, Gunnar Dybwad played a very large role in this development, at least as far as the field of mental retardation was concerned. He promoted a rights orientation and judicial recourse for years, and all this work suddenly erupted into fruition with an avalanche of litigation in the late 1960s and early 1970s, most of it successful. In almost all the early cases, Dybwad was involved behind the scenes, exhorting and/or consulting. The "rights" thinking first rested on two rationales. One was to finally achieve the old goal of "more money" by having certain services defined as a legal right. The second rationale was the removal of the social stigma that went with selective, arbitrary, or charitable funding. We now know that rightful funding does not necessarily accomplish this. The early rights movement focused on one big goal, and several smaller ones. The big goal was rightful funding of schooling for handicapped children, but the movement might at first have settled for such funding for most rather than all children, and would certainly have settled for segregated education. Smaller goals included less compulsion in institutional settings, less compulsory drugging, and so forth.

In my opinion, the rights orientation would have had different, and less favorable, outcomes than it did if the lawyers had not begun to draw on the Normalization-related writings as soon as these came out. In fact, the lawyers often incorporated material from the Normalization-related literature within weeks or months after it appeared and used this material very well.

Altogether, if one had asked people active in mental retardation specifically during roughly the years of 1965–1968 what it is they wanted, one would generally have found a terrible impoverishment of concepts. For instance, most parents were so worn out battling the school system that they could hardly see around the corner of the next small step forward. ... Just how pessimistic and outright nihilistic people tended to be about the mentally retarded in the 1950s, and to a large degree the 1960s, and how modest the aspirations of even most advocates for the retarded were, is difficult to imagine by people who were not there at that time.

Because of the widely prevalent sense of futility about the retarded condition, expectations were low, and the more retarded a person was, the less was expected. The term "incurable" was also closely linked to mental retardation. Even people like Edgar Doll, one of the grand old men of mental retardation, who, as far as I know, was very kindly toward retarded people, insisted to me in 1961 or 1962 that "a mongoloid is a mongoloid is a mongoloid" when I argued on behalf of the 1959 definition of mental retardation of the American Association on Mental Deficiency that left open the possibility that a retarded person might become unretarded.

The attitude of futility was also dominant, and exemplified, at the Plymouth State Home and Training School in Michigan where I assumed the position of director of research and training in 1963. There were only one teacher and one teacher's aide for the whole institution. From the rest of the staff, there was hardly any engagement with residents, even though a very large proportion of them were children and adolescents. ...

So, in my opinion, if Normalization had not come along when it did, and possibly even if it had come along but not been interpreted in a convincing fashion and on a massive scale, we would have seen mental retardation develop in the following directions:

1   There would have been massive investments into building new, smaller, region-alized institutions. This trend was already underway from the late 1950s on.
    ...
2   There would have been many more states pursuing the regional center model. ... Giant California committed itself to a regional center scheme, and many other states might have followed these leads if Normalization ideas of community-dispersed services had not become available as an alternative. The university-affiliated mental retardation centers, with their expensive clinical components that were beginning to bloom then, were playing right into the "center" concept. ...
3   A third thing that would have happened is that group residences would have developed, but they would have been very large and very abnormal. This is

what was happening in Connecticut in the late 1960s and was considered a model. … Some states still have these to this day. …

4   A fourth thing that would have happened would have been vastly more segregated education. Again, some states were well on their way toward segregated schools, and even segregated school districts, that is, school districts only for handicapped children.

5   A fifth thing that would have happened is much slower expansion of the education of the more severely handicapped children.

Without Normalization, many of the positive things that have come about would have come about anyway, but many of them anywhere between 10–20 years later, and some of the more subtle corollaries of Normalization would not have come about to this day. In fact, some corollaries of at least the Wolfensberger formulation are still normatively rejected even on the conceptual level, to say nothing of the implementive one.

This brief sketch of selected ideas that constituted people's major "hopes" in regard to human services or major human service sectors, or in regard to social changes that would have a bearing on human problems and human services, reveals the poverty of truly high-order ideas, and especially ideas that were not outright utopian or divorced from practicality, as Marxism has always been. …

Influences on service reformers and Wolfensberger that prepared them for the Normalization idea

In this section, I will review some of the major influences that predisposed me to be receptive to the Normalization principle. This coverage not only sheds light on why I embraced and promoted Normalization, but also why many other persons who had similar experiences became disposed in the same direction.

First of all, a new generation of people might easily forget that, at least in North America, the evolution and acceptance of the Normalization principle was deeply rooted in efforts at reforming institutions – mostly those for retarded people… . Had institutions not been so awful, even people with a sense of justice and compassion would probably not have felt a great need for a radical alternative.

However, we also have to call to mind that until the late 1960s, there was only an occasional outcry about an institutional scandal or atrocity here and there, but very little protest about the normativeness of bad institutional conditions, and hardly any opposition at all to institutionalism *per se*. …

My own odyssey toward Normalization started in 1956, when my sense of justice was outraged by the conditions in the so-called "back wards" of a mental institution in which I was then working as a clinical psychology trainee (at the Norfolk State Hospital, Norfolk, Nebraska, 1956–1957). [See Introduction – Ed.] This outrage was fueled in subsequent years by additional tours of, and episodes of work in, several other institutions of different kinds.

Another thing that laid important groundwork for Normalization and SRV in my mind from my earliest days in human services in the 1950s was that I found it easy to evoke positive behavior from devalued people through my positive expectations of them and my expressions of trust in them. As early as 1956, while still working on my master's degree, I conveyed expectations and trust to inmates of the most violent and locked ward of a large state mental institution (the one mentioned above) in such a fashion that I was never attacked, though many other people were. Similarly, despite being present in all sorts of violent situations in human service contexts since, I have never been attacked myself, and have attributed this at least in part to the positive role expectations that I conveyed to potential attackers. (Strangely enough, while I found it relatively easy to convey positive expectations to wounded and devalued people, I have always found it very difficult to do the same to imperial people.)

For the rest of this section of his paper, Wolfensberger refers to publications which affected his and others' thinking at this time, in particular Goffman and Vail, referred to in the Introduction and the *New Society* article in Extract 3. He also speaks of the implications of interpreting 'retarded people' as 'human, citizens, and capable of further development' which had come, at least in part, from Bank-Mikkelsen in Denmark, and led to the 'developmental model' of the above article. Finally the influence, from sociology, of the concept of 'deviancy', clearly revealed in the extract from the *Normalization* text in Extract 4, is discussed, together with the experiential development of Wolfensberger's visit to Europe, described in the Introduction, the conclusion of which is the first extract of Chapter 1. This then leads to the next section of the address.

...

The history of intercontinental exchange in human services that was the context for the transfer of Normalization from Scandinavia to North America

Next, I want to make a further contribution to an understanding of the socio-historical context that facilitated the transfer of Normalization ideas from Denmark and Sweden to North America. ...

What laid the groundwork for this transfer was, first of all, the long tradition of people from North America visiting human services in Europe, and then telling and writing about it back home, and of outright importing new ideas and practices that they had learned abroad. Sometimes, they even recruited European practitioners of new developments and established them in NorthAmerica. [Various examples are then given, which are omitted here – Ed.] ...

Of course, the information flow was not all one-way. At a certain point, it became more reciprocal. For instance, many eugenic ideas that had originated in Britain, and then had been taken up and implemented in the US, began to be carried back to Europe as Europeans began to take intense note of these developments and to cite them in support of the promotion of parallels in Europe – and, in the case of the Nazis, surpass them (e.g. Kevles, 1985; Proctor, 1988).

During the 1950s and 1960s, there had been a slow but influential trickle of American visitors (many from the mental health field) to Europe that included – perhaps for the first time – Scandinavia as a major source of noteworthy innovations. Coverage of mental retardation services was often a secondary aspect of their visits because, in those days, mental retardation services were generally administered by mental health services and professionals. However, what did intrigue visitors was that starting around 1960, a good number of institutions were built in Sweden that were not only "better institutions," but came close to being "best institutions." They were small and anticipated later Normalization formulations by having small sleeping spaces (instead of dormitories), small and diversified social spaces (instead of "day rooms"), a culturally normative internal decor (in fact, they were often breathtakingly beautiful), being well-staffed, and increasingly locally administered. (See also Grunewald, 1969.)

Then follows an extensive descriptive list of publications cited by Wolfensberger of accounts by visitors to and from Europe that would have been available to contemporary readers, and would have played their part in the 'transfer of ideas'. This includes his own reports and articles on personal exchanges with the key group of academics and service planners described in the Introduction, and leads to the conclusion that such exchanges constituted 'fertile soil' for such a transfer. He adds a concluding note, however, with typical forthrightness

... There are four points I want to add before going to the next topic.

1   When I toured services on the European mainland in 1963, one thing that struck me was that the leaders I met were rather smug about what they were doing. They felt that they had a good angle on their field and had little to learn from what was going on elsewhere – even elsewhere in Europe. The United Kingdom and Eire were different, with much orientation to the US. Especially in Eire, many service leaders in the early 1960s had been in the US, or were planning to go... .

2   One remarkable thing about so many American visitors to other countries is how little they perceived of what they saw that was good or even exemplary (at least for its time), and how often they interpreted as old hat good things that they had probably never seen. By the time I went to Scandinavia in 1969, I was already on the leading edge of reform thinking in North America and well prepared by my earlier exposure to Normalization and the editing of *Changing Patterns*. Nonetheless, where so many other visitors came away with an "isn't it nice" response or "we are already doing this or that," I came away with my mind blown, as they say these days. But then, we had the same experience with visitors to our Nebraska services between 1969 and the mid-1970s who could look at things they had never seen and go away without a conversion experience, perhaps allowing that "this is nice" or even muttering "this is old hat"!

3   There was one kind of reverse visiting that is relevant to the transfer process, and that is the one that consisted of several trips each by Niels Erik Bank-Mikkelsen, Karl Grunewald, and Bengt Nirje to the US between 1967 and 1971. At that time, Bank-Mikkelsen was head of the Danish mental retardation service, Grunewald was his counterpart in Sweden, and Nirje was executive director of the Swedish parents' association in mental retardation. They toured and spoke widely, a lot of what they spoke on reflecting Normalization thinking, and they received a great deal of press when they expressed their disgust at what they saw in US institutions. ... In late 1967, Bank-Mikkelsen made national news in the US when he said that in Denmark, cattle were better kept than retarded people in US institutions such as Sonoma State Hospital in California. All three visitors got so burned by the negative reactions of institution defenders to their comments that they became very reticent to use strong language (as I can document from my correspondence files).These visits and the press they got also contributed part of the background for the transfer of Normalization to North America. ...

4   It is my impression that until the early or mid-1970s, the Americans were indeed primarily the learners in this travel exchange, but that then the balance began to tip the other way, with Europeans beginning to fall all over themselves to visit North America – mainly the US – and transfer developments from there to Europe. This was partly just one element of the Americanization of the developed world, but part of it had to do with the explosion of human service ideas and practices in the US, including those in response to *Changing Patterns*, the Nebraska mental retardation service system model, the Normalization principle, and the legal rights victories. [See Introduction – Ed.] ...

The production of Changing Patterns in Residential Services for the Mentally Retarded

The next section is introduced with the already noted key events of the Nebraska service model and the production of *Changing Patterns in Residential Services for the Mentally Retarded* (Kugel and Wolfensberger, 1969). Wolfensberger emphasizes the mutually reinforcing effect of these events and begins his account of the former with a recollection of his first meeting with Bengt Nirje when he came to speak in Nebraska, where Wolfensberger was working.

...

According to my diary, I met him first when on one of these trips, he spoke about Normalization at the North Central Regional Convention of the National Association for Retarded Children in March (10–11) 1967 in Lincoln, Nebraska. What made Nirje's presentations so impactful were two things: (a) While he had stage fright before presentations, once the curtain went up – so to speak – he was a charismatic, electrifying speaker with great rapport with his audience. He later reported that he got his first standing ovation in the US in Nebraska in 1967. (b) He had more and better illustrative slides than anyone else and interpreted them very well. I found a note in my diary that I should recommend to Dr. Kugel, my dean, to spring the expenses to invite him to give a seminar in Omaha sometime.

... I met Nirje again at the September 1967 conference of the International Association for the Scientific Study of Mental Deficiency in Montpellier, France. There, he introduced me to Karl Grunewald. I also met Bank-Mikkelsen there, who invited me to Denmark – an offer I was to take up less than two years later.

Dr. Robert Kugel joined the faculty as head of pediatrics soon after I arrived in Omaha, and became dean of the medical school not long after that. He had an established history of involvements and publications in mental retardation, and had been appointed by President Johnson to the President's Committee on Mental Retardation (PCMR). The PCMR was the successor to President Kennedy's extremely influential President's Panel on Mental Retardation that had produced an epochal report in 1962 (President's Panel on Mental Retardation, 1962, with several subcommittee reports: 1963a, 1963b, 1963c, 1963d, 1963e, 1963f, 1964a, 1964b).

In September 1967, the PCMR sent a subcommittee, including Kugel, to Denmark, Sweden, Britain, and France (Humphrey, Jones, & Kugel, 1968). Later that year, the PCMR commissioned Kugel to compile a resource package on residential services for the mentally retarded in the US so that the committee could draw on it for formulating recommendations, and gave him a grant to cover expenses. In turn, Kugel enlisted me to do the bulk of the hands-on work of the project. Somewhere along the line, the decision was made that the compendium should not merely be an in-house resource, but a book, and about halfway through the project, when it became clear how much editing I had to do, I requested to be a co-editor instead of only the major staff worker on the book.

Our basic plan for the book was to first document compellingly just how awful institutions were, then to sketch some alternatives and positive models, and then come up with an integrative chapter that would point to the necessary action measures.

The significance of that part of the book that documented the bankruptcy of the institution system can hardly be appreciated any more these days, because until then, hardly any criticisms of institutions – or even institutionalism – had appeared in the *professional* literature, in part because it would simply not be permitted by those in power and in part because critics who were professionals figured that they could kiss their careers good-bye. ... To the best of my knowledge, Blatt's *Christmas in Purgatory* (Blatt & Kaplan, 1966) was the first book-length institutional exposé by a leading professional. I suspect that the publication of this book facilitated the appearance of subsequent critiques of the mental retardation institutions. Prior to Blatt, I barely managed to get away with a few critical comments in my three 1964 and 1965 articles ... that reported on my more noteworthy observations of mental retardation programs in Europe. [See extract 2 – Ed.] ...

One issue that became totally clear to us right away – in good part because of my concurrent involvement in the reform of the Nebraska mental retardation services – was that it would be impossible to come up with a meaningful proposal for residential services outside the context of the total service system. But since our mandate was focused on residential services, we did what I have always done: "Give them not what they say they want, but what they really need," and we used the reference to residential services in the book title as a cover for addressing the total service system.

Kugel and I came up with a list of chapters we wanted and their potential authors, which included some authors whose work we already knew to be relevant. One problem was that the PCMR wanted to get the work done in very short order because it had been charged by the President to come up with concrete recommendations within a year. Nonetheless, when we contacted the potential contributors, almost all agreed right away, which was amazing considering how prominent some were and how busy they all were. Grunewald was the only invitee who at first declined but eventually yielded to some arm-twisting by Nirje and me. Also, once most contributors were aboard, the National Association for Retarded Children chipped in a small but crucial amount of money to help a few of the contributors with their expenses. Who and why some contributors were solicited is almost self-evident. The reason for others I can only imperfectly reconstruct, but "political" considerations played a part in one or two cases. …

By the end of January 1968, we not only had all contributors aboard, but one, Michael Klaber, had already sent in a first draft of his description of the mental retardation system in Connecticut, which was then considered a model. However, what later turned out to be the biggest conceptual contribution of the book – namely, the Normalization principle – was hard and late to come by; in fact, it was a heart-stopping cliff-hanger. To begin with, we had not even asked Nirje to write on Normalization, but an evaluation of the US institutions for the retarded that he had visited in 1967, and we planned to put this in the section entitled "As Others See Us." Nirje indicated that he would evaluate these institutions in light of "what we mean here by Normalization." As late as January 24, 1968, I wrote to Nirje that "the presentation and elaboration of the concept of Normalization strikes me as particularly appropriate," showing that I perceived it as a good idea to include, but not as yet as the centerpiece of the book, let alone as the cornerstone of the reform movement.

Furthermore, whether we would ever actually get a manuscript from Nirje was very iffy. Believe it or not, our deadline was the end of February 1968. In March, Grunewald wrote us that Nirje was stressed, had not yet begun to write, but had said that he knew very well what to write. In turn, I conveyed to Nirje that I knew he was stressed and hoped he would stay stressed until he was done, since he was legendary for performing best when under stress. By late May, we not only had many final chapter drafts in hand, but preliminary drafts from all the remaining authors – except Nirje.

But while he had difficulty writing the paper, he had no difficulty writing us long, literate letters, apparently meant to be reassuring, with messages such as the following: "I am still alive and aware of the fact that you are waiting for my paper … I realize that you are pressed for time, and I am writing this to confirm that I am aware of the lack of time now … I am now taking out a week vacation to be able mentally to concentrate on the paper. To be on the safe side I will leave the country for a week." Nirje may well have been stressed, but my own stress level was astronomical, and I found his reassurances not very reassuring. On June 8, 1968, he wrote, "My paper is still not written, and I feel very bad about it. I can too well imagine your disappointment and irritation."

However, that month, he also came on another trip to the US, and so we arranged for him to be virtually taken prisoner in Washington and locked up with some secretaries at the President's Committee office for three days – and this worked! He dictated to them at a furious pace, and, by June 20, he had his first draft completed there and sent it to us. We recognized quickly that a section of his chapter had something that we had come to realize that the book lacked. Namely, despite the presence of several chapters on services that were exemplary for their time, the monograph did not contain a clearly stated unifying idea for an alternative to the prevailing institutional scene. In fact, until we got Nirje's chapter, we considered the chapters by Tizard and Dunn to be the pivotal ones. So we divided Nirje's chapter into two: one chapter early in the book on how bad US institutions were, and another one late in the book sketching Normalization as one of the major alternatives. Within days after Nirje got back home to Sweden in late June, he had our proposed revisions in hand, and he was actually quite ecstatic about how well they read. Amazingly, Nirje's (1969) Normalization chapter consisted of less than eight pages of text, plus an appendix of less than seven pages summarizing the Swedish law on "provisions and services for the mentally retarded" of 1967 that reflected Normalization thinking, though at least the English translation did not actually mention "the Normalization principle," much as the Danish mental retardation "care" law of 1959 reflected the idea without giving it a name.

Anticipating skepticism and resistance from opponents to reform, Nirje made two observations in a July 1968 letter. Namely, even in his few visits to US institutions, he (a) had already seen worse things than those shown in Blatt and Kaplan's (1966) *Christmas in Purgatory*, and (b) he underlined something that Grunewald had said earlier, which was that the services in Sweden "are not dreams in the blue but actual accomplishments of 'hard-headed' and penny-pinching appropriation committees of the county councils."

The last chapter on action implications was to be authored by Gunnar Dybwad, who was given much less time to work on it because he had to see everybody else's work first. According to my correspondence, I proposed to Dybwad on June 21, 1968, that the cardinal features of future trends in mental retardation residential services [be] four basic and highly interrelated components:

1   *Integration* of the retarded with the non-retarded, which implies location of services in population centers.
2   *Dispersement*, implying smaller units and achieving closeness to family and community.
3   *Specialization*, which also implies smaller units and individualization, but which calls for reduction in closeness between resident and family in some cases. (This was the seed of the later construct of "model coherency," elaborated in Wolfensberger and Glenn, 1975.)

As Wolfensberger notes, the concept of 'specialization' was developed at some length in publications around the 1970s. Essentially it derived from the notion that services could not adequately try to serve all functions that had been combined in the institutions, e.g. residential care, work, leisure, health care, etc., and thus would need to address only specific needs of specific types of clients. Though possibly co-ordinated within one agency or one service system, such services would therefore have 'specialized' purposes. The construct of 'model coherency' was then spelled out in PASS (referred to above), and further elaborated in both written form and in teaching events.

4   *Continuity* between residential and other services, resulting in less fragmentation, more individualization, and economy. Of course, this concept of continuity was not at all the one against which the post-Normalizationists these days have been railing.

The reason I suggested to Dybwad to work these concepts into his chapter, which he did, was that they had already been evolved in connection with, and written into, two sets of Nebraska's mental retardation reform plans... .

However, before this chapter came about, it became clear that Dybwad had a Nirje problem in brimming with insights but having difficulty staying put in front of paper and pen. By late June, we had finals of many chapters and advanced drafts of all the others except Dybwad's, and by early August all the advanced drafts had been finalized and distributed to all the PCMR members for review, but we still had no draft from Dybwad.

Then Dybwad did another Nirje on us. With everyone on pins and needles to get his chapter, and us not even having a draft, Dybwad took off on a world tour, leaving a string of forwarding addresses where he generally could not be reached by our mail. And then in early August, Kugel received a sorrowful letter from Dybwad dated August l: "I am now in my 60th year ... all alone here in my sickroom in Adelaide" (Australia!), "weak ... weary ... with plenty of time to think and worry" – especially about what he called me later in the letter, "an editorial aggressopath." "... That's why I am writing to *you*, Bob," expecting Kugel to protect him from me. But Kugel also took off on vacation, so I had to write Dybwad a long letter.

With time running out on us, and having learned a lesson from Nirje, we did to Dybwad as we had done to Nirje, except more so. After his recovery and return, we got him to fly to Omaha on several weekends in a row and locked him up in my office suite with secretaries or myself by his side virtually around the clock for days to write or type everything he thought, said, dictated, or wrote by hand, with mountains of food always close at hand. When he was not in my office, he was in our home sleeping, but he also often slept in my office. This also worked very well, and he produced a great chapter that recapitulated, elaborated, and extrapolated certain Normalization issues, also incorporating some of the ideas already developed in Nebraska at that time, such as elements of the above-mentioned construct of "specialization" of services.

All chapter drafts underwent at least one editing by me, and a critique by Kugel, and some underwent very extensive editing and revising. Also, all chapters were reviewed and commented on (sometimes with implications for yet further revision) by several members of the PCMR, and also by several of the expert consultants of the PCMR... . On February 16–17, 1968, the PCMR had also held a national conference in the Washington area for 25 or so selected leaders and consultants to take a preview at the direction of the monograph, with Kugel, Gunnar Dybwad, and myself as major presenters.

Actually, the final decision whether the PCMR would officially sponsor the publication of the book was not made until all the members had reviewed the manuscript in its totality later in 1968. Around early December 1968, the final version of the monograph went to the US Government Printing Office and appeared in print within weeks in January 1969. (Nirje (1992) recalled January 10 as the publication date. In a 1997 personal communication, he also claimed that the PCMR hurried *Changing Patterns* into print before Richard Nixon was inaugurated in February, lest his administration interdict the printing.) Both in its mode of coming into being and in the reaction to it, one could characterize the book as having had a caesarean birth. It soon became known as "the blue book," and sometimes as the Kugelberger book, as a lot of people began to refer to either Kugel or myself as Kugelberger, some in jest and some from temporary disorientation.

Of the first printing run of 5,000 copies, 2,160 were immediately distributed, free of charge, with a cover letter, to all state governors, all members of the US Congress, all state mental retardation coordinators, all 450 superintendents of public institutions for the mentally retarded and "mentally ill," 550 directors or operators of private residences for the mentally retarded, all leaders of the National Association for Retarded Children (NARC) and of the American Association on Mental Deficiency, all leading figures of all the state units of the NARC, and miscellaneous others. There were at least two more printings, for a total of over 20,000 copies, and when these ran out (sometime between 1972 and 1974), the Pennsylvania State Office of Mental Retardation paid to have facsimile reprintings done, again with very wide distribution, especially all over Pennsylvania because it was then in the forefront of reform.

In his 1983 text on the history of mental retardation, Scheerenberger (1983) called *Changing Patterns* "one of the most consequential and successful publications of the reform era" (p. 227) and of a quarter-century. Among the likely reasons for this, we can point to five.

1 Unbeknownst to most people today, the book contained the first published explicit formulation and description, of any length in any language, of the Normalization principle. This is the reason why portions of it got so quickly translated back into Swedish (Grunewald, 1971) and Danish (Grunewald, 1972), and soon after into German (Kugel & Wolfensberger, 1974).

2 However, not only was Normalization presented in its clearest form to date, but it was presented in stark contrast to the devastating institutional realities and their history. It is well known that a change agentry effort is vastly more likely to succeed if the inadequacies of a prevailing pattern are exposed... .

3 A great many of the recommendations incorporated into *Changing Patterns* had begun to be implemented in Nebraska, even before the book was published, via a virtual service revolution. This implementation took place both on the level of systems organizing, and on the programmatic and clinical level. The principle of specialization was demonstrated by the initiation of a wide variety of services. Also, all this began to be sketched in various publications (e.g., Wolfensberger & Menolascino, 1970a, 1970b), and was otherwise widely disseminated. People came from all over the world to see for themselves, and many experienced a mental paradigm shift. This lent credence and power to *Changing Patterns.*

4 By a fortuitous coincidence, three of the contributors to the book (Cooke, Bank-Mikkelsen, and Tizard) were announced in spring 1968 as winners of the Kennedy Foundation International Award – at that time, the closest thing to a Nobel prize in mental retardation – for achievements prior to their contributions to the book. (Gunnar and Rosemary Dybwad were to receive the award belatedly in 1986.)

5 The strategy of massive distribution of the book by the PCMR must also have played a big role. ...

In retrospect, I have marveled that as extensive a work as *Changing Patterns* could attract so many senior and competent people as authors on such a rapid schedule of production. The prestige of the President's Committee on Mental Retardation probably had much to do with it, plus the attraction of being part of an extensive reassessment of the field. One reason that motivated many invited contributors to participate was well expressed in Lloyd Dunn's acceptance letter of December 15, 1967: "All I need is another assignment as I attempt to get my affairs in order for my leave of absence from the United States. However, the business of residential facilities in this country is such an important matter that I cannot refuse your kind invitation. ..."

...

I do not want to leave readers with the impression that all the contributors to *Changing Patterns* agreed with its major conclusions. Far from it: Some have continued to champion institutions to this day; I believe that some never came to understand systemic diversified community-dispersed services; some never did anything to promote Normalization; even some who liked Normalization understood it incompletely and/or did not embrace some of its implications. ... Some contributors dropped off the cutting edge of reform into the human service woodwork; some, though they eventually approved of the work, engaged themselves in other pursuits and were for all practical purposes no longer involved in the reform struggle. But then – as I will show later – the PCMR itself never endorsed the book either. The contributors most prominent in continuing the war joined by *Changing Patterns* in North America on an ongoing basis were – in my opinion – Nirje, Blatt, Dybwad, and I, and even we either continued to have differences on some important issues, and/or developed such as time went on. Also, all of us who did embrace Normalization still had incomplete and still-evolving notions of it. ...

The elements of Normalization that initially were novel or highly controverted

This section begins with a recapitulation of the 'bankrupt' state of services when normalization came on the scene, then gives some examples of small-scale results in early normalization-based services, that in Wolfensberger's view, caught people's imagination. It then goes on to broader issues.

...

Against the background of the "bad old days" conditions, the poverty of higher-order ideas for proper services, and the little things that blew people's minds as revolutionary, we can now appreciate much better certain concepts or implications that were associated with either Nirje's and/or my Normalization formulation. I will only briefly sketch those that one would not have encountered as popular at the time, either because these things were novel, or because they had not been widely disseminated previously, or because they had been forgotten or outright rejected. It seems to me that 11 things can be put into this category.

1   The idea of applying normative conditions to deviant people ... before people learned to think and talk of normalized residential settings, they sometimes did talk of "homelike" ones, but the term was almost always applied to institutional settings since the vast majority of people had never seen other kinds of residences. ... Also, "homelike" largely meant "less institutional" rather than normalized. After all, such settings were literally thought of as similar to a home, but not truly like an ordinary home.

2　Striving beyond normativeness toward the societal ideal for vulnerable persons, i.e., what I later called the conservatism corollary. (See Wolfensberger, 1998... .)

3　The notion that a single theory or principle could be applied not only to all retarded people, and not only to all handicapped ones, but to all deviant ones.

4　The delineation of major historic deviancy roles and their impact on "models" of (a) social interactions, and (b) human services.

5　The power of role circularities.

6　The concept of a "developmental model."

7　The concept of (deviancy) image juxtaposition, its components, and its importance.

8　The concept of age-appropriateness, and the distinction between age-appropriate and culture-appropriate phenomena. ... The term "age-appropriate" is now encountered in generic public discourse.

9　The separation of certain service and life functions from each other; "specialization," later "model coherency."

10　The dispersal of services, in order to achieve the five desiderata of (a) avoidance of negative dynamics within larger groupings of deviant people, (b) "specialization," (c) not overloading social assimilation potentials, (d) avoidance of deviant-person and deviant-group juxtapositions, and (e) easier access by users and the public.

11　The distinction between physical and social integration, already greatly elaborated in Wolfensberger and Glenn (1973).

In regard to numbers 7 and 10(d), the phrase "juxtaposition of deviancies" is already found in my work-related diary as early as October 1970, but its most systematic formulation came in the 1975 edition of PASS (Wolfensberger & Glenn, 1975). The person who gave me the most decisive help in spelling out this construct was Dr. Bill Bronson, who had been sentenced by the New York State Department of Mental Hygiene to a year of penal servitude under Burton Blatt and me at Syracuse University for his role in bringing about the Willowbrook exposé.

The concept of "service specialization," which eventually became model coherency, evolved from an idea apparently first presented in 1959 by Lloyd M. Dunn, chair of the Department of Special Education at George Peabody College for Teachers (since become part of Vanderbilt University) in Nashville, Tennessee, in an advanced graduate course on social and educational aspects of mental retardation which I attended. He proposed that "omnibus" institutions for the mentally retarded be replaced by smaller, more dispersed specialized institutions for specific subgroups of different identities and needs. ...

Among the reasons that Normalization was so powerful were three interrelated ones. (a) It enabled people to put together, into one unified mental scheme, so many things that they had seen here or there, that had positively impressed them, and that previously they had not known how to connect to each other. (b) It often told them something that they had known "inside," and to which they could now explicitly assent. (c) It gave them an idiom that enabled them to discourse explicitly and effectively on these things. So, for instance, if they had seen persons with severe behavior problems occupy spaces that contained many breakable items and had ordinary glass windows, and own some personal possessions, who were not being unnecessarily locked up, who had some beauty in the environment, and so forth, people could now subsume all this under the "aha" idea, "why, yes, these are normal things, and these are human beings, and if one treats people more normally, that will get them to act more normally."

The sections so far extracted at length have been selected in an attempt to provide the reader with insights into the radical nature of the principle of normalization, and the tenuous (and humorous) beginnings of what became a mass movement. The paper then goes on with more historic detail of immediate developments following the publication of *Changing Patterns*, including a degree of backlash and diversion by the PCMR, widely acclaimed public presentations by the core group and then some others of the implications, and the first edition of what was to become an important tool in both evaluation of services and the teaching of normalization, the PASS instrument (Wolfensberger and Glenn, 1969). Then, in the section leading up to the production of the 1972 *Normalization* text, the story of Wolfensberger being extruded from his job in Nebraska and moving to Toronto, noted in the Introduction, is combined with his various attempts to get an assembled set of papers on normalization published. That he did, and what this meant in two specific aspects of the levels of implementation and of social integration, will be covered in extracts later in this chapter. The edited extract from the Ottawa paper, however, ends with two further pieces from the closing sections. One looks to differentiate between Wolfensberger's developing formulation of normalization and that of others, and the other to summarize reactions to normalization in the late 1960s and early 1970s. The first comes from Section 9 of the paper (p. 91).

...

In connection with the production of the 1972 text on *The Principle of Normalization in Human Services*, it also seems appropriate to say something about the difference between Nirje's Normalization formulation, my own, and for that matter, anybody else's. ... In order to have a rational and productive discussion about the definition of Normalization (and later SRV), it is essential to keep in mind four tenets of the philosophy of science: (a) all definitions are arbitrary, (b) they should have clarity so that people can discourse on a defined entity without projecting conflicting meanings into it because of a definition's lack of clarity, (c) a definition should have utility, and (d) much like classification schemes, a definition that conforms to Occam's razor (i.e., "one should not multiply entities without necessity") and has parsimony is generally to be preferred. It is doubtful whether any definition other than a parsimonious one will earn the accolade of being called elegant, which is a term used for theories that economically and harmoniously have a lot of explanatory power.

We can now see that there could be many definitions of Normalization that meet the first three criteria, in being clear and useful despite their arbitrariness. However, different definitions relating to a topic are extremely unlikely to have the same degree of parsimony, and, most likely, no more than one – if any – will be deemed elegant. Thus, when it comes to definitions of Normalization, one should ask which – if any – meet the criteria of clarity, utility, and parsimony, and which does it best, and it is these aspirations that led me to depart in some very significant ways from the definitions formulated by Bank-Mikkelsen and Nirje. ...

I want to point to three ways in which my Normalization formulation, even from its primitive divergence from Nirje's starting in 1968, accumulated parsimony credits.

1   If one combs the writings of Bank-Mikkelsen and Nirje prior to 1973, one will note that they had only or primarily mental retardation applications on their minds. Even Nirje's (1992) revised 1992 definition of Normalization only expanded it to other handicaps. In contrast, I felt as early as 1968 that Normalization could and should be generalized to all conditions considered to be deviant by society, that is, to people who are rejected and devalued by their societies for other reasons, such as appearance, nationality, race, age, or whatever; or who are in devalued states (such as that of sickness) or devalued roles (including that of hospital patient).

2   In human services, goals and means are very intertwined. My formulation not only speaks to both means and goals, but also has things to say about which of multiple competing means are preferable.

3   The more other meritorious pre-existing or later arriving lower-order concepts, theories, or service means can be subsumed by a theory, the more parsimonious it is, and my Normalization formulation – and SRV even more so – subsumes a zillion ideas and measures on many levels that have been, and will be, promoted in human service and human relationships. ...

Parsimony is one of the great attractions of Normalization, as Lakin and Bruininks (1985) noted in reference to Wolfensberger's formulation: "Normalization as a concept has endured primarily because it is elegant in its simplicity, yet it provides both a utilitarian and an equalitarian guide against which to measure the coherence of programs and services for handicapped citizens" (p. 12).

Then from the conclusion to the paper, Wolfensberger reflects on five different reactions to the normalization principle (p. 95).

...

1   Benevolent and polite rejection, derived from the conviction of the listeners that the speakers simply did not know the relevant realities about the lives of

handicapped (mostly retarded) persons, because if they did, they certainly would not be making such outlandish claims and proposals. This kind of response was particularly apt to be forthcoming from parents of retarded persons, who were pleased that someone was well-intentioned toward people such as their children, even though ignorant or misguided.

2   The grossest kind of hostile rejection, which came almost entirely from service professionals. In the early years of teaching Normalization, the teachers would often get into the nastiest arguments with hostile listeners or entire audiences, and sometimes even the smallest and most obvious elements of Normalization were vehemently contested.

3   Noncomprehension, in that what was presented was simply not grasped because it was so remote from what people knew and were able to conceptualize. However, in that case, the response did not tend to be hostile but bland, often of the nature of "What else is new?"

4   An "aha" response, when what we were teaching made profound sense to people but they had never heard it stated before, or never in a way in which they could understand it. This latter response most likely was emitted by ordinary citizens who were neither human service workers nor parents of handicapped persons.

5   Finally, there were people who were open to learning about Normalization but who did not agree with at least portions of it because they held high-order beliefs, perhaps of a religious, political, or socioeconomic nature, that clashed – or seemed to them to clash – with Normalization. Many persons in this group found that the more they understood our Normalization formulation, the less conflict there would be in implementive measures. However, there often was also agreement on many implementive measures – but not for the same reasons. For instance, it was not unusual for services of Christian bodies to get higher scores on the PASS instrument than most other services, but not necessarily for reasons that would have derived from Normalization.

This pattern of five kinds of response continued pretty much the same throughout the 1970s, except that in the early 1970s, several additional ones gained greater ascendancy.

1   One came almost exclusively from human service workers. Some concluded that Normalization was the craze of the moment and they did not want to be left behind or appear outdated, but they really had no commitment to it. They figured that they had better learn the Normalization idiom and its superficial notions lest they be viewed as archaic, or lose prestige or positions, especially if they worked in settings where Normalization had been mandated from the top. Some people went on doing whatever they had been doing or wanted to do and simply called it "Normalization." These people of empty minds and often weak service souls almost all jumped off soon and onto whatever other popular and "safe" crazes came into vogue.

2   There were people who had opposed Normalization from day one but were embarrassed to admit it once so many Normalization corollaries became everyday conventional wisdom. Instead, they continued their opposition by calling for going "beyond Normalization." For instance, Rosen, Clark, and Kivitz (1977) issued a "beyond Normalization" call as early as 1977, and one has heard that phrase ever since, and often from people who never were "in Normalization" enough to go beyond it.

3   Another group also consisted largely of the same old enemies of Normalization who now began to shift their arguments into the form that Normalization lacked research evidence. These people are still with us, and probably always will be, since they continue to stutter the same argument despite mountainous supportive evidence from both formal research and other forms of empiricism – and this group of largely social science academicians can generally not relate to the latter.

4   As the years passed by, we also had to begin increasingly to combat not merely opposition to Normalization, but also all the misconceptions or wrong teachings about it. That became increasingly a problem until SRV began to be formulated in 1983 (Wolfensberger, 1983a [see Chapter 3, extract 10 – Ed.]). Relatedly, there were the well-intentioned people who either (a) thought they had understood Normalization but had not, and therefore applied the term "Normalization" to non-normalizing practices, or (b) subscribed to one of several competing formulations of Normalization. With the latter group, one might be in very extensive agreement – perhaps on 80% of the relevant measures, but even then not always for the same reason.

It was only around 1980 that a distinct change set in, apparently for four reasons. (a) Many ideas that had been taught in connection with Normalization became more widely known and accepted. (b) Particularly with the evolution of SRV, striking improvements took place in our teaching. (c) Certain ideas arising from other sources, such as the civil-rights movement, were sufficiently concordant or overlapping with Normalization or SRV to make these latter appear reasonable. (d) More and more, people began to actually see instances of implementation of what had been taught, and saw that it either worked or was better than what went before. ...

---

7   From: 'Typical programmatic and architectural implications of the normalization principle', 1972, Chapter 4 of Normalization: The Principle of Normalization in Human Services, 31–42, Toronto: National Institute on Mental Retardation.

The next extract deals with an issue that became crucial in the misinterpretations of normalization and SRV, as noted in the closing remarks above. This is, of course, the matter of implementation, and in particular what is implied by normalization in terms of who does what to whom. Many of the criticisms over the years imply, or even state as fact, that normalization is about imposing changes on individuals so as to conform them to society, with little attention being paid to changing society or subsections thereof. The extract below puts that particular record straight, in particular the table and subsequent discussion, which reveal the different levels of action proposed in the 1972 *Normalization* text, including action at the societal level. That table has, of course, been clarified and updated in later teaching materials on normalization and SRV (see Wolfensberger, 1998 for an updating and expansion in social role terms). The extract also contains the basic structure of issues that normalization would apply to service systems at various levels, which was being developed at the same time into the various versions of the evaluation instrument PASS (*Program Analysis of Service Systems*, Wolfensberger and Glenn, 1969, 1973, 1975), and subsequently used to great effect in the teaching of normalization.

...

The levels and dimensions of the normalization principle

One can conceive of the implications of the normalization principle as falling into two dimensions and three levels of action (Table 2.1). One dimension is concerned with the structure of interactions that involve deviant or potentially deviant individuals directly, while the second dimension is concerned with the way such persons are interpreted to others. Another way of putting this is to say that both dimensions deal with the structuring of a deviant person's environment, one dimension involving the person directly, the other involving the way this person is symbolically represented in the minds of others. Of great importance to the latter are labels, concepts, stereotypes, role perceptions, and role expectancies that are applied to a person, and that often determine the circularity between his own self-concept, the way others react to him, and the way he is likely to respond.

Role perceptions and stereotypes are known to exert considerable influence on behavior. ... However, only through some very recent research has the full power of the feedback loop between role expectancy and role performance been brought into sharp focus. The work of Rosenthal and Jacobson (1968), which suggests the power of role perception in the development of children, is one of the more spec-tacular examples. It is consistent with and explains a number of other research findings. For example, it appears quite consistent with the well-documented fact that retarded children who are placed into special classes underachieve grossly when compared to their retarded peers who are carried along in regular classes, even without any special attention.

The immediacy of contact with, or interpretation of, (deviant) individuals can be divided rather meaningfully into three levels. The first level involves individual human managers with individual (potentially) deviant persons. The second level is concerned with the immediate (primary) and intermediate social systems that act upon a person; such systems include the (deviant) person's family, peer group, classroom, school, neighborhood, place of work, or service agency. The third level

Table 2.1 A schema of the expression of the Normalization principle on three levels of two dimensions of action

Levels of action	Dimensions of action	
	Interaction	**Interpretation**
Person	Eliciting, shaping, and maintaining normative skills and habits in persons by means of direct physical and social interaction with them.	Presenting, managing, addressing, labeling, and interpreting individual persons in a manner emphasizing their similarities to rather than differences from others.
Primary and intermediate social systems	Eliciting, shaping, and maintaining normative skills and habits in persons by working indirectly through their primary and intermediate social systems, such as family, classroom, school, work setting, service agency, and neighborhood.	Shaping, presenting, and interpreting intermediate social systems surrounding a person or consisting of target persons so that these systems as well as the persons in them are perceived as culturally normative as possible.
Societal systems	Eliciting, shaping, and maintaining normative behavior in persons by appropriate shaping of large societal social systems, and structures such as entire school systems, laws, and government.	Shaping cultural values, attitudes, and stereotypes so as to elicit maximal feasible cultural acceptance of differences.

concerns itself with the larger relevant societal social systems, such as the school system of an entire province, state, or nation, the laws of the land, and the mores of a society. Below, implications in each of the six categories summarized in Table 2.1 will be discussed. [For clarity tables are numbered within each chapter of this book – they therefore may differ from the numbering in the original articles – Ed.]

Normalizing action on the personal level

THE INTERACTION DIMENSION

On the first level of the interaction dimension (i.e. the person level), the normalization principle would dictate that we provide services which maximize the behavioral competence of a (deviant) person. Indeed much of the programming offered by human management fields and agencies would fall into this general category.

However, we appear to be much more effective in shaping skills to be physically adaptive than in shaping them to be socially normative, or in shaping their *habitual* normative exercise. ... Too often, we may content ourselves to teach a handicapped child to walk, but we may be relatively unconcerned when the child develops a quite preventable idiosyncratic gait which elicits or reinforces a perception of deviance. We may teach a retarded young adult how to use a deodorant – but then fail to convert this skill into the adaptive habit. ...

Obviously, the design of a human management-related building can have much to do with the shaping of both skills and habits of its users. For instance, buildings can make, or fail to make, developmental challenges and demands; they can elicit adaptive decision-making and enhance independence, or impose dependency. Life space should be zoned so as to encourage rather than discourage individuals from interacting in small groups at least part of the time, in contrast to space which implies interaction in large groups only, or which discourages almost all interaction. Even in the presence of other design elements which permit use of the building by the severely physically handicapped, many residential and educational human service buildings should have stairs and not merely ramps, and residential facilities generally should provide residents with access to the controls that adjust room and water temperature; turn lights on and off; open and close windows, blinds and curtains; and flush toilets. To do otherwise deprives residents of culturally normal opportunities, restricts their range of learning opportunities, and fosters non-normative dependency.

THE INTERPRETATION DIMENSION

The interaction dimension just reviewed implies that we teach a person to habitually exercise those behaviors which elicit social judgment even if they have little practical problem-solving value. These behaviors include etiquette, and may be related or attached to other normative skills of dressing, grooming, walking, talking, eating, etc.

However, there are situations where a person's public image does not (alone) depend on what he is or does, but on how those around him 'present' him. In either case, a person's image depends greatly on the actions of those who exercise 'managerial' controls over him, and therefore the manager should take steps to minimize the probabilities that the person for whom he has responsibility presents himself to the public in a fashion that is apt to lower what we might call the 'perceived deviancy threshold'. For instance, while a moderately retarded adult can be taught to dress himself habitually in a normative fashion, a moderately retarded child still has to be dressed by others, or told what to wear. A retarded adult living independently in society may indulge himself and become deviantly obese, and there may be little we can do about it. However, a mildly retarded adult in a community hostel or supervised apartment will usually still be under agency management, and his diet can be regulated to some degree.

Similarly, where a person's appearance is less determined by himself than by the manager, it is important to attend carefully to such things as the grooming and hairstyle that we might confer upon such a person. ... In other words, the probabilities should be minimized that a citizen can identify on sight, as being different, a person who is already deviant, or who is apt to be so labeled in the future.

Labels can be as powerful as appearances. The type of public response to a young man with Down's syndrome will depend significantly on whether we introduce him to the public as 'Mr. Smith' or 'Joseph Smith'; somewhat condescendingly as 'Joe'; perhaps derogatorily as 'Joe, the mongoloid'; or contemptuously as 'a mongolian idiot'.

The question may be raised why it is so important to reduce the perceived deviancy of a person who may already be clearly identified as deviant. The answer is that there are degrees of deviancy, and every additional measure of deviance becomes an additional social handicap, further reducing a person's self-image, and increasing the likelihood that he will emit non-normative maladaptive behavior.

Normalizing action on the level of primary and intermediate social systems

THE INTERACTION DIMENSION

On the level of primary and intermediate social systems in the interaction dimension, we would not work with (deviant) individuals directly, but through those social systems which act rather closely upon them. The importance and cost-efficiency of shaping social systems can not be over-emphasized. If the system is maladaptive, all the efforts of the clinicians interacting with clients on the person level can be vitiated. This has often been the case in residential institutions where the systemic structure has vastly reduced the effectiveness of dedicated workers. ...

Examples of working through a social system rather than with the afflicted directly would include counseling the family of an impaired person; or performing environmental manipulations of his family social system, as we would if we helped the family obtain a home that was physically more suitable for the rearing of a handicapped child. We might help his school to start a special class into which he might fit, counsel his teacher, or prevail upon some appropriate governing body to replace (with a new and more competent director) the director of an agency that had served the person poorly in the past.

Similarly, in order to accomplish the greatest amount of normalization, both by encouraging deviant persons to imitate nondeviant ones, as well as by shaping the stereotypes held by the public of various deviant groups, deviant individuals should have maximal exposure to the nondeviant, and minimal exposure (or juxtaposition) to workers, volunteers, or other individuals who are perceived as deviant themselves by a significant proportion of the public.

In typical community life, social interaction with one's everyday contacts brings with it innumerable occasions and role expectancies that have implications to the normalization process. Unfortunately, a person identified as deviant is often further 'dehabilitated' by being deprived of these normalizing social contacts, or by being cast into social roles where he is actually expected to act deviantly. For instance, by placing a deviant client among other deviant clients, we may reduce his social contacts with nondeviant persons. Often, we compound this problem by permitting some or even most of the staff working with a deviant group to be deviant. Thus, a common phenomenon in human management is for deviant persons to drift into employment where they work with clients who are deviant themselves. ...

Usually, human managers defend such juxtaposition practices on the grounds that the deviant worker can make a contribution by such an arrangement, that he can be habilitated by it, etc. However, when a person is perceived somewhat (or definitely) as a deviant 'reject' by society, and is then placed into a position where he administers services to other persons similarly perceived, it is inevitable that members of the public conclude consciously or unconsciously that the deviant individuals who are being served are of low value. ... Thus, a juxtaposition of deviant workers with deviant clients devalues both of them, but particularly so the client. Inevitably, this devaluing perception will induce the public to emit behavior toward the deviant client group that is more likely to be 'dehabilitating' than normalizing. ...

Normalization principles would thus not only argue against the juxtaposition of deviant workers with deviant clients, but would demand that as much as possible, deviant individuals be surrounded by non-deviant ones. By the same logic, those who serve a group of deviant clients should meet at least the same standards of qualification as are applied to persons who work with comparable non-deviant groups.

Buildings should be so designed and located as to be physically integrated into the community, encourage maximal social integration of the persons served in and by them, and provide client-users with a wide range and large number of normalizing experiences. Since a neighborhood or community can only integrate a limited number of deviant persons at any one time, the size of a facility should be such as to congregate no more deviant client-users than can readily be absorbed in and by the surrounding area, services, resources, social life, etc. This means that hostels and other group residences have to be small, and in most cases, several residential units of small size should not be placed too close together. For instance, instead of putting two sheltered hostel-apartments for four retarded adults each in one apartment house, more integration would be achieved by placing the apartments into separate apartment houses some distance apart.

Smallness of size, in turn, dictates that residential services should be specialized for specific types of problems and/or groups. Unlike the all-purpose institution, a small group residence is usually incapable of rendering appropriate services simultaneously to infants and the aged, the near-independent and the totally dependent, the well-behaved and the uncontrolled, the blind and the deaf, etc. At any rate, services for children and adults ordinarily should be physically separated anyway, both in order to reduce the probability that children will imitate the deviant behavior of their elders, and because services to adults and children are generally also separated in the mainstream of society. ...

Normalizing dispersal of specialized residences generally means that the location, distribution, and concentration of facilities should follow the prevailing population distribution. Thus, service facilities, and even group residences, must not only be dispersed across communities within a region, but also within specific communities. For example, one of the first comprehensive community service plans based on the normalization principle (Menolascino, Clark & Wolfensberger, 1968, 1970) envisioned as many as fifty small, dispersed, specialized residences, hostels, and apartments for the mentally retarded of Douglas County in Nebraska (an urban area containing the city of Omaha and a population of about 400,000). By means of such a specialized dispersed system, it is planned to eliminate entirely the need for traditional institutional residences, even for the most severely impaired.

In regard to size of a facility or client group, it is important not merely to consider the ability of the surrounding social systems to absorb deviant individuals, but also the size of a grouping that tends to create clannishness, exclusiveness, and inward-centeredness. Members of small groups tend to gravitate outward and to interact with other social systems; as group size increases, this tendency diminishes. The sheer size of the group may create mutual barriers of attitudes; and a person in a large group may find too many of his social needs met too conveniently to motivate him to reach out for normalizing socialization.

In regard to the physical and contextual separation of age groups, strong rationales can be derived from both the interaction and interpretation dimensions. First of all, in regard to the juxtaposition of children and adults, we must remember that many normative services for children in the mainstream of society are separate from services for adults. Furthermore, deviant adults are only rarely and in limited ways appropriate role models for children. Often this is true because today's adults did not receive the kinds of services we can offer to the children of today and tomorrow. Thus, we do not want the children to acquire some of the less adaptive characteristics of the casualties of yesteryear, but want them to be exposed as much as possible to healthy normal children of their own or similar age, or to adults who are appropriate models for their development.

Additionally, when a service for children and a service for adults are placed in close context to each other, they are often under the same administrator, and/or experience a lot of social interactions of each other's staff. A common example is a sheltered workshop in the same building and under the same management as a program for children. In such situations, the director usually will be either adult- *or* child-oriented, and the program toward which he lacks proper orientation suffers. If he is adult-oriented, the children's program will suffer, as it has typically to this day in psychiatry generally, which is overwhelmingly adult-centered. If he is child-oriented, the adults will be apt to be cast into children's roles. Similarly, the virtually unavoidable close interaction between the staff of the children's program and the adult clients will tend to denormalize the adults by imposing the eternal child role upon them. As a result, the adults in such a setting will be perceived by the public to be little differentiated from children. Finally, the optimal physical locations and juxtapositions of children's and adult services are often quite different. By selecting the same site for both, one of the services is often disadvantaged in regard to the most normalized location for its particular mission and identity.

For the sake of continuity, one of the principles relevant to the juxtaposition of aged with mature or young adults will here be drawn forward from the interpretation dimension in the next section. If we place impaired adults in a setting or grouping perceived to be specific to the aged (such as a nursing home), it is virtually inevitable that in the perception of many – if not most – observers, the younger impaired adults will be identified with the aura of hopelessness that is unfortunately imposed upon the aged ones. This means that it is much more adaptive to integrate one or a few aged persons among younger ones (in order to acquire their aura) than vice versa.

The underlying principle to all of the above juxtaposition issues is that any negative aura (identity, role expectancy, etc.) attached to a setting or a particular group will be transferred upon a minority within that setting or group. The aura can rarely be reversed by adding a valued minority to the setting or group. It is much more powerful both in terms of public perception and direct behavior modification to include a devalued person or minority in a mainstream (or even valued) majority, than to mix devalued groups with each other, or to place a valued minority with a devalued majority. One of the recurring and stronger findings of social psychology is that deviant members of a group are much more likely to change their behavior to meet the standards and norms of the group and especially its model members than the other way around (Berelson & Steiner, 1964).

THE INTERPRETATION DIMENSION

On the same level, in the dimension of interpretation, considerable thought must be given to how service facilities, and the groups of clients they serve, are named or labeled. ... The name of a possible facility should be carefully considered so as to promote a role perception of its client-users that is non-deviant, or at least minimizes the perceived deviancy. Thus, even words such as 'retarded', 'crippled', 'handicapped', etc. should probably be avoided in facility names. In fact, some facilities might fare better staying unnamed altogether, perhaps being referred to informally according to the street or area in which they are located, e.g. the 'Harney Street Hostel', or the 'Bellevue Heights Workshop'. Similarly, the labels applied to groups of clients by an agency are very important. For instance, adults should not be referred to as 'children', 'kids', or 'inmates'; but as 'men', women', 'clients', 'citizens', 'trainees', 'workers', 'residents', or 'guests', as the case may be, all these latter terms lacking stigma, conveying respect, and being more normative. The term 'patient' should only be used in contexts that are unequivocally medical, and in which the various obligations and privileges of the sick role are appropriate for the persons served (Parsons & Fox, 1958).

Even the symbols surrounding a potentially devalued person or group should be carefully considered. These symbols may be both transmitted and received unconsciously, but nevertheless tend to suggest or perpetuate social perceptions. … An implication of particular poignancy is that contrary to common belief, a staff-to-client ratio that is any higher than necessary is undesirable. A high staff ratio can imply an interpretation of the client as being more deviant than he is, and can thus be denormalizing under certain circumstances. This is also one of the reasons why service facilities (especially residences) should 'specialize'. We should group clients so that each group can be served with the minimum feasible number of restrictions and personnel.

In many instances, a normalizing measure falls into both dimensions of the person level, or into both the person and primary-intermediate level of the interaction dimension. In consequence, a measure may serve the function of shaping a normative skill while simultaneously creating a normative role perception in an observer which, in turn, elicits additional normative behavior from the deviant client in a beneficial circularity. Some examples of management with such dual impact follow.

Normalization means living in a bisexual world. This has differing implications in different service settings. In children's programs, it means that men as well as women should be involved. For adults, especially in residential services, it usually means that the building and the social structure should produce at least as much mingling of sexes as in a hotel. There are only a few contexts – many of these in adolescence – where activities are normally sex-segregated.

The daily routine of clients as well as client groups should be so structured as to be analogous to that of comparable non-deviant persons of the same age. A physically or mentally handicapped adult, even if severely impaired, should be engaged as much as possible in work that is culturally normative in type, quantity, and setting. Even if conducted in sheltered settings, work should be culturally typical adult work, rather than involving activities commonly associated with children, with play, with recreation, or with leisure; and sheltered workshops should resemble industry.

An important aspect of normalization is to apply health, safety, comfort, and similar standards to human management facilities and programs as they are applied to comparable settings for other citizens. This has implications primarily to residential facilities, such as institutions; and even more particularly to publicly operated services which, in many jurisdictions, may and do operate below the standards prescribed by law and/or regulation for private facilities. However, it also has implications to clinics and other settings. For instance, reception and waiting areas should be as comfortable, attractive, and private as typical citizens might encounter in comparable community services.

Also, in regard to physical facilities, thought must be given to the 'building perception', i.e. the way the physical facility is likely to be perceived by the public. The external appearance or context of a building, even if it is perfect in terms of internal arrangements, can exert a detrimental effect upon citizens' response to the persons associated with this building. For instance, a building that looks like a prison or that was recently used by disturbed individuals is apt to elicit associations not conducive to integration of subsequent client-users of the building. Positive or negative associations affect not only outside observers, but also those who work with the client who is being perceived.

Architecture speaks a powerful language, and can shout out loud interpretations of the client-users of buildings. For instance, putting a drain in the middle of a living room floor (as in some institutions) interprets the person who lives in such a room as an animal who must be 'kept' and cleaned as in a zoo. A non-enclosed toilet says that its user has no human feelings of modesty. Bars on the windows, or even an isolated location of a building, suggest that the building's inhabitants are a menace to society. However, since group residences in particular imply an agency context, and since buildings generally interpret their users almost invariably in a social-systemic rather than individual context, the architectural implications on the person level are virtually indistinguishable from those on the level of primary and intermediate social system.

Normalizing action on the societal level

THE INTERACTION DIMENSION

On the societal level of the interaction dimension, we might work to change the entire school system of a province, state, or even nation, rather than merely changing one class or one school. For instance, many authorities have stated that our present school system unconsciously encourages teenagers from lower class and disadvant-aged backgrounds to drop out. To change such practices, we may have to change laws, perhaps reform teacher training institutions, revise funding and taxing patterns and priorities, etc.

THE INTERPRETATION DIMENSION

Perhaps the major challenge in the interpretational dimension of the societal level is to achieve a redefinition of deviancy, and to foster greater acceptance of some behaviors or characteristics considered deviant today. Normalization can be enhanced by encouraging currently normative citizens to broaden the range of what they consider to be normative. To cite a simple example: to wear a business suit [rather than a formal suit such as a tuxedo – Ed.] to an important reception or social affair would probably have been perceived as deviant behavior in the past; however, if a number of prominent individuals or a significant minority of persons wore business suits or other more casual attire to such events, such behavior would no longer be considered deviant. Thus, citizens in the mainstream of a culture can do much toward the eradication of harmless deviancy by adopting habits and lifestyles which arc somewhat more tolerant and casual than some of those of the past, many of which have been entirely due to historical accident and convention, and are entirely neutral from a moral viewpoint.

Teaching, exhortation, demonstration, and life-style modeling may be necessary to convince the public that deviancy is of our own making, and is often harmless.

We should work for greater acceptance of differentness of modes of grooming, dressing, speaking; of skin color, race, religious and national origin; of appearance, age, sex, intelligence, and education. Also encouraged should be greater acceptance of the physically and sensory handicapped, the epileptic, the emotionally disordered, and perhaps the sexually unorthodox. Here, it is important to recall that societal response to deviancy tends to be general, rather than specific to a particular deviance. By furthering societal acceptance for one type of differentness, we are also and indirectly gaining increased acceptance for a group in which we have a particular personal or professional interest.

Concluding comments on the normalization principle

There are, of course, innumerable other implications from the clinical level to the level of large social systems. The examples given here represent only a selected and arbitrary sampling. However, they underline that many major and minor practices that are currently accepted and not found objectionable by proponents of other human management systems are, in fact, quite inconsistent with the principle of normalization.

The normalization principle has powerful theoretical force *vis-à-vis* other human management systems, and despite its late emergence, considerable empirical evidence – primarily from social psychology and related fields – can be marshaled in support of it. However, upon first superficial exposure to the principle, one may well ask how it differs from a number of other approaches.

The difference lies in the simplicity, parsimony, and comprehensiveness of the principle. It subsumes many current human management theories and measures but goes beyond them in stipulating other measures that have been neglected so far. And the principle is easily understood once one has opened one's mind to it. …

---

8 From: 'Societal integration as a corollary of normalization', 1972, Chapter 5 of *Normalization: The Principle of Normalization in Human Services*, 44–54. Toronto: National Institute on Mental Retardation.

Having established its applicability at all levels of human service systems, the next chapter in the *Normalization* text, and the next extract, goes on to deal with the issue of integration. Though one of the key components of normalization, it was often the one that was most often ignored, or at least the subtleties of full integration were most ignored. As the previous extract noted, even a physical presence of an extraordinary building in a community setting, though giving more opportunities for people to interact with that community, still marked them out in the public mind as 'users of services' and thus reduced the perception of the public that such people were those with whom they might like to interact. The next extract elaborates the thinking behind this key issue, again one which holds as a theme throughout the development of normalization and SRV. Readers (and some critics) might also note the examples of integration given at the end of this extract. On the one hand, some of the issues discussed are now part of the underlying assumptions of services, whilst on the other, some remain obstinately resistant to the hopes expressed by Wolfensberger. His caveat at the end of the extract, and other, broader issues, discussed elsewhere in this book in other extracts would seem to have a deal of relevance here.

Societal integration as a corollary of normalization

...

Integration can be achieved in many areas, and in many ways. One major paradigm is to obtain services from generic agencies which serve the general public, rather than from specialty agencies which serve only or primarily groups of individuals perceived as deviant.

For instance, visually limited children were once educated almost entirely by special schools or at least special classes. Today, they are increasingly educated in the regular classroom by regular teachers who receive special orientation and support from resource rooms and resource teachers. In their general practice, general medical practitioners handle psychiatric problems which were formerly the almost exclusive province of specially-designated mental health personnel. Retarded children who were once placed into special institutions are increasingly placed into ordinary foster homes. The list could go on at some length.

In the past, generic services were often denied to special groups on the basis of two arguments. One was that since the generic agency did not possess the necessary specialized skills and resources, the person with a special condition would be *better served* by a special service. The second argument was that certain deviant individuals *should* be segregated from the mainstream of society, and be served apart – even if not always expertly. People who were different should remain 'with their own kind' – to use the popular expression. It is important to recognize that the first argument was primarily an empirical-technical one, but that the second one was largely value-based.

Today, we can marshal powerful empirical and programmatic arguments in favor of the tenet that segregated services, almost by their nature, are inferior services. This holds true not merely for racial segregation, where this principle was most forcefully promulgated by the courts; it also holds true for segregation of other minority-deviancy groups.

Programmatically, segregation is particularly self-defeating in any context that is claimed to be habilitational, which includes special education. If we are serious about working for the goal of preparing a person toward independence and normative functioning, then we must prepare him to function in the context of the ordinary societal contacts which he is expected to have and to handle adaptively in the future.

One of the basic principles of education, in the broad sense, is to 'educe' (lead forth) the learner stepwise into the context in which he is to function; and to bring about this education as early as possible, because the earlier a behavior is learned, the more likely it is to persist. Also, early learning is usually easier than later learning.

Here is where much of our habilitation, human management, and especially traditional special education and rehabilitation, have been weak. Too often, training took place in one context, which was an artificial, segregated, and non-normative one; and at the end of the training period, there came a precipitous transfer into realistic normative societal settings. Perhaps our so-called 'corrective' services are the most extreme example of this practice. The fact that our failure rates have not been higher than they have been is more due to the resilience of man than the merit of our practices. ...

This much for the programmatic-empirical argument. However, the arguments involving primarily issues of values have also changed, as our conception of the privileges and obligations of citizenship have changed in recent years. Indeed, we have seen develop almost a preoccupation with issues of right and justice. ... One of these is of prime relevance here, and that is the new belief that unless a person is a proven menace, he cannot be separated from society by fiat, perhaps merely because his presence is inconvenient or unpleasant. Our society is becoming more pluralistic, and even the armed forces have had to accept a soldier's right to wear sideburns and peace medals. Also, that a deviancy is harmful and warrants denial of societal participation must now be painstakingly proven – individual by individual; such a judgment can no longer be imposed upon a class of persons. Admission, and even commitment, to an institution can no longer be equated with loss of citizenship rights, as was almost universally the case in the past, especially in the field of mental retardation. Even the fact that parents can no longer be held responsible for the support of handicapped children who have attained the legally-defined age of adulthood bespeaks subtly of a new legal interpretation of the handicapped adult as an adult rather than an eternally-dependent child – even if he should require legal guardianship throughout his adult life.

It is apparent that today, neither programmatic nor value-based rationales are sufficient to justify a segregationist service structure. However, it has not always been the majority that has excluded the minority; on many occasions, a minority has deliberately cut itself off from the mainstream. Such self-elected segregation may have been motivated by the fear of mainstream demands; by the desire to continue an established power and bureaucracy structure that might become redundant through integration; and by the fear of change and of rejection. For instance, many leaders in mental retardation have been afraid to give up their special programs and merge their clients into generic and/or public programs for fear that once their special program was discontinued, the other program might begin to exclude the retarded clients who would then be without service altogether. In some version or other, fears like this are encountered again and again – and they are often justified. ...

The two integrations: physical and social

If integration is one of the major means for achieving and acknowledging societal acceptance, as well as for accomplishing adaptive behavior change, then we must distinguish between and elaborate upon its dimensions and components. First of all, let us define integration as being the opposite of segregation; and the process of integration as consisting of those practice and measures which maximize a person's (potential) participation in the mainstream of his culture.

For a (deviant) person, integration is achieved when he lives in a culturally normative community setting in ordinary community housing, can move and communicate in ways typical for his age, and is able to utilize, in typical ways, typical community resources: developmental, social, recreational, and religious facilities; hospitals and clinics; the post office; stores and restaurants; job placements; and so on.

Ultimately, integration is only meaningful if it is social integration; i.e. if involves social interaction and acceptance, and not merely physical presence. However, social integration can only be attained if certain preconditions exist, among these being physical integration, although physical integration by itself will not guarantee social integration.

Physical integration

Social integration takes place on the 'person level' and involves the close interaction of (potentially) deviant individuals with those who are not so perceived. However, physical integration generally involves buildings or at least 'settings', i.e. a physical setting which permits or facilitates social interaction. In the context of this discussion, the building will probably be one in or through which human services are mediated.

Physical integration (or segregation) of a service facility is determined primarily by four factors to be discussed below... .

LOCATION

The center and emphasis of services generally should be at the community level where the persons are to be served, and the structure such that they may remain in or be absorbed into the prevailing social, economic, educational, etc. systems. Unless it is distinctly desired as part of an appropriate human management model or rationale, as perhaps in the case of a retreat camp, physical isolation of settings is one of the conditions to be avoided.

PHYSICAL CONTEXT

The type of area in which the program is to be located should be consistent with the type of service to be provided, e.g. vocational services in industrial park areas, hostels in residential areas, etc. Services in upper lower-class neighborhoods of medium density population with a large array of resources (post office, stores, restaurants, libraries, churches, play grounds, movies, etc.) will, in all likelihood, be capable of absorbing deviant persons at a relatively high rate, while thinly-populated upper-class suburban areas beyond walking distance from community resources would probably be less suited.

ACCESS

It should be kept in mind that elements in addition to distance can determine access. Among these are availability and convenience of transportation means and routes, and other circumstances which can be highly specific.

SIZE OR DISPERSAL

...

Every effort should be made not to congregate deviant persons in numbers larger than the surrounding (community) social systems can absorb and integrate. This principle implies that instead of single large facilities, a larger number of modestly-sized facilities usually permit greater normalizing dispersal within as well as between population centers, especially so in the larger communities. Dispersal is particularly important for the numerically most-needed programs, and especially for residential services.

Services should be dispersed across a region consistent with population patterns, and so located as to enable all clients to take full advantage of other existing community resources. Programs should be so developed as to break up, or prevent the establishment of, excessively large service facilities.

While the four elements of location, relationship, access, and size (dispersal) tend to be related to each other, there can also be some independence among them. For instance, a facility could be very close to other resources, and yet access to it may be very difficult to attain. Conversely, a physically distant facility might be close to several major means of access such as expressways, rail transportation, etc.

Social integration

Integration can be facilitated (or inhibited) not only by physical but also by social circumstances. A service could conceivably be optimally integrated physically, and yet suffer from extensive social segregation. For instance, despite optimal location, such factors as agency policy, service structures, and/or social circumstances might still keep a deviant person out of the cultural mainstream, and segregated from normative and normalizing social intercourse. Thus, a person needs not only to be *in* but also *of* the community.

It would appear that once physical integration exists, social integration (or segregation) will be determined by at least four factors: program features affecting social interactions; the labels that are given to services and facilities; the labels and terms applied to the clients; and the way in which the service building is perceived. ... The four factors ... affect not only outside observers, but also those who work with the client who is being perceived.

Current integrative opportunities

Below, I will briefly discuss some program areas (especially education, work, and housing) in which the time appears to be propitious in North America for major normalizing restructuring of prevailing service patterns, via the process of integration. There probably are other areas, but the ones discussed here can serve as examples.

Integration in educational programs

For a long time, the idea has prevailed that special education is and must be synonymous with segregated education. The realization is now growing that this need not be so. Indeed, we are finding, on the one hand, that segregation often brings with it a lowering rather than an improvement of standards; and on the other hand, that by the very nature of things, integrated education has certain normalizing features which can make it better than segregated education. ...

INTEGRATION IN EARLY CHILDHOOD EDUCATION

In this area, particularly, we are used to thinking mostly in terms of day care centers, nurseries, kindergartens, etc. which either serve only the handicapped, or at best have special and segregated sections for them. And yet, it is probably on this very level that integration should be achieved most urgently, and can be most easily.

Early integration is relatively easy because: very young children are less perturbed by individual differences; early education programs tend to be more apt to have groups of mixed ages and sizes anyway; and such programs are oriented to more individualized handling than the regular schools are for older children. Among major benefits of early integration are the breaking down of social barriers and stereotypes, not only in our young future citizens, but even in our current fellow-citizens – their parents.

Already, one can see many early education programs which have included small numbers of handicapped children – although sometimes more by oversight than by design. In almost every instance of early integration that I have encountered, I have been impressed with the smoothness of the integration process and the amount of progress made by handicapped children involved. Particularly at this age level, normal peers seem to constitute non-threatening models from which the handicapped (especially the retarded) children learn much more than they typically do from their impaired peers.

MAXIMAL INTEGRATION IN TRADITIONAL EDUCATION

On this topic, so much has been said that only brief recapitulation is necessary. Most of the mildly impaired and retarded can function in regular grades if special additional services (e.g. resource rooms, resource teachers) are provided. This is also true of many severely handicapped children, such as the deaf or blind, and others who may have some very severe and rare handicaps (e.g. Mullins, 1971). Other severely impaired children, such as the severely retarded, can function in special classes that are integrated into regular schools, rather than in special classes grouped together and/or placed in separate wings or even separate schools. Secondary work-study programs, which often use only in-school or sheltered workshop assignments for their work training, need to emphasize assignment in business and industry instead.

INTEGRATION IN VOCATIONAL EDUCATION

Legislation as well as attitudinal changes are presently opening up new integrative vistas in vocational education. These opportunities need to be pursued vigorously. There exists now the option to do – within the mainstream of the rapidly expanding vocational education field – much of what was previously done in the specially-designated and stigma-attached field of rehabilitation, or on the side-tracks of secondary special education.

CONCLUDING COMMENTS ON INTEGRATED EDUCATION

It is both salutary and gratifying to note that in the future, integrated special education will become better, and easier to accomplish, as all education becomes special education, i.e. as we move more and more from lockstep teaching to individualization of the learning-teaching process. Vast improvements in the educational manpower structure have already taken place, and such improvements make for better and more individualized education. Other developments – almost certain to be even more significant – will be the increased availability of new and better educational aides, the routine use of computer-assisted and computer-managed instruction, and new administrative methods of structuring the educational process. As all education becomes special, grade leveling and grade grouping of children – as we now know it – will disappear, and integration will no longer present the problems it does today.

Industry integrated work stations

For many years, we have aspired to the establishment of more vocational service centers ('workshops') which would offer vocational evaluation, training, long-term employment, and possibly other vocation-related services, either to the handicapped in general, or to special handicapped groups. For instance, it was widely felt that the problems of the retarded were such as to require separate (segregated) work centers. ... From a normalization (though not always economic) viewpoint, there is little to be gained by favoring a generic (i.e. all-handicapped) over a specialty (e.g. all-retardation) workshop. In the generic center, a deviant person would still be grouped with others similarly perceived (e.g. the retarded, blind, deaf, physically impaired, emotionally disturbed, alcoholic). On the other hand, integration of a deviant worker or work trainee with typical workers in business and industry would constitute a major normalizing advance.

The time has come to establish the functions of the 'sheltered workshop' right in the work community, right within the confines of specific firms, right on the work floor. Service systems can rent floor space from factories, often for nominal sums. 'Segregated' work space can serve for initial placement of trainees or workers, with integration being restricted to space and functions associated with the time clock, the toilets, and the cafeteria and/or canteen area. After a period of transition, some handicapped workers can be integrated into the midst of the work floor. Many such workers eventually will achieve a normative level of production, and will become eligible to be hired by that firm or elsewhere in the job market. Establishment of work stations in industry can reduce the need for special and segregated services considerably. ... Industry-integrated work training and/or sheltered work is not new. It has been practiced successfully – though only sporadically – in the past, both in North America and elsewhere. But now, the time has come to implement this option systematically and massively.

Integrating residences for special needs groups

Where possible, the utilization of the much-neglected options of adoptive, foster, and boarding placement for handicapped children (even the profoundly retarded) is most desirable. These various approaches have been extensively discussed in the recent literature. However, in addition to these opportunities, much community integration of the retarded, the emotionally disordered, etc. can be achieved by developing small group residences, such as home-like hostels and highly dispersed special apartments.

Even where community-integrated group residences are considered and established, the possibility is seldom considered that in addition to integrating the group residence into the community, integration can also be achieved *within* the residence itself (e.g. Colbert, 1969). Such internal integration can be brought about in a number of ways. For instance, two or three mature college students might share an apartment with two or three retarded persons who are working in competitive industry or in sheltered situations. A college might lease some rooms or a wing of a dormitory, to be used by retarded young adults on a temporary basis while they are under training in a vocational center. Hostels might serve both handicapped and homeless non-handicapped children, instead of only the handicapped. Public housing might be designed from the very beginning to accommodate both the impaired and the unimpaired (e.g. Klein & Abrams, 1971). Finally, there is little reason why many of the institutionalized aged cannot be placed into ordinary (but good) nursing homes.

The objection is sometimes heard that the handicapped do not want to live integratedly. Often, this is a defensive claim, advanced to avoid having to pursue such integration. A recent survey of 658 handicapped persons (Columbus & Fogel, 1971) certainly suggests that lack of opportunity is a larger factor than lack of desire.

Miscellaneous areas ready for integration

It is absurd to build expensive dental suites and surgical operating theaters specifically for the retarded or emotionally disturbed, as is done in so many institutions. Teeth and appendices can be excised just as readily in ordinary community hospitals and dental offices if a little care is taken in the planning and social interpretation of such procedures.

Today, we conduct special camps for the handicapped, reserve bowling alleys for occasions when the handicapped bowl by themselves, and reserve swimming pools on a similar basis. Other examples of segregation in recreation can readily be cited. Often, such segregation is practiced not intentionally or from lack of alternatives, but from a neglect to pursue a strategy of integration consciously and systematically. ...

Nowhere is integration more appropriate than in those atmospheres where the essence rather than the accidents of man's nature is emphasized, and where man is even interpreted as possessing similarities to God, i.e. in religious worship and instruction. Here, much integration can be accomplished by thoughtful planning. ...

Cautions

Sometimes, integration is easier than we think, and sometimes harder. For instance, we thought we had achieved a great deal of integration in our first hostels for retarded adults in Omaha. Each hostel was ideally located in lower middle-class neighborhoods, near community resources and transportation routes. The residents took the public bus to the workshop, and went to ordinary neighborhood and community recreation sites and events. However, in the hostel, all residents were retarded; on the way to the workshop, they went together in groups, which had an isolating effect; at the workshop, the fellow-workers were retarded; going in small groups to recreation was, again, isolating; and the same was true for church. Thus, the residents still ate, worked, played, worshipped, and slept primarily in contact with other retarded persons. They were integrated physically, but not socially. ...

9   From: "The definition of normalization: update, problems, disagreements and misunderstandings," 1980, in R.J. Flynn and K.E. Nitsch (eds) *Normalization, Social Integration and Community Services*, 71–115, Baltimore: University Park Press.

The next extract takes us forward some ten years, and is a response to the considerable impact of normalization in the 1970s described earlier. The earlier extracts largely concerned the USA and Canada, though in Australia, New Zealand and the UK influence was felt at least in public discussion of services. The impact also, of course, brought out a reaction, both from within the service world and academia, and, as we saw earlier, the origins of the term in Scandinavia and their interpretation in service terms provided a somewhat different model for services to examine. The chapter from which the extract below is taken first of all goes into this issue, with largely the same story as told in the opening part of this chapter. Similarly, the categories of controversy bear some resemblance to the 'reactions' identified earlier. Since this chapter appeared shortly before the reformulation of normalization as SRV (presaged in the opening remarks below and dealt with at length in Chapter 3), the extract will be relatively brief, being focussed on its discussion of the range of ideas around values and norms of societies.

Chances are that before 1968, very few people in North America had heard the term *normalization* used in a human services context. The majority of those who are now familiar with the term have probably encountered it some time since 1972. Thus, as far as word use in human services goes, the term is quite new – although many people dispute the newness of the theoretical concepts that underlie it.

Today, we are confronted with confusion about the meaning of normalization. Neither ardent supporters of the normalization principle nor its impassioned opponents can agree among each other as to what it is they agree with – or even what they disagree on – in either their support or their opposition. So, when someone either advances or opposes the principle of normalization, one now has to ask the question, "normalization according to whom?"

This chapter addresses the meaning of the term *normalization*. Unfortunately, the term is derived from the culturally common and familiar word *normal*, which already has well-established meanings in the minds of practically every citizen. For this reason, it was probably a rather serious strategic error to use this term in the first place, rather than a less familiar term or neologism that would not have evoked familiar, but inaccurate, perceptions and meanings.

After a review of early uses and the Scandinavian formulations and their differences with Wolfensberger, the chapter goes on to discuss the Wolfensberger formulation and the issue of societal norms.

...

For the purposes of a North American audience, and for broadest adaptability to human services in general, I proposed, in 1969 (though not published until 1972), that the definition of the normalization principle be: "Utilization of means which are as culturally normative as possible, in order to establish and/or maintain personal behaviors and characteristics which are as culturally normative as possible." I have slightly changed this definition in my teachings so that, today, I use the formulation: "Utilization of means which are as culturally normative as possible, in order to establish, enable, or support behaviors, appearances and interpretations which are as culturally normative as possible." For less formal teaching purposes, I also often use a less awkward phrasing: "Use of culturally normative means (familiar, valued techniques, tools, methods), in order to enable persons life conditions (income, housing, health services, etc.) which are at least as good as that of average citizens, and to as much as possible enhance or support their behavior (skills, competencies, etc.), appearances (clothes, grooming, etc.), experiences (adjustment, feelings, etc.), and status and reputation (labels, attitudes of others, etc.)." When I am asked to explain normalization to a lay audience in a few seconds, I sometimes refer to "the use of culturally valued means in order to enable people to live culturally valued lives."

... Perhaps one of the most common misconceptions about the principle of normalization, at least as formulated here, is that it implies that a person should be fitted to the statistical norm of the society. In other words, some people see normalization as having been achieved when a person is or does something the way most people are or do. However, this is a naive and invalid interpretation of the principle as I have formulated it.

In order to understand this issue clearly, three phenomena are of importance.

1   The phenomenological and expectancy norm in a society is not necessarily identical with the statistical norm. In other words, what people would not be surprised to encounter in society, or what they would highly value but rarely encounter, may not be what actually prevails. Thus, a phenomenon may fall well within the range of that which is normative, even though it may only be rarely encountered in the culture. ...

2   Some of the above phenomena can be explained simply by the following fact: that which is expected is quite often that which is valued, even though that which is valued is not necessarily expected statistically and may not necessarily occur very often. Similarly, the concept of the "norm," even in its common sense, applies not only to the statistically common, but also to that which may be uncommonly encountered, but which is internally idealized.

3   A phenomenon that is both very common and generally valued can actually be *de*-normalizing when it occurs in the life of a devalued person. For instance, family homes or ordinary apartment houses adjacent to cemeteries are not only fairly common in our society, but they are also quite often valued because

Table 2.2 A clarification of some of the determinants of normalization

Cultural values	Process of socialization →	Cultural norms	Process of internalization →	Statistical-behavioral norms
Constitute a society's idealized standards of the desirable		More specific rules based on values		Empirically-observed, regular patterns of behavior, traits, and appearances
Highly general		Infused with a moral imperative or "oughtness"		Produced because most people believe in, approve of, or conform to most cultural norms most of the time
Derived from broad human experience and specific historical development		Prescribe generally expected behaviors, traits, or appearances for specific situations		
Invested with a "sacred" character		Sanctions are either positive (honor) or negative (opprobrium)		
Rarely attained by any one person		Include folkways, mores, and laws		

of their quiet location and the fact that many of the cemeteries resemble (or perhaps even are) parks. At the same time, however, it is devastatingly de-normalizing for an elderly person to have to live in a special residence that is adjacent to a cemetery. ...

Some of the above issues become clearer upon examination of Table 2.2. This type of schematization was not present in the 1972 *Normalization* text, an omission that has permitted the excessively statistical interpretation of normalization. However, the 1973 edition of PASS corrected this problem, although critics have tended not to take note thereof. I hope that this chapter clarifies 1) that measures under any of the three columns, not only those in the statistical norms column, of Table 2.2 would be normalizing, and 2) that for people who are already devalued, or at risk thereof, a measure generally becomes more normalizing as it moves to the left of the table. Some key assumptions (with extensive empirical support, however) include the following: that a person will benefit maximally from those measures that reflect and/or capture his/her highest values and ideals; that a person will relate optimally to that other person whom he/she perceives as representing, embodying, or carrying his/her idealized values; and that most people in a culture agree, at least to some extent, with a majority of other members on at least the theoretical desirability of certain idealized norms. For example, even people who practice oppression will generally idealize liberty; even people who practice deception will idealize truth.

Chapter 3

Social Role Valorization

Introduction

As the previous chapter indicated, the late 1970s saw the beginnings of dissatisfaction by Wolfensberger with the many variations and controversies arising from the widespread implementation and subsequent reaction to his, and others', formulations of normalization. After the attempt, in the book from which the extract that ended the last chapter was taken, to deal with these whilst retaining the term 'normalization,' he was to reformulate and reconceptualize the ideas as Social Role Valorization (SRV). We shall see, in the extracts which follow, the connectedness to the roots of normalization in a variety of ways. The whole notion of devaluation, and its origins in deviancy theory and the historic roles; the 'wounds' which were beginning to form a vital part of the teaching culture around Wolfensberger's Training Institute; and the structure that the PASS instrument had brought to the analysis – all contributed to an evolving construct.

10 From: 'Social Role Valorization: a new insight, and a new term, for normalization', 1985, *Australian Association for the Mentally Retarded Journal*, 9(1), 4–11.

In the extract which follows, the issues covered above have been edited, but the key new insights presented more or less in full. PASSING was published in 1983 (unfortunately still using the term normalization), and between 1983 and 1985 three articles appeared announcing SRV. This extract is from one of these. It is significant that it comes from an Australian journal, as that country was probably the least equivocal in taking up the new term, and being part of the SRV teaching culture generated from Wolfensberger's Training Institute. It is also the paper in which the aim to move towards SRV as a social science theory is most clearly articulated.

...

Ever since 1969, I have attempted to convert the early formulations of normalization by Bank-Mikkelsen (1969) and Nirje (1969) into a scientific theory that is universal, precise, and congruent with social and behavioural science. Although I retained the term "normalization" in my series of elaborations and systematisations of the principle ..., I was never satisfied with it. The major reasons for my dissatisfaction were that different people attached different meanings to it; and a great many people thought that because the word was so simple and straightforward, they knew exactly what it meant, could expertly converse upon it and even critique it, and therefore did not need to read the literature on it – though, of course, they were usually wrong in these assumptions. Thus, even though the principle of normalization had been elaborated into a tightly-built, intellectually demanding and research-anchored over-arching human service theory, very few people in the academic and research culture took it seriously.

This is why I suggested with grim humour in the normalization update book by Flynn and Nitsch (1980) that a totally unfamiliar word might have been preferable, and I whimsically gave "orthofactorization" as an example. (This word might be taken to mean "making things right," or "doing things correctly".)

Despite these serious problems with the word "normalization," I resisted a change in name for two reasons. (a) I was unable to think of a superior choice. I carefully examined the various alternatives which different people proposed (such as mainstreaming and humanization), but each one had problems that were probably greater, or at least as great, as those associated with 'normalization'. ... (b) Because by early 1970 the term "normalization" had acquired so much momentum, simple wisdom dictated that no name change be attempted unless an unequivocally superior term could be identified.

Explicit goal identified

With the advent of two recent developments came the long-awaited opportunity. One development was the recent insight (Wolfensberger & Tullman, 1982; Wolfensberger & Thomas, 1983) that the most explicit and highest goal of what has been called normalization must be the creation, support and defense of *valued social roles* for people who are at risk of social devaluation, because if a person's social role is a societally valued one, then other desirable things will be accorded to that person almost automatically, at least within the resources and norms of his/her society. Indeed, attributes of the person which might otherwise have been viewed negatively by society would come to be viewed positively. For instance, we know that many members of society try to become more like those people who fill highly valued roles. ....If a stuttering person were king, many courtiers might develop at least a slight stutter. Along these lines, for over 300 years, first men and then women across the whole world have worn quite inconvenient and unhealthy high-heeled shoes in imitation of Louis XIV – who introduced them because he was short. ...

All of the above illustrates that a judgement about whether or not a person or group is valued is not so much determined by who and what the person or group is, as by how others *perceive* that person or group, by the social roles accorded to them, and by the value that others attach to the social roles that the person or group is seen as filling.

Devalued social role

People who are not seen as having valued social roles are considered to be of low value. We know that among other things, people who are seen as devalued have very different life experiences from those in valued roles.

1   Devalued people almost certainly will be badly treated. They are apt to be rejected, even persecuted, and treated in ways which tend to diminish their dignity, adjustment, growth, competence, health, wealth, lifespan, etc.
2   The bad treatment given to devalued persons will largely express and reflect the devalued societal roles which they are perceived as "playing". For instance, if handicapped children are viewed (consciously or unconsciously) in the role of animals, then they may be segregated into settings that look like cages and animal pens, that are located close to zoos or animal laboratories, and their service may be given an animal name. ...
3   How a person is perceived and treated by others will determine strongly how that person subsequently behaves. Therefore, the more consistently a person is perceived and treated as being in a negative role, the more likely it is that s/he will conform to that expectation and actually will behave in ways that are not valued by society. On the other hand, the more a person is encouraged to assume roles and behaviours which are appropriate and desirable, the more will be expected of him/her, the more s/he is apt to achieve, and the more s/he will live up to those positive roles. ...

Goal and strategies organized

In attempting to attain the goals of socially valued roles and life conditions for (devalued) people, any number of things can or must be done which, for practical and problem-solving purposes, can be divided into two large classes: (a) enhancement of people's *social image* or perceived value in the eyes of others, and (b) enhancement of their *competencies*.

In our society, image enhancement and competency enhancement can be assumed to be generally reciprocally reinforcing, both positively and negatively. That is, a person who is competency-impaired is highly at risk of becoming seen and interpreted as of low value, thus suffering image-impairment; a person who is impaired in social image is apt to be responded to by others in ways that impair/reduce his/her competency. Both processes work equally in the reverse direction; that is, a person whose social image is positively valued is apt to be provided with experiences, expectancies, and other life conditions which generally will also increase his/her competencies, and a person who is highly competent is also more apt to be imaged positively. ...

With regard to human services specifically, one can now conceptualise Social Role Valorization as implying a hierarchical arrangement of implications, which can be summarised as in Table 3.1

New conceptualisation leads to new terms

This first development – that is, the insight that the epitome of normalization was the creation of valued social roles for people at risk of social devaluation – occurred shortly before the second development relevant to this new conceptualisation, namely, my discovery that in modern French human service contexts, people had begun to use the word *valorisation* in order to signify the attachment of value to people. In Canadian French, the term *valorisation sociale* has been used in teaching the normalization principle since late 1980. This discovery led to the conclusion that the perfect French term for normalization might be something like *la valorisation du rôle social*. Ordinary French dictionaries do not carry this term in relation to human services, and if one asks French people with no human service connections, they are apt to say that there is no such word, at least not one that would apply to people. However, the fact that French human service circles have been using this term in recent years certainly pointed out its potential utility and broader adoption. As is readily apparent from its root in both French and English, which goes back to Latin, the term is derived from a word meaning courage – *valor*, and from one for value – *valeur*. Even for the word "valor" (sometimes spelled valour, at least in British usage), Webster's Dictionary gives three meanings, the *first* of which is value or worth. Similarly, "valorous" is defined *first* as having value or worth, and only secondly as meaning brave.

In combination, the above insights and discoveries suggested that an eminently suitable English term for normalization would be "Social Role Valorization." Valorization is found in many dictionaries as meaning "attempting to give a market value or price to a commodity." This arcane meaning is a drawback, because it implies the attachment of value to objects instead of people, but this dictionary definition is not familiar to most people, nor does it appear to constitute a compelling negative image juxtaposition. Further, the word "valorization" has, or elicits, very strong positive meanings that correspond to what we have been trying to convey, even though it is at the same time unfamiliar to most people. Therefore, unlike the word normalization, people are more likely to listen to definitions and explanations of it, rather than attaching to it their own preconceived notions. Considering what happens to people's minds when they encounter the simplistic sounding term "normalization," we can see that it is actually an advantage that the term "valorization" either (a) is devoid of meaning to most people, (b) carries the meaning of value, or (c) evokes an unrelated technical concept that is relatively meaningless to most people, and is recognized by the few people who know it as inapplicable to the context to which it is here being applied. ...

Table 3.1 The hierarchical structure of social role valorization (formerly known as the principle of normalization)

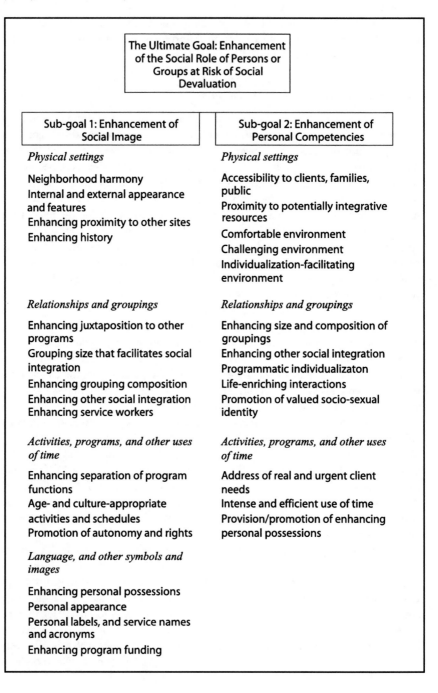

The Ultimate Goal: Enhancement of the Social Role of Persons or Groups at Risk of Social Devaluation

Sub-goal 1: Enhancement of Social Image	Sub-goal 2: Enhancement of Personal Competencies
Physical settings	*Physical settings*
Neighborhood harmony	Accessibility to clients, families, public
Internal and external appearance and features	Proximity to potentially integrative resources
Enhancing proximity to other sites	Comfortable environment
Enhancing history	Challenging environment
	Individualization-facilitating environment
Relationships and groupings	*Relationships and groupings*
Enhancing juxtaposition to other programs	Enhancing size and composition of groupings
Grouping size that facilitates social integration	Enhancing other social integration
Enhancing grouping composition	Programmatic individualizaton
Enhancing other social integration	Life-enriching interactions
Enhancing service workers	Promotion of valued socio-sexual identity
Activities, programs, and other uses of time	*Activities, programs, and other uses of time*
Enhancing separation of program functions	Address of real and urgent client needs
Age- and culture-appropriate activities and schedules	Intense and efficient use of time
Promotion of autonomy and rights	Provision/promotion of enhancing personal possessions
Language, and other symbols and images	
Enhancing personal possessions	
Personal appearance	
Personal labels, and service names and acronyms	
Enhancing program funding	

Within this new conceptualization, something would now be said to be "social role-valorizing" rather than "normalizing." However, the term "normative" still has selected utility, but users need to be aware that the term has two meanings, a sociological and a statistical one. [See last extract of Chapter 2 – Ed.] ...

The person and the role

However, I believe that it would be a theoretical error to use the term "valorization" by itself to replace "normalization", because valuing a person – "person valorization", so to speak – has to be distinguished from according to that person a valued social role. It seems to me that as long as we remain within a scientific-theoretical frame of discourse – which is where Social Role Valorization theory largely is – we can only speak of the valorization of a person's role. When we speak of valuing a person, we step at least partially outside a scientific-theoretical framework that is profoundly anchored to empiricism, and into the realm of supraempirical value systems, such as religions, world views, and other belief systems. Furthermore, people might very well value a person, but still not construct valued social roles for that person in society. For example, one may truly love an elderly person – perhaps one's grandparent – yet do nothing to prevent that person from being cast into the role of a child, or of a sick or diseased organism that is interpreted as being near death. In fact, it has not been uncommon for people who do love individual devalued persons to actually *participate* in casting them into negative roles.

Furthermore, one sometimes hears it said (especially from people with a religious perspective) that if one values the person, it is irrelevant whether that person is valued in the eyes of others and of "the world." Thus, nothing may be done to enhance the competencies of a devalued person or group, to help them overcome infirmities or acquire habits of socially valued grooming, to reduce the negative images attached to these persons, and so on. These things may be dismissed as unimportant by the one who positively values such persons, perhaps even with the argument that these things are ultimately unimportant before God. Such an orientation often results in a defiant challenge to "the world" to similarly value the persons at issue regardless of their identity and characteristics.

Such an appeal does have merit, but is almost totally ineffective in bringing about the desired goal. Any unbiased reading of history will reveal that social devaluation and division are so thoroughly a part of human identity that people need all the help they can get to overcome their baser inclinations to reject and devalue others. Furthermore, genuine personal valuation cannot be merely a verbal abstraction, but must manifest itself in behaviour *vis-à-vis* people at risk of devaluation. One of the first steps in getting other people to be less devaluing is to get them to approach the person with devalued characteristics in a non-destructive fashion. In most instances, people only will be brought to do that if they can be helped to see the person in positive ways, which primarily means in positive roles. One can also identify other ways of influencing people's perceptions, as by value purification and consciousness-raising activities, but the former strategies may involve appeals to people's highest values and religious beliefs, and go far beyond human service contexts.

Now in use

I have begun to use the term Social Role Valorization routinely in lieu of normalization, and call on others to do the same, but one should be aware that more than just a name change is involved. Rather, the new term also captures the fact that the things we previously considered to be normalizing really contribute to the enhancement of the social role(s) of a person or group in the eyes of others. Even by itself, this insight can remove a great deal of misunderstanding and controversy that has surrounded normalization (Wolfensberger, 1980a).

---

11 From: 'A brief overview of Social Role Valorization', 2000, *Mental Retardation*, 38(2), 105–23.

After its introduction into the literature and to the teaching culture supported by Wolfensberger's Training Institute, the notion of SRV had a mixed history in various countries. As far as written material goes, Wolfensberger produced three monographs, in 1991, 1992 and 1998, with revisions for foreign language translations in between, but though these had a wide circulation within the teaching culture, their private publication meant that the more general academic literature, especially in certain countries such as the UK, did not discuss or debate the theory to any great extent. The latest published version for a wider audience forms the basis for the next extract. The 'wounds', which we have covered in greater depth in Chapter 1, are the major editing reduction from the extract, along with the basic definition and its derivation, and the elements of role theory covered in the 1985 Australian paper. Despite its relative currency, the SRV concept is still evolving, and so more may be expected before this book is published, but this extract clarifies a number of key issues, particularly the wide applicability of SRV to all devalued groups, its empirical base, and suggestions for implementation. Issues concerning the interpretation of SRV, its place within a political discourse, and its relationship with ideas of 'empowerment' will be covered in the three extracts which follow this one.

...

In the context of SRV, it is the valorization of social roles that is at issue.

A major corollary of this ... is that one needs to be clear whose role-valorization of whom one wants to obtain. (In the rest of this paper, I will sometimes use the word *party* when a statement can apply to any two, or all, of the following referents: an individual, a group, or an entire class.) After all, different reference targets may hold different values. This implies that one's role-valorizing actions may have to be different for different reference targets, so as to recruit their values to the role-valorization of some party that had been, or was about to be, devalued by them.

This fact demands many value decisions. However, because by its very nature science cannot provide answers to value questions (such as whether anyone should hold valued or devalued roles; or should or should not be valued or devalued, and in whose eyes; or should or should not be afforded the good things of life), one must derive answers to such questions from one's value system; that is, from one's de facto religion (Wolfensberger, 1995).

In this treatise, my primary focus is on *societal* (rather than only personal) devaluation, on such devaluation in *our* society, and how such devaluation could be combated via SRV. In order to evolve this exposition, I first sketch a few important realities and facts: (a) who the classes of people are who are widely devalued in our society, (b) some of the bad things that are likely to happen to them, and (c) some facts about social roles and social imagery.

The classes of people who are widely devalued in Western society today

In our society – and indeed in much of Western societies generally – the following classes of people are apt to be devalued by a significant proportion of society.

1   People who are impaired in some way, as perhaps in their senses, bodies, or minds.
2   People who are seriously disordered or unorthodox in their conduct or behavior, including (a) those who are either excessively active (the hyperactive) or not active enough (the lethargic, the lazy); (b) those considered disordered or unorthodox in their sexual identity and/or conduct; and (c) those who are self-destructive, including those enslaved to alcohol and other drugs.
3   People whose visible bodily characteristics are viewed very negatively, such as those who are very disfigured, obese, short, tall, etc.
4   People who rebel against the social order, which might include political dissidents, those who refuse to work, and those who violate the law.
5   The poor, who have been very devalued in our society since at least ca. 1500.
6   People who have very few skills or whose skills are not wanted or useful to society, such as the illiterate and unemployed.
7   People who are unassimilated into the culture for any number of (other) reasons. Historically, this has included (a) members of racial and ethnic minority groups; (b) members of religious minorities, particularly if these also take a stance against the political and/or value system of the culture; (c) those who do not know or use the prevailing tongue; (d) illegal immigrants and/or immigrants of a devalued ethnic group; and (e) migrant laborers. Lately, this has also increasingly included (a) people at the extremes of the age spectrum – the elderly, the unborn, and the newborn; and (b) teenagers. Of course, some devalued classes are much more devalued than others and, hence,

at greater risk than others, including people who fall into several of these categories.

The paper then goes on to lay out the 'wounding experiences' of devalued people, and to make some basic points regarding role theory, which have been covered above. We pick up the paper at the end of the section on role theory, where Wolfensberger identifies some reasons why social roles are so important, with four key points being made.

Why social roles are so important

...

1   Roles give a person a "place" *vis-à-vis* others and in society, and it is largely via their roles that people define and situate themselves in the world. For instance, almost all of one's relational behavior is profoundly informed and shaped by the roles one holds. As well, it is largely via roles that people define and situate others in the world, in that roles give people at least a preliminary mental "handle" as to who a person is and how they should relate to that person. This is why people typically seek role-related information about a person they encounter: age, sex, marital and family status, education, nature of employment, etc. All this explains why it is outright difficult to talk about specific individuals without invoking social roles, as one will discover if one tries to do so.

    One phenomenon that underlines the importance of social roles is what Lemay (1999) has called "role avidity" – i.e., "role hunger," meaning that people very much want to see themselves in socially recognizable roles. Role avidity explains many (usually maladaptive) phenomena, such as people ludicrously expanding a minor role into a life-consuming one, preferring even devalued roles to no roles at all, or preferring a big devalued role to several small valued ones. It follows that role avidity is apt to be highest in those people (e.g., many retarded ones) who want more social relations, but do not inhabit roles that lend themselves well to establishing or maintaining such relations.

2   In their totality, the roles that people fill affect just about every aspect of their lives (e.g., what relationships the person will have with others, or will even be permitted to enter into); who the person will (be permitted to) associate with; where and with whom the person will live; what sorts of things the person will do during the day; what the person's schedules and routines will be; what sort of economic status and income the person will have; the degree of respect the person will be accorded by others; the kind of autonomy the person will enjoy; whether and how much the person will participate in community affairs; even such things as health, health care, diet, and what clothes one wears – and more – will be strongly influenced, or even determined, by one's roles. However, there is also a two-way relationship between a person's real or attributed

characteristics and a person's role: one may end up in a role because of one's characteristics, but whatever roles one is placed into for whatever reason also tend to strongly shape one's characteristics, one's behavior, and even one's identity.

3   The more a person holds "big" roles that are highly valued, the more are other people likely to put up with the person's other negative roles, characteristics, or behaviors, or even reinterpret these as being not so bad. In other words, holding big positive roles is a strong defense against being devalued on account of other reasons.

4   Altogether, it is a major thesis of SRV that, at least on a probabilistic and long-term basis, society will extend whatever good things it has to offer to people in valued roles and may even push these on such people, but will do bad things (or little or nothing that is positive) to those in devalued roles.

These four points imply that people who have some kind of impairment, but who occupy valued roles – and especially "big," many, and highly valued ones – are much more likely to (a) be spared some of the bad things that are likely to befall impaired people in negative roles, and (b) be beneficiaries of the good things that are commonly afforded to people in valued roles.

...

Fortunately, there are many positive roles that are potentially available even to already devalued people. ... Particularly in some domains, such as that of economic productivity, the number of potential positive and more specific roles is virtually infinite.

A table is then given in the article at about this point, being a particular version of one used in SRV teaching. Given the context of the journal *Mental Retardation*, the focus of this table is not as general as the one from which it is derived and therefore for the purposes of this book, and with permission of Professor Wolfensberger, we include the more general version as Table 3.2 below.

The relationship between social roles and social images

The previously mentioned construct of "imagery" plays a prominent part in SRV. Images are mental pictures ... that are commonly evoked in response to, or in connection with, or as the result of a juxtaposition to something else: a stimulus, an event, a perception (of people, places, objects, etc.), a memory or an idea, a social stereotype, etc. ... If in the mind of an observer, two or more entities somehow have gotten associated with each other, and one of these entities has certain images attached to it, then in the observer's mind, these images will tend to be transferred, and attached, to the other entities as well. Such image transfer can occur from entity A to entity B, from B to A, and from each to the other simultaneously. Many

Table 3.2 Major role domains, with positive and negative examples

Common role domains	Positive role examples	Negative role examples
Relationships	Wife, husband, parent, grandparent, friend, brother, sister, son, daughter, aunt, uncle, fiancé	Old maid, orphan, black sheep of the family
Residence, domicile	Home- or land-owner, building superintendent, good neighbor, tenant	Homeless street person, vagabond, hobo, bad neighbor
Economic productivity, occupation	Worker, employee, apprentice, expert, breadwinner, union member, wage-earner, customer, employer, boss, business owner	Idler, loafer, union-buster, informer, ne'er-do-well, scab
Education	Teacher, professor, scholar, student, peer-tutor	Dunce, special class student, slowest member of the class
Leisure, sports	Athlete, competitor, champion, coach, fan, booster, cheerleader	Oaf, klutz, loser, sore loser, bad sport
Community/civic identity and participation	Public official, citizen, voter, taxpayer, community activist, board member, jury member, patriot	Foreigner, stranger, subversive, dissident, traitor, welfare recipient, "sponger", prisoner
Religious and ethical belief and practises	Pastor, philosopher, thinker, deacon, sexton, acolyte, cantor, chorister, parishioner	Sinner, lost soul, faddist, apostate
Culture	Arts patron, music-lover, book-lover, dancer, (amateur) musician, literatus	Philistine, illiterate, boor

factors affect what associations get thusly transferred in people's minds, into which direction they are transferred, and whether the implied message is positive or negative.

Important to our context is that images that are conveyed about people can communicate both role messages and value messages; and, in turn, roles can convey images and value messages. In fact, it is hard to think of a social role without all sorts of images coming to mind that pertain to that role. ...

When positive images are attached to a party, that party is more likely to be first viewed positively, and then to be accorded or afforded positive roles. Negative images associated with a party are more likely to result in that party being first devalued and then cast into negative roles. And all this is apt to get done with little or no consciousness, because a major portion of human perceptual learning, and even cognitive processes – not to mention social interactions – is unconscious. Therefore, much in the domain of imagery, expectancy, and roles is also unconscious, and particularly so are one's social devaluations and one's attachment of negative image to people whom one devalues. The reason is that at least in Western cultures, such actions are judged to be unworthy, so one feels guilty about them and, therefore, represses what they really mean, or that one is even complicit in such devaluations and corresponding actions.

However, how a particular message about a party is interpreted by perceivers will often depend on who the message is about. People are known to tend to interpret messages as confirming their pre-existing positive or negative stereotypes of a party. This implies that although negative value could get transferred to anyone who engages in a negatively imaged activity, behavior, or juxtaposition, it can wreak vastly more damage if it plays into already pre-existing negative stereotypes about them. Also, it takes vastly more evidence to overcome a negative stereotype than to confirm it. ...

In respect to low intelligence specifically, the negative images it has been apt to evoke have been those of childishness, gaping, ... drooling ..., slowness and clumsiness of movement, distractibility, slow and indistinct speech, inappropriate affect, being inappropriately dressed, etc. Because such images are found in innumerable cultures around the world and across historical eras, one can call them archetypal. Furthermore, many roles associated in people's minds with low intelligence are negatively valued, such as the eternal child; the village idiot; the performer of very lowly and unskilled work tasks, ... Historically, there have also been some positive images about, and roles for, retarded people: child-like innocence, joy in simple things, gentle and loving consoler, forthrightness, ice-breaker at social gatherings, conscientious worker, devoted follower of a religious faith, other people's moral conscience, etc. Some of these images and roles have been sketched in Wolfensberger (1988) [See extract 32 – Ed.].

The avenues for conveying either value-laden image messages, role messages, or expectancies about people can be classified into the six categories sketched below.

Physical contexts and environments

Where people are and get put can carry very strong images as well as role and value messages. For instance, if one encounters a place that is called a hospital, one expects to find sick people and medical personnel in it. This can be a problem if the "patients" there are really not sick at all but have merely been interpreted that way and cast into the sick patient role. ... A dirty environment reflects negatively on the people in it, above and beyond whatever role messages it may convey.

All this means that impaired people are apt to be image- and role-enhanced if they live in the same kinds of places, and are schooled in the same settings, as valued persons; ... if their settings are comfortable and beautiful, clean and well-kept, and blend harmoniously with their neighborhoods; and if their environments convey accurate and positive messages about their age and optimistic messages about their capacities for growth and development.

Social contexts and associations

Social associations can strongly convey role messages. There are innumerable folk sayings about how one is defined by the company one keeps. More specifically, when persons with the same impairment are juxtaposed to each other, the idea that all such people "belong together" is conveyed to, or reinforced in, observers. Relatedly, the idea can easily take hold in an observer's mind that the less impaired persons in such a juxtaposition are actually as impaired as the more severely impaired ones. Further, when people who have one kind of ... "wound," are juxta-posed to people who have another kind, observers also commonly get the idea that both parties are somehow the same. ... For instance, if mentally retarded people are all mixed in with cerebral palsied people, the retarded people are apt to be assumed to be physically impaired, and the cerebral palsied people are apt to be assumed to be retarded, even if neither is the case. ...

In contrast, mentally handicapped people are apt to acquire – or retain – positive imagery and role expectancies by being associated with people who are perceived as competent, vigorous, moral, distinguished, etc., and who occupy positive roles. However, in order for such positive image transfer to take place, it is generally important that only a small number of devalued persons be associated with, or juxtaposed to, a much larger number of valued ones, because it is the majority – and even predominant – identity of any social grouping that is apt to define its individual members in the eyes of observers.

Behaviors and activities

Behaviors, activities, and how these are carried out and timed can also convey positive or negative images and messages about people and their roles. For instance, vigorous activities carried out over normal or even long periods of the day, week, or year convey images and messages of strength, persistence, commitment, competency, etc. Negative messages are apt to be conveyed if people engage in activities or schedules that are viewed as negatively atypical, either for people of their age (and thus being age-inappropriate) or for anyone in their society (and thus being culture-inappropriate). ... Certain activities, settings, and social juxtapositions tend to go with each other, and these typical combinations can have characteristic positive or negative valence. For instance, if one attends a college, one is apt to carry out one's activities in juxtaposition to faculty members, custodial staff, librarians, and other students, with the overall valuation of the combination usually being a positive one. In contrast, a negative valuation is apt to be incurred from the larger culture if six college students go joyriding in a red-light district at 2 a.m.

Language used with or about people, or about anything associated with them

Language can powerfully communicate about people in a number of ways. About people of low intelligence specifically, many languages have hundreds of words or phrases, almost all of which evoke negative images and role ideas: eternal child, dumb ox, blockhead, village idiot, vegetable, low-grade, and so on. When people are addressed with value-degrading language, it may hurt their feelings; but if the same language is used to talk (or write) about them, then negative ideas and feelings about them get planted or reinforced in the minds of others, who are highly apt to convert these sooner or later into behavior that is vastly more damaging than hurt feelings.

But language can also be used to convey positive messages about people, as by addressing them, or speaking about them, in ways that dignify them or imply positive roles: Mr. or Mrs., our guest, employees, chairperson, athlete, a good worker, my brother, etc.

In addition to terminology, there is tone of voice and gestures. So often, impaired adults and aged people are spoken to in high-pitched melodic voices – the same tone most people use with children and pet animals. This is "the child role voice".... . Also relevant are the names, acronyms, and logos adopted by organizations and agencies concerned with (devalued) people. A logo that looks like a child's stick figure suggests that the adults with which the organization is concerned are child-like.

Personal appearance

A person's appearance ... can send out strong positive or negative messages. So commonly, the appearance of mentally impaired people does not project a positive image. They may wear clothing that is ill-fitting, out-of-fashion, worn out, torn, dirty, or immature for their age; they may carry themselves awkwardly, having never been taught graceful movement and good posture; they may have poor hygiene habits and, hence, bad body odor; and no effort may be made to help them look attractive or even elegant.

Also, much as certain activities and social juxtapositions tend to go together ... so do personal appearance and the physical context. Thus, a person's appearance may be very positive – but only if it accords with a certain setting (e.g., leisure clothes do not go well with business settings, business clothes look weird on a beach, etc.). ...

Miscellaneous role and image communicators

There are several other channels that can convey role, image, and value messages. One is the funding that supports a person or service. For instance, the image of an impaired person is not enhanced if the person's pension or health coverage comes from a funding category for the "totally and permanently disabled" ... .

Very important in the application of SRV is that people will accord roles to others on the basis of what information they *believe* they possess about them and consider to be relevant ... in other words, on the basis of whatever messages have been conveyed via the various role and image communicators. ...

The relationship between social images and competency within a Social Role Valorization framework

Although both competencies and images will affect people's roles, we also need to appreciate that a complicated feedback loop exists ... among competencies, images, expectancies, roles, and opportunities, and that this feedback loop can work to the benefit or the disadvantage of a party – perhaps decisively so, because the feedback effects are very powerful. On the one hand, if some party possesses a positive image, this almost always motivates others to either accord that party positive roles, or at least to afford that party greater opportunities to move into more valued roles and/or to acquire competencies needed to fill valued roles. ... In turn, the acquisition and possession of most competencies tends to enhance a party's image in the eyes of others. ...

On the other hand, if a party has a negative image, then others are not likely to afford to that party the opportunity to gain competencies, or even to exercise the competencies already possessed. For instance, if an individual is imaged as an eternal child who will never grow up, other people are less likely to give that person the chance to show that he or she can in fact grow and mature, or has grown and matured. ... Even if a party is attributed with competencies that it does not really possess, the party may still benefit from this feedback loop, in that its image is apt to be enhanced – in the same way that a party assumed not to possess certain competencies that it does in fact possess can suffer image harm and denial of opportunities.

A practical step-wise regimen for applying Social Role-Valorizing measures to a specific party

When one is ready to apply SRV to a specific party... then one can vastly increase one's chances for success by adhering to a six-step regimen sketched below.

Step 1. Becoming familiar with a party's wounds

If one is dealing with a party that has been wounded because of its devalued status, then it is absolutely necessary to deeply familiarize oneself with those wounds.

Step 2. Knowing a party's risk factors

In addition, one needs to know in what respects a party is vulnerable (i.e., what the areas of high risk are for that party). For instance, elderly persons are at higher risk of developing health problems, elderly women specifically are at risk of breaking bones ... . Mentally retarded persons are at risk of being taken advantage of by people who are smarter and unscrupulous, and of being expected to fail at tasks that require learning or competency ... . Among the mentally retarded, two risk points have recently become more common. One is with retarded children who are doing well in an integrated schooling situation but who may drop back into much less favourable circumstances when they "age out" of school. Another is with many mentally retarded adults who enjoyed 10 or 20 years of reasonably good living and working situations, but whose circumstances can rapidly deteriorate already in their mid-years. Altogether, failure to take risk factors into account often has devastating consequences.

Step 3. Inventorizing a party's current roles

One makes an inventory of both the positive, the negative, and the in-between, ambivalent, or mixed roles that the party currently holds.

Step 4. Explicating a party's current societal standing

In part with the help of the above inventories, one forms an overall idea of the party's current social standing and value in the eyes of society. Is the party highly valued, of average standing, marginally on the positive or negative side of neutral, deeply devalued, of equivocal value standing, or what? The previously mentioned risk analysis will be very informative here, because it is conceivable that a party – even if currently valued – may have a higher-than-average risk of a particular kind and may need more than ordinary safeguards in that risk area against role-degradation and loss of social value.

Step 5. Reviewing certain practical realities about image versus competency measures

Four overall considerations about roles, images, and competency will be helpful as one applies SRV.

(a) One needs to form a judgment as to whether – in the case of a particular party – the enhancement of competency or of imagery would be more likely to be effective. For instance, a competent person released from prison can be expected to benefit most from image enhancement, while for a person who recently lost competencies due to an accident, restoration of the lost competencies may have primacy. The image problems of mentally retarded persons are usually secondary to their competency deficits, which may have certain action implications.

(b)   At the same time, one also needs to form a judgment about whether the most desirable measure is also reasonably feasible. For instance, with severely mentally impaired persons, competency enhancement may be the theoretically most effective measure, but image enhancement may be the only thing that may be practical to accomplish. Also, in many people's cases, image enhancement is the first and easiest thing one can do, whereas competency enhancement may be a long and drawn-out process. In contrast, children tend to absorb age-appropriate competencies like a sponge, so competency enhancement may be highly feasible with them.

In regard to both (a) and (b), the fact is that the less accessible any competency-related roles are, the more important become attributed or ascribed roles, and often specifically relationship-based ones.

(c)   The more that a party who is already in devalued roles, or who is at significant risk of role-degradation, is seen by others (i) in places frequented by valued people in society, *and* (ii) in actual association with valued people, *and* (iii) in activities that are valued, the more are role-valorization benefits apt to accrue to that devalued party, often first in the image domain and sometimes also, and derivatively, in the competency domain. This is especially apt to be true if the valued people who associate with the persons at issue do so without being coerced, or feeling resentful about it. In contrast, if even one of these three positive elements is missing, then people's image certainly, and sometimes their competency as well, are apt to suffer. ...

(d)   It is very important that in efforts to enhance the image of a devalued person, one does not become deceptive. If one projects onto a person images of competency or positive roles that the person does not possess, this could have devastating consequences: (i) observers may expect something that the person cannot do, which in turn could endanger the person, could confirm such a person's failure expectancies, and/or could confirm observers' negative stereotypes about such persons, and (ii) the parties who conveyed the false messages may lose all credibility.

Step 6. Identifying the currently held, or desired, roles that one wants to valorize or change to a party's advantage (i.e., the role goals)

Leaning again on the earlier inventories, it is now time to begin to select one's role goals, and there are up to six types to select from. However, at least the first four of the five steps reviewed earlier must be taken before one is in a good position to decide which of these goals to pursue. The fifth of the above steps (with its four considerations) can be incorporated into the design of any of the role goals that follow.

VALORIZING THE POSITIVE ROLES A PARTY ALREADY HOLDS

If the previously established inventory has identified any positive roles a party already holds, then one relevant measure is to explore what can be done to further valorize one or more of these roles. This is particularly important if the party at issue does not hold many valued roles or also holds some devalued ones. There are two distinct subgoals here.

(a) The first one is to enhance – perhaps by enlargement – one or all of the valued roles already held. An example of an image measure would be to upgrade the title of a person's valued role. An example of a competency measure would be to help a person to acquire new skills so that he or she can perform additional valued functions within one or more valued roles already held. ...

(b) The second sub-goal is to defend the valued roles already held against losses, diminishment, or degradations. This is particularly important when a party is at distinct risk of losing one or more of its valued roles, for example when an individual's job is in jeopardy or a person acquires a chronic bodily affliction or becomes elderly. There are often things that can be done to prevent, delay, or reduce such role losses. It is important to practice high consciousness of these risks, how they commonly lead to wounds, and to counter them as early and vigorously as possible. ... Sometimes, the preservation of even a single valued role can be life-deciding to a person ... [see Chapter 6 – Ed.].

AVERTING ENTRY INTO (ADDITIONAL) DEVALUED ROLES

Regardless of whatever valued roles they may hold and be able to maintain, some people are at high risk of entering, or being cast into, new roles that are devalued, perhaps even in addition to whatever devalued roles they already hold. It is usually much easier to prevent such entry than to reverse it. High consciousness is of crucial importance here, particularly about which devalued roles a party is at risk of being thrust into. Thus, the previous inventory of risk factors once more becomes very helpful. For instance, impaired persons are often at risk of entering the sick role or chronic patient role. Such roles might be staved off by such competency-supporting measures as good health regimens, proper diet and exercise, and being cautious about taking recourse to certain health and mental services that are apt to ensnare a person into long-term patienthood. ...

ENABLING EITHER ENTRY INTO POSITIVELY VALUED NEW ROLES OR THE
REGAINING OF VALUED ROLES PREVIOUSLY HELD

Often, it is possible to enable people to enter new roles that are valued (role acquisition) or to regain valued roles they had once held but have since lost (role recovery), Such a valued role may be an addition to one or more valued roles already held, or it may be a replacement for one or more valued roles already lost or about to be lost. However, for some people, it could be the first or even only valued role! ...

Many actions in this category will involve both image- and competency-enhancement, such as enabling a child to take on the valued role of student, an adult to enter the role of worker or employee, or someone to enter the role of church choir member. ...

Sometimes, a person can recapture a valued role once held but then lost. ... Very relevant to many retarded people is that valued family roles may have been lost, perhaps because of discontinuities in family contacts or break-up of the family, institutionalization, or imprisonment. But it is often possible to restore a person's family ties and roles, so that the person becomes once again a valued brother or sister, aunt or uncle, grandparent or grandchild ... .

In regard to this role goal, and the first one of valorizing the positive roles already held, it is not always possible to craft what I had called a "big" positive role for devalued people, or it may take a long time to do so. Generally, it is much easier to craft small positive roles, and it may even be possible to craft several of them in relatively short order.

EXTRICATING A PARTY FROM CURRENTLY HELD DEVALUED ROLES

There are all sorts of things that can be done to help people to escape whatever devalued roles they are in. Actually, this is a function that is explicitly claimed (though rarely in role theory terms) by many human services ... . For instance, where an impaired adult is caught in an eternal child role, one might be able to help that person to escape that role by engaging in adult activities, developing adult interests and hobbies, etc. ...

REDUCING THE NEGATIVITY OF A DEVALUED ROLE CURRENTLY HELD

Most people occupy some – usually small – negative roles at least at some time during their lives, even if these negative roles are overshadowed by the positive ones they hold. For instance, we are all lawbreakers at various times, or dawdlers, or in a sick role ... . Unfortunately, devalued people often have not only mainly negative roles, but these may also dominate their lives. So aside from whatever other role goals might be pursued, the negativeness of one or all of a party's negative roles might also be reduced. This is not as good as fully extricating a person from a devalued role, but it is an improvement. Indeed, in a great many instances, a party is so deeply embedded in major negative roles that the best that one may be able to do is to take some of the negativeness out of one or some of them. ...

There are innumerable instances in which the acquisition of a new competency can diminish the negativity of one's devalued role. For instance, the more a person with a major medical condition, and clearly in the role of a sick patient, can learn to self-administer the required treatment and to take care of his or her condition, the less dominant will the sick role be in the minds of observers.

EXCHANGING CURRENTLY HELD DEVALUED ROLES FOR LESS DEVALUED
NEW ONES

Different from upgrading a devalued role is to enable a party to exchange one devalued role against a new one that is less devalued. For instance, a retarded person who is presently seen in the very negative role of a menace, an animal, or otherwise as nonhuman, would be vastly less endangered by being seen in the less negative role of an eternal child. ... In regard to this strategy, and the previous one of enabling entry into new valued roles, it is very important to note that there are innumerable valued work roles for adults that are not paid, but, nonetheless, status-improvement and other benefits can be achieved through them. Of course, one should not aim to exchange one devalued role for a less devalued one if one can do even better and escape the devalued role altogether, or exchange it for a valued one.

Pointers about the pursuit of any of the role goals

One can now say some more things about the pursuit of any and all of the aforementioned role goals, and the respective means for pursuing them.

1   One will often want to pursue several of the role goals at once.
2   Holding one valued role often leads to others, a small valued role can some-times serve as a springboard to a bigger or larger one, and relational roles often serve as mediators to other (including competency-exercising) ones.
3   However, one trap to avoid is trying to inflate small positive roles already held into grotesque proportions, perhaps also at the expense of enabling entry into new positive roles. For instance, a small positive role (such as storyteller) that the person has been holding may get enlarged beyond its normative prominence, so that the person becomes obnoxious to others or an object of ridicule by telling stories all the time. ...
4   Selecting the most role-valorizing measure can be very tricky when either different SRV goals or means compete with each other, or an SRV goal based on a certain value competes with another goal that has its rationale in other values. In fact, it is not uncommon for an image goal to compete with a competency goal, as when a competency-enhancing prosthetic device detracts from a person's positive image. Although there are principles for resolving such conflicts, these situations can be complicated and can scramble people's minds. A very common example of a clash of goals (and possibly values) occurs when a measure that would role-valorize a party within that party's larger society would not do so within that party's racial, ethnic, or religious subculture, or vice versa. This can be particularly wrenching when a person

wants to belong to one (sub)culture but then would have to be and do certain
things that draw devaluation and wounding from the other.

5   In regard to most of the above strategies, it is crucially important that the
positive roles that a person holds are made known, or better known, to others.
After all, the benefits of SRV depend first on how other people perceive a
party, and derivatively, based on these perceptions, what they decide to do to
and for that party. If they do not know the valued roles a person holds, then
they may not accord certain positive things to the person.

6   Similarly, it can be of decisive importance that observers *perceive* a party's
valued *activities* or *functions* in terms of very clearly established, identifiable
and positive social role identities and concepts. Otherwise, the perceivers
may not respond in a way that brings benefits to the party at issue. And in
order for other people to thusly perceive, they may first have to have such
activities translated to them into valued role terms. For instance, people will
be much less impressed when they are told that an impaired person grows
flowers (which is phrased in terms of an activity) than if they are told that
that person is a rose-gardener, a member of a gardening club, and a flower-
seller to a local market – all things that are roles. Of course, in the translation
process, one needs to keep in mind the earlier caveat about not being deceptive.

The potential contribution of different parties to the role-valorization of devalued people at various levels of social organization

I have said very little about who might do the work of role-valorization, but the
fact is that almost all involved parties can do some of it: devalued people themselves,
their families, other personal associates, advocates and allies, servers, service
agencies, government, the media, etc. Where the intended beneficiaries are not in
a good position to act effectively on their own behalf (usually because of impaired
competency or reduced standing), then actions on their behalf by others become
especially important. Also, different parties may be particularly well-situated to
take actions relevant to either imagery or competency and/or on one or more of
four distinct levels of social organization: that of the individual person, the levels
of primary and intermediate social systems, and the societal level overall, as charted
out in Wolfensberger (1998) [and also, in terms of normalization, in extract
7 – Ed.].

In the pursuit of even a very specific image or competency enhancement, one
may be able to do things on several or all levels of social organization, and even
without requiring any changes from the intended beneficiary – a fact that many
people fail to understand. For example, adding raised letters and numbers, or Braille
signs, to the control panel in an elevator enables blind people who can already
read Braille to be more competent using the elevator and getting about. ...

In this brief presentation, relatively little has been said about the vast number
of measures one could pursue on higher systemic levels, especially the societal
one. However, two things should be clear. (a) There is a strong feedback loop

between changes in or by individuals, groups, and classes and changes in and by society. (b) Efforts to change larger social systems may have more pay-off but could take a very long time – and could fail, whereas one has vastly better prospects at early success on the scale of individuals, groups, specific agencies, etc. Also, if societal change is one's goal, one should use appropriate, and multiple, social change strategies, only some of which are SRV measures. ...

Conclusion

Role theory can be an extremely powerful tool for analyzing and explaining what happens to impaired and/or devalued people and for crafting action measures to protect them from all sorts of bad things being done to them. Surprisingly, role theory and its findings had only been moderately exploited to this purpose prior to the advent of SRV.

There is much controversy about the valuation of roles, of persons or people, and of the religious or philosophical construct of personhood. However, one thing is patently obvious. Being in roles valued by a perceiver makes it more likely that this perceiver will do good rather than bad things to and for one. Thus, all that has been covered boils down to putting good things – or at least, less bad things – about some person, group, or class into the minds of those others who are in a position to do good (or less bad) things to them. If people have and hold good things in their minds about others, they are more likely to do good things to them, just as if they hold bad things in their minds about and towards others, they are likely to do bad things to them. Relatedly, one could view SRV as a way of helping people to do what they really should want to do, and as a way of working toward a society in which (in the words of the French personalist Peter Maurin, 1997) it is easier for people to be good. The widespread practice of SRV would accomplish this by making it easier for people to value others, or to at least devalue them less.

However, one could take away some wrong ideas from this extremely short presentation. For instance, although SRV is a rather high-level conceptual scheme, and a parsimonious one at that (in being able to point to a vast number of actions on all levels of social organization and to incorporate the theorizing and findings of many other empirical theories), it has its limitations as do all schemata. These are not detailed in this short article, but no one should be surprised that SRV will not prevent wars, defeat disease, eliminate poverty, correct all invalid stereotypes, heal all wounds, or even eliminate mental retardation or make it a valued condition.

Finally, I want to emphasize again that even though SRV is the practical applica-tion of the knowledge of social science, such an application must be guided by values, and therefore some form of de facto religion. Social Role Valorization mines a wide range of sociology and psychology, it explains an entire range of phenomena around social valuation and devaluation, it predicts what will happen to people when they are subject to certain valuing or devaluing conditions, and it offers guidance as to what one might be able to do about any of this if one so chooses. But whom one decides to value or devalue, and for whom one decides to seek more positive roles, valuation, and life experiences in society, and how far one wants to pursue this – these are all de facto religious decisions, not scientific ones, as explained in more detail in Wolfensberger (1995).

The last reference in the extract above, referring to 'de facto religious decisions' brings out issues which have figured prominently in various critiques of SRV (though still, sometimes, largely in the UK under the name of normalization). These are issues which also concerned normalization, of course, but as Wolfensberger has attempted to refine SRV into a social science theory, identifying its links with empiricism and its predictive power, rather than its political 'stance', such critiques have largely failed to distinguish the two, or acknowledge the development of SRV. In attempting to clarify these issues, at least from the perspective of SRV, Wolfensberger has written a number of papers, four of which are extracted here.

---

12   From: 'An "if this, then that" formulation of decisions related to Social Role Valorization as a better way of interpreting it to people', 1995, *Mental Retardation*, 33(3), 163–9.

This extract proposes a way of using SRV as a guide to decision-making, and the distinction between the likely outcomes of actions, which SRV can predict prob-abilistically, and the desirability of actions, which needs to be clearly articulated as a values decision.

...

SRV is in the class of overarching meta-theories that are empirical in nature. ... As an empirical theory, it states a certain number of what appear to be facts (e.g., about how human beings relate to each other and behave). It then makes assertions about how various presumed acts are ... related to each other. This means that SRV theory makes assertions about what can be expected to happen *if* a certain course of action is, or is not, pursued. It *then* presents people with one or more action decisions ..., based on their view of what is needed for and by the party at issue. ...

Somewhat simplified, these relations based on social laws of how humans individually and collectively behave can be stated as "if this, then that" formulations ..., elaborated below. ...

1. If X is done, then one must expect that Y will occur

For instance, *if* one relentlessly says bad ... things about Group A to Group B, *then* many members of Group B can be ... expected to end ... up believing what is said, to think badly of Group A, and to do bad things to Group A as a result. ... Or, *if* one ... engages handicapped adults in childish activities and routines, *then* they will be probably viewed ... as overgrown or eternal children, and be denied appropriate developmental challenges or adult roles. ...

2. If Y has occurred, then it is quite likely that X has been done earlier

For instance, *if* Group B has done dirt to Group A, *then* ... many people in Group B had a lot of bad things conveyed to them ... about Group A. Thus, to continue a previous example, *if* certain people view and treat handicapped adults as eternal children, *then* such handicapped adults had probably been interpreted as big children, observed in childish activities and routines, perhaps been clothed and groomed as children, or been heard addressed as children.

3. If one wants Y to occur, then one will have ... to do X

For instance, ... *if* one wants Group B to do good things to Group A, *then* one will ... have to communicate a lot of good things about Group A to Group B. ... *If* one wants handicapped adults to be seen and treated as adults, then ... one must ... engage them in adult activities and routines, ... to the maximum degree possible.

4. If one concludes that doing X is too costly, ... then one may have to modify, or even sacrifice, one's goal Y

Thus, *if* one is unwilling to say a lot of good things about Group A to Group B in order to get Group B to do good things to Group A, *then* one has to accept ... that Group B probably will not do good things to Group A. ... *If* it is judged to be too demanding or difficult to arrange a handicapped adult's life so that the person is engaged in adult routines and activities, and is addressed and presented as an adult, or *if* it is judged that doing so is too cruel to an adult who has been used to a childish world and likes it, *then* one has to accept that at least some other people are not going to see and treat this adult as an adult, but will instead perceive and treat this adult as a child. ...

Some additional examples may also help illustrate this fourth formulation. Suppose an agency's name and logo convey negative ... messages about the service and the people served. The name and logo could be changed to be more positive, but this might require ... a great deal of time and effort by a lot of people, and would mean that the agency would have to re-establish a public name and visibility. Agency personnel might ... decide that changing the name and logo is not worth these efforts and costs – but *if* so, they should *then* accept the image loss to clients (and ... other people similar to the clients) that is apt to come with maintaining the current name and logo.

Or suppose a person has a very... visible facial malformation that elicits ... rejection and distantiation. *If* many more people are to be more accepting of that person, *then* the malformation will have to be addressed, perhaps by cosmetic means ... or even surgery. ... Suppose the ... person is not willing to undergo it (surgery). ... Then that person ... must be prepared for the rejection that will almost certainly come. Such rejection cannot be talked and exhorted away. ...

I believe that interpreting SRV as an "if this, then that" set of propositions is a better and more accurate way of teaching the theory than to present it to the effect that SRV "dictates" that something must be done. The "if this, then that" formulation ... presents ... an audience with the types of decisions they have to make, namely, determining what they would or would not like to see happen to or for devalued people, ... and then deciding whether that which is required ... to achieve or avert these outcomes can be done, whether they are prepared to do it, or whether they will do something else on the basis of competing theories, higher values, etc. ...

---

13   From: 'Social Role Valorization is too conservative. No, it is too radical', 1995, *Disability and Society*, 10(3), 245–7.

The next explanatory extract takes up the issue of whether SRV is inherently conservative, as some critics have alleged, or whether by exposing the nature of devaluation, it draws forth the possibility of radical action. As before, however, the political beliefs or values of the actors are highlighted by SRV, not dictated by it. It comes from a UK-based journal, and one which had published a number of the criticisms discussed below.

A common criticism of Wolfensberger's formulation of normalization ... and Social Role Valorization (SRV) ... is that it endorses contemporary social values and socio-political power arrangements that oppress all sorts of people. Of course, this criticism comes from the left. Yet it is amusing that at the same time, normalization/SRV are criticized by the right as radical, subversive, and a foil for left-wing ideas. Who is correct?

Both – and neither, as I will now explain.

As regards the criticism that SRV just upholds and perpetuates the status quo, and is therefore conservative: on the one hand, normalization – and SRV perhaps even yet more clearly – have made the point that if one wants good things to happen to people already devalued, then one should not put them into yet additional value jeopardy. Among other things, this means that one should try to associate to devalued people those things that are currently highly valued in the larger society, so that the devalued people will come to be associated with things that society holds dear, aspires to, values deeply. It is this capitalization upon existing values, and particularly the so-called 'conservatism corollary' of SRV, that critics from the left single out. The very name of the conservatism corollary is also – so to speak – a red flag to them. (The conservatism corollary, explained further in Wolfensberger (1992), says that if one wishes to prevent, reduce, or compensate for devaluation and wounding, then one should enable devalued people to have, be, or be associated with those things (including people) that are at the highly valued end of a societal value continuum, rather than those which are 'merely' ordinary, typical, tolerated, or even marginal.)

As regards the criticism that normalization/SRV is radical and subversive: from the first, normalization has emphasized the importance of working to change those values of society which push certain parties into devalued identity, and keep them there (e.g. Wolfensberger, 1970a, b, 1972). What the right does not like about normalization/SRV is its implicit or explicit accusation that prevailing cultural values and arrangements are oppressive of certain classes, and that unless at least some of these values are changed, large numbers of people will be made and/or kept devalued (often for no fault of their own), and in most cases also oppressed. The right is first of all embarrassed that SRV shows its values and structures to cause and maintain devaluation; and secondly, it does not like the idea of making structural changes in society. Yet further, the right has never been particularly sympathetic to the lowly or weak, and especially not people whom it perceives as having brought their troubles on themselves; and to the degree that any devalued groups are so perceived, then to that degree the right resents the idea that society should do good things to and for them, especially if these things are costly and demanding.

The critique of SRV from the left has been (a) vastly more explicit than that from the right, and (b) vastly more visible, including in this journal. One reason is that so many people in human services, and especially in academic roles related to human services, lean to the left. ... The critique from the right has been less explicit: it really did not have to be, since the right's identity in many countries has been so heavily and 'successfully' bound up with prevailing structures, law, funding and service control, and that in many instances even when more left-leaning governments were in control.

After all, since the late Middle Ages, the bulk of human services has been allied with the powers and authorities in society, and has therefore participated in, and perpetuated, societal devaluation. With the exception of Scandinavian societies in recent years, human services have not embraced normalization/SRV, notwithstanding shrill cries ... that services have sold out wholesale to normalization/SRV.

That services have really not embraced normalization/SRV is strikingly clear from the relentless evidence of thousands of service evaluations since 1969, with first the PASS tool (Wolfensberger & Glenn, 1973, 1975) and then the PASSING tool (Wolfensberger & Thomas, 1983, 1989), which have rarely found services that were of high quality. (See the research conducted by Flynn, 1975, 1980, 1994; Flynn, La Pointe, Wolfensberger & Thomas, 1991; on British services specifically, see Williams, 1987).

Normalization and SRV theory have always been clear (though sometimes those who have taught and promoted these have not) that they emphasize *both* capitalizing upon cultural values, *and* the need to change at least some of them; therefore, any *unnuanced* criticisms that normalization/SRV are allied to the status quo, or that they are subversive of it, are both faulty. But critics from both camps would do well to take note of the greatly clarifying 'if this, then that' way of formulating

SRV issues that evolved between 1992 and 1994 (Wolfensberger, 1992, 1995 [see previous extract – Ed.]).This formulation brings out clearly that it is those values one holds, or decides to bring to bear, that are above the level of at least the social science theory of SRV, that will … tell one whether certain people ought to be valued or devalued and why, whether all human beings are equal in value or not, and whether treating anyone badly (which almost always happens when devaluation is present) is justifiable, and under what circumstances.

… One's values will determine whether one believes that in regard to any devalued group, only society should have to make any changes or accommodations, but not the devalued party or those who may have control over the lives of the devalued party. It is also one's values that tell one in which direction societal values should be changed, if one believes they should be; i.e. whether to be more or less tolerant than they are, whether to be more 'inclusive' or more 'exclusive', etc.

… One's values may tell one the opposite …, namely, that society is fine the way it is, and therefore the only parties that need to change are the devalued people and those around them, their allies, and perhaps services to them, by accommodating themselves to society – as, for instance, by bringing themselves more into alignment with what society values positively – and not the other way around.

… An additional question to resolve is to what degree human services do or do not reflect societal values and policies. For instance, some people may believe that because human services serve upon the very people that society most disdains and rejects, such services therefore are opposed to societal devaluations, and instead highly value those devalued people who are their clients. Other people may believe that services – being structured, sanctioned, and largely funded by society – are a means of enacting societal policies of devaluation and oppression, though perhaps under the guise of benevolence, care, and beneficence. To what degree services are, in fact, a reflection of societal values and policies should be an empirical question, but will probably be judged in light of one's values, and therefore, the conclusion is not apt to be purely empirical. However one resolves the question, it will determine to what degree one thinks that human services should accommodate themselves to society and its values, or should be structured in contradiction to these.

… SRV as a social science theory can tell one a great deal as to which measure is apt to bring about which outcome, such as what is likely to result in greater valuation of a person or group, and what is likely to result in greater devaluation. Thus, in this sense, SRV can inform one what 'works' But it is only one's values that may inform one that even something that 'works' should not be used, e.g., because it is immoral or wrong, or because it is not good for some affected party or actor, such as the implementer.

Similarly, one's values may inform one that doing other things are more important than that certain people gain societal valuation and acceptance, and that one should therefore put one's energies into those other things that are deemed more important.

14   From: 'Social Role Valorization and, or versus, "Empowerment"', 2002, *Mental Retardation*, 40(3), 252–8.

This next extract expands still further on the notion of SRV and values positions, by its address of the relationship between SRV and a philosophy which today dominates much discourse in human service academic circles (though, as Wolfensberger notes above in relation to claims for SRV dominance, its effect in practice is far more problematic). This is the discourse on rights and self-determination of oppressed groups. This has so taken up the academic 'airwaves' in the UK as to be considered the 'accepted wisdom', certainly at the expense of SRV (Race, 2002b). In other countries the picture is more mixed; although the dominance of the self-determination culture still exists, especially in disability circles, there appears to still be a place for SRV where normalization existed before, with some countries managing to find some common ground. This extract is the most recent of Wolfensberger's writings appearing in this book.

One socio-political ideology that in the last two decades or so has been on the rise in the service and advocacy culture is that of conveying to bodily or functionally impaired people, and to members of other societally devalued classes, power (as expressed in "empowerment" language), self-determination, and choice (as in "freedom of choice" language), even to the point of unbridled license to do whatever they want. Sometimes, this strategy is specifically alleged to be a superior or preferable alternative to Social Role Valorization (e.g., Branson & Miller, 1992; Chappell, 1992; Perrin & Nirje, 1985). Some people have also claimed (e.g., Nirje, 1992; Perrin & Nirje, 1985) that the original formulation of the normalization principle had been all about rights and empowerment, and that this emphasis has been ignored, left out, or overridden by later formulations of the principle by Wolfensberger..., and possibly by others, and by its reconceptualization as Social Role Valorization ... [see earlier in this and the previous chapter – Ed.], all of which these critics consider faulty. However, such claims constitute a historical revisionism, because early formulations of normalization (e.g., Nirje, 1969; Wolfensberger, 1972) were only partially concerned with rights, and although the power idiom and thinking began to infiltrate from the political arena into the human service and advocacy culture in the 1970s, it did not become commonplace there until the late 1980s.

Once the empowerment construct and idiom became popular, it was applied not only to traditional ways of discoursing about power, but to almost anything. Perceiving the appeal of a power construct and idiom, people began to incorporate it indiscriminately and almost everywhere, and issues that once would have been framed in very different terms began to be widely framed as issues of power. Even issues of competence are now commonly framed this way.

Then follows a voluminous list , which Wolfensberger claims is itself only a selection, of issues being taught or interpreted as empowerment, of which space permits only a couple of the more bizarre – 'searching for the historical Jesus' and 'practising polygamy.' After this list, Wolfensberger concludes:

...

Obviously, a term or construct that can mean anything eventually will mean nothing.

Confronted with the vast popularity of the self-determination and power ideology in recent years, some parties sympathetic to Social Role Valorization (SRV) have claimed, implied, or assumed that SRV is congruent with this ideology, and perhaps even that "empowerment" and self-determination are or should be the ultimate goal of SRV. However, even if one discounts most of the shallow and silly interpretations of empowerment, and conceptualizes power in more conventional ways, there are a number of important differences between SRV and ideologies of empowerment that will now be explained.

Some important differences between Social Role Valorization and the ideology of empowerment

Coercive vs. persuasive change strategies

The empowerment ideology relies a great deal on coercion, and/or a conflict model. One gives people powers to compel other people to do something, or not to do something. In contrast, SRV relies largely on educational and persuasive strategies that change people's mind content about certain classes of other people by changing their perceptions, expectations, and attitudes.

Ideology or religion vs. empiricism

One thing that all the ideologies of power, autonomy and choice have in common is that they are based on *de facto* religion (i.e., on ideas of what "should" be), rather than on science which – at best – can describe what is and predict what will be.

Because people's minds tend to get scrambled the moment they hear the word *religion*, it is very important to understand what I do and do not mean by it. I mean the term to be understood the way many philosophers of science and epistemologists do, namely, as *any* supra-empirical or extra-empirical belief or belief system, or worldview. Accordingly, capitalism, communism, fascism, democracy, the hope that science or technology will save the world, and thousands of other beliefs are religions, *including* belief systems that have been formally defined as religions, such as Judaism, Christianity, Islam, Buddhism, ancestor worship, voodoo, and so on. In fact, epistemologists have made the convincing point that even atheism is a religion, as much as theism or deism, because it too is based on an assertion that can never be empirically disproven by appeal to the laws of nature. Insofar as every person capable of some thought holds to beliefs that are not empirically falsifiable, each such person has a religion – in fact, many people incoherently have several religions. ...

While in the above sense then, ideologies of autonomy, empowerment, and self-determination are de facto religions, SRV is an empiricism-based body of theory (actually, an amalgam of multiple theories) that can describe, explain and predict phenomena, but that does not prescribe, even though SRV was created with the hope that it would be used as a basis for role-valorizing actions. For instance, like all moral "shoulds," statements as to how much power *anyone* should have, or which rights should be given to or withheld from which people, must come from the supra-empirical level, and thus from above SRV. However, SRV can only inform us – actually or potentially – on an empirical basis how the restricting or according of power, autonomy and rights is likely to impact on people's social image, their competence, their roles, and how others will perceive them and relate to them. The reason this kind of information is crucially important to SRV implementation is that, as I explained in this journal (Wolfensberger, 2000 [see extract 11 – Ed.]) within the SRV framework, imagery and competency are seen as the two major strategies for attaining valued social roles, and SRV posits that people in valued social roles are apt to be accorded the good things in life, while people in societally devalued roles are apt to get mistreated. Since these assertions by SRV are within the realm of empirical falsifiability, they are in the domain of science.

Both Nirje's (1969) and Wolfensberger's (1972) formulations of normalization did promote *normative* autonomy and rights for people, but this is no longer true of SRV. The reason is that while normalization was a mixture of ideology and empirical social science, SRV aspires to base its claims entirely on empiricism and on social science – though at a high and overarching level – that inform one what will happen to people if one does this or that, what will happen if one does not, and what may have happened in the first place to bring about certain situations that one may want to change (Wolfensberger, 1995, 1998, 2000).

Also, since SRV aspires to be no more than an action scheme based on social science, it cannot inform people whether they should or should not value all, some, or no humans, but it can give very powerful rules as to what one would have to do *if* one wanted people to occupy roles that are valued by others (Wolfensberger, 1995). Also, SRV posits that people will be vastly more likely to become valued as persons by those others who perceive them to occupy valued social roles. Note however that while SRV can speak of valuing people or humans, it cannot speak of valuing persons if by "persons" is meant anything other than human beings. The reason this bears saying is that "persons" have traditionally been defined in philosophical, ethical, legal or programmatic terms that are derived from de facto (even if not explicated) religious (i.e., supra-empirical) beliefs, and often coincided with definitions of *humanhood*. More recent definitions of *personhood* ... are often no longer synonymous with traditional scientific definitions of humanhood.

Claims regarding how the good things of life are to be achieved

One of the big differences between SRV and the self-determination and power theories, strategies, or paradigms really boils down to how any of these would answer the following question: are people more likely to get the good things of life by occupying social roles that are valued by others (which presumably will also be translated into more general social valuation), or by the exercise of power, autonomy and self-determination in and over their lives, and of power over, or *vis-à-vis*, other people? SRV proposes the former, the empowerment ideology seems to propose the latter. The power ideology appears to claim that having or not having power not only determines how one will be treated, but also whether one will get the good things of life. But the SRV literature and its oral teaching culture propose that in the end, what ultimately determines how a person or group will be treated, and what others will afford to such a party in life, is what is in the minds of those who do the treating and affording, and most specifically, whether and to what degree they perceive the party in valued social roles. Usually, the "they" consists of the majority of society; sometimes, "they" may be only its ruling minority, or the members of a societal subculture of close relevance to the party at issue.

For its position, SRV can cite much evidence that people will be granted by others the good things of life to the degree that (a) they occupy valued roles and/ or are more generally valued, and (b) those others have it in *their* power to grant the good things at issue. In regard to the latter, we should note that human collectivities sometimes are in such extreme straits that they have little to offer to even their most valued members other than positive regard. But putting aside such extreme situations for the moment, both history and knowledge of human nature inform us that people can be – and often have been – valued, protected, and freely afforded a good life even though they are/were totally powerless, especially in the material sense in which the empowerment cultus usually employs the term *power* (e.g., Brown & Smith, 1989; Chappell, 1992; Branson & Miller, 1992). Conversely, people who have a great deal of power to do and get what they want are not necessarily highly valued, even many of their roles that carry power may not be valued, and they may not be *freely* accorded all sorts of good things by *many other people*, even though there may be certain good things that powerful persons may be able to procure for themselves, or wrest away from others by means of power, though usually only if they are quite competent people. Under extreme conditions especially, this wresting can be of a Nietzschean nature, where raw power is exercised by the stronger over the weaker in disregard of any legal or moral law, as we have seen in recent civil and international wars – and there are always stronger and weaker parties. No religious, social, psychological, political, or economic cultus has ever succeeded in equalizing power between stronger and weaker parties, only in reshuffling who is stronger versus who is weaker. Any claims that some scheme some day will achieve equalization is utopian, and if it were not, it would probably be maladaptive and undesirable.

Having power is definitely not the same as being either valued, or even accepted, by others. Nor is the accumulation of enough power to intimidate others always a particularly successful way to win positive valuation and acceptance from others. We can see this, for instance, when crime bosses and drug lords definitely do acquire and wield power, and thereby cow others into submission and win their obeisance through bribery or intimidation – but then are loved, admired, or valued by few people. Also, once their power is somehow lost, so will be most of the submission, obeisance, and "respect" they once had, and they will probably be valued by yet fewer people than they were before they acquired power. Crime bosses who wield much power may be devalued even by those who depend on them, and when they lose their power, they may not only be fallen upon, but there may be no one to stand by them.

We can further understand that power is not necessarily the way to positive valuation when we consider that many people with very little or no material power, or even no power whatsoever, can nonetheless be highly valued. For instance, many valued moral leaders (such as Gandhi) have held and exercised at least no material power; similarly, most newborns are highly valued by their families but possess zero power in any ordinary sense.

Yet another question, though a secondary one, is what happens when people are *de facto* reduced in power and autonomy, regardless of how much one might like them not to be? For instance, when a person is in a coma, otherwise very ill, or profoundly mentally retarded – what then? It seems impossible to deny that then, what happens to the person will depend almost entirely on how others around the person perceive him or her, and whether they value him or her positively and deeply.

Thus, one might say that although powerful people can wrest from others some of the good things of life for themselves by their exercise of power, their ability to do so will largely or entirely desert them as soon as they suffer an appreciable loss in that power – which may happen to them (or anybody) at any time. At that moment, their fate will be determined by other factors, and one of the biggest such factors is the degree to which others feel positive about them, and hold them in positive regard.

It is, of course, understandable that people – especially devalued ones – would deeply resent the fact that others are making value judgments about them, and that these judgments affect their social status and well-being in a negative way. Although this could be considered one of many sad facts of life – an expression of the imperfection of human nature – people imbued with modernistic values are no longer willing or able to see it this way, but believe that there is a brute-force solution to this problem, much as they believe that there is to virtually any problem. To the degree that this belief is resistant to empirical evidence about the cosmos and human nature – as it commonly is – it is in the de facto religious realm, as noted earlier.

Differences in the relevance accorded to personal competency

The more a person is impaired in normative competencies (and particularly in normative mental competency), the less a person will be able to exercise normative autonomy and "self-determination," and the higher becomes the risk that attempts at such exercise will cause harm – possibly of major extent – to self, and usually also others. This is why in apparently all cultures in the past, and many still today, a person known to be competency-impaired usually either was/is not asked to perform certain functions and fill certain roles, or was/is even outright forbidden to do so. SRV acknowledges both the reality and the relevance of such competency impairments, emphasizes the importance of competency-enhancement, and predicts that to the degree that a party's competency impairments limit its ability to wisely make life decisions, and to understand and constructively deal with the good or bad consequences of those decisions, then to that degree things will go ill with that party *unless* other people with good sense, good judgment, wisdom, and positive feelings for the party are willing and permitted to make decisions for that party – again, to the degree the party is impaired in a particular competency at issue. This assertion is especially likely to be true if the other people will make the decisions in a way that is not unnecessarily image-degrading to the party. But, in its emphasis on granting people full "choice" and self-determination in all things, the power ideology trivializes, or even denies, the relevance or legitimacy of issues of competency in any such decisions.

Further, if the idea of "choice" and self-determination in all things were taken at full face value and to its extreme, it would de facto result in what has come to be called "dumping," i.e., in handicapped people not only being set into society free from all constraints or supervision, but also without the supports that they *do* need to live safely and decently. After all, many such persons (or people who claim to speak for them) say that this is what they want, and commonly these days, this is what they get. Again, SRV itself cannot tell us whether people *should* be thusly dumped, but it can inform us of what this entails in the lives of dumped people, and that this is largely bad things, and often even death. Yet these days, this course of action is widely defended, justified – or even applauded – by empowerment ideologues who interpret self-determination as the highest good in life, and who exalt an allegedly "empowered" state above all other issues of personal welfare.

In those instances where what a competency-impaired party wants or even demands is not in its best interests, then other parties on the scene that have a caring, or even responsible, relationship with the competency-impaired party can become very conflicted, especially so if what the person wants or demands has also been defined as a legal right. However, at least SRV does not place an obligation to accede to the impaired party's demands onto those who are in a position to make such decisions. This is because, as noted earlier, SRV can only inform people how valued social roles for people can be either procured and protected, or degraded and diminished, but does not dictate any value stance. Social Role Valorization informs us that where a measure would harm a person in competency or image, it is also extremely unlikely to lead to more valued roles for the person – if anything, such a measure apt to lead to the degradation or loss of valued roles. ...

Historically, cultures have always legitimized certain people to impose restrictions on certain others, and/or to see to it that impaired persons get what they need, even if it is not what such impaired persons say they want. However, SRV itself cannot generate dictates as to what constitutes legitimate authority for making such decisions for others, because the legitimization of such authority is ultimately based on societal values, and therefore on de facto religion. What SRV, or at least social science, can do is inform us of what happens when society does not legitimize the above authority functions. However, the empowerment ideology would reject any or most impositions or unasked-for intervention by others, and would even encourage and "egg on" competency-impaired people to demand whatever they want as their "right," regardless of what the consequences might be to them or others of either demanding such rights – or receiving them. In fact, such "egging on" is a major reality in the praxis of the contemporary empowerment cultus.

Another problem with the power ideology is that humans in general are very confused and inconsistent about what they want and how this relates to what they need, and they often say they want one thing when they really want or need another, or do not know what they want. Because this seems once again to be a part of human nature, or at least is an almost normative reality for humans, we live with it (and often die from it), but the problems this creates are vastly magnified when people are impaired in mental competency, and perhaps already deeply wounded. An aged person who changes his/her will every day for 30 days in a row – especially if the person's estate is appreciable – is extremely likely to be declared incompetent rather than to be accorded "choice" and self-determination.

Conclusion to these important differences

...

In regard to how a party's welfare and power are related, it is strange that one rarely hears three potentially relevant rationales spelled out as being very distinct: first, that power would be merely an instrumentality through which people would get the good things of life, rather than ... an empowered life being defined as the good life; second, that autonomy may not be the same as self-determination; and third, that either the autonomy or self-determination gained by empowerment would make the empowered people feel good and contented. Yet even the most casual observation of the lives of devalued people will reveal that these three alleged goals, benefits, or connections are neither at all the same, nor all true. For instance, people with great autonomy may have extremely few discretions available to them; and furthermore, all sorts of impaired people who have been dumped out of institutions into "independence" have gained autonomy, enjoy this autonomy greatly, defend it fiercely – but live miserably, often under material conditions vastly inferior to those they lived under in institutions.

Indeed, over and over, one gets the impression that the power ideology/lobby simply does not appear to recognize, or deal with, or even care, what happens to people who are already devalued by society when they do things that deeply offend the values and sensibilities of the valued (and usually powerful) sectors of society:

commonly, such perceived offenders *will* end up even more rejected, abused, violated, and brutalized than they are already, and perhaps even get made dead. They may even be given their autonomy and self-determination – but not any of the other good things in life. ... The fact is that so many people these days are obsessed with the self-determination of impaired or devalued people, but not equally obsessed – if at all – with their welfare, so that ... horror stories abound of how vulnerable people get egged on into situations in which they experience disaster, perhaps even are "made dead," [see Chapter 6 – Ed.] with the eggers-on nowhere in sight to either protect them – or share their fate.

One clash between SRV and an empowerment ideology becomes apparent even in the very language that names these schemes. Social Role Valorization is an overarching conceptual and action scheme that informs one how one may be able to enhance people's social roles if that is what one wants to do. ... But empowerment or self-determination schemes seek *only* power and autonomy. *Never* outside of Nietzschean thinking have I seen an analysis accompany demands for power and autonomy that has gone beyond an assertion that these things are a right, or should be a right. *Never* outside of Nietzschean thinking have I seen an analysis of what would happen if *everybody* were powerful and exercised all their power – or even only all their rights – all the time. ... Nor have I ever seen in any of the promotions in recent decades of religions of radical individualism, self-determination, empowerment, "choice," and rights in the context of deviancy/social devaluation, human impairment or human services, an analysis of any length or depth of how these alleged goods *should* be linked to things such as duties, mercy, forgiveness, forbearance, virtues of self-denial, etc., or even competency.

In fact, when the power ideologists these days speak of empowerment and self-determination, they often root these ideas in a construct of rights, but hardly ever spell out whether this is to be a legal rights construct, or a human rights construct that transcends human and governmental law; and in the latter case, which the transcendent rather than human rights are, and what the source of such rights is. Also complicating is the fact that (especially since the time of Nietzsche) some people have promoted a power construct that is not rooted in law of either kind, but in the individual will (as in "the will to power" of Nietzsche).

Altogether, and actually quite obviously, the vast majority of the recent discourse on empowerment is based on a mentality that rejects or ignores age-old teachings that there are deep problems with power, and that often, the challenge is to curb one's will to power rather than to grab more power .

Conclusion

The promotion of empowerment and total self-determination for impaired people comes at the worst possible time, namely, just as humanity is beginning to be beset by environmental catastrophe and the return of an age of plagues, and as both Western societies and the world order – such as it was – are collapsing (e.g., Wolfensberger, 1994; note also that the above was written *before* 11 September

2001). Human decency and so-called natural law (rather than SRV) inform us that impaired people need to have competent advocates at their side who, if the occasion requires it, are willing and able to make wise decisions on their behalf even if these do not always please a person of limited, disturbed, or diminished mentality.

Of course, it is quite possible that even when confronted with the above considerations, some people will nonetheless embrace a rather naked and unnuanced empowerment and self-determination position as a religion – in which case it is clear that what they want really *is* power, and *not* valuation and acceptance by and from others, or perhaps even from themselves. Thus, one would not be dealing with an empirical controversy over what does and does not work, but with a controversy at the level of fundamental values and religious beliefs. In a free society, people should have the right to pursue ("choose") – up to a point – conflicting goods, provided such people are mentally competent enough to have at least a modicum of understanding of the decision, and the cost to themselves, both now and in the future. But to demand that one single value and accompanying lifestyle should be thrust on others who do not share the same religion – let alone the competencies to live accordingly – is a form of religious dictatorship.

Further, to the extent that the disagreement is about religion rather than what works, there is a lot of deception on the part of the power lobby, in that it fails to reveal to people at risk in society what it is that *does* work even when power fails. Another truth that the power lobby is withholding from its audiences is that there have never been, and never will be, social systems of any longevity at all that are not stratified. Of course, one reason this truth is not revealed is that the power people either do not believe it despite the weight of historical evidence, or do not want ... to believe it. Very naively, they believe (or at least talk as if they believed) that what others consider to be human nature is only learned, and that one of the most self-evident and true universals of human history can be abolished – as long, of course, as *they* are on top with the power. ... So yet another generation of gullible or vulnerable people is being misled by an intellectual, ideological and professional elite, much as previous generations of such elites taught their versions of false religions. ...

---

15 From: 'Some of the universal "good things of life" which the implementation of Social Role Valorization can be expected to make more accessible to devalued people', 1996, SRV/VRS: The International Social Role Valorization Journal/La Revue Internationale de la Valorisation des Rôles Sociaux, 2(2), 12–14.

Given the controversies over what SRV does and does not 'say', and whether or not it takes a 'stance' (or should do), the final extract is an attempt to outline (in an article written with two colleagues, Susan Thomas and Guy Caruso) what Wolfensberger means by the 'good things of life', mentioned several times in the previous extracts. For all its place as a social science theory, and however much academic debate can take place about it, the roots of SRV in the ideological movement that was at the forefront of the implementation of normalization inevitably means that questions are asked about the *goals* of SRV. This paper answers those questions, and in doing so gives for many a reason to go beyond those academic debates and attempt to put SRV into practice.

Ironically, it is also a set of goals that are claimed to be behind many service agencies and service training courses, though as we have seen, a number of these have rejected SRV, whilst an increasing number of others are unaware of it. Readers from human services might like to examine the aims of their agencies and training courses, and reflect on the similarities and differences from those contained in this extract. We pick it up after the reminders by the authors of the previously discussed issues of values and decisions in SRV, and in particular the notion that SRV 'imposes' on people a lifestyle and circumstances that they would not choose. After referring to the *If this, then that* paper, the authors go on to consider what people would be likely to choose.

...

There is … a great deal that one can say on the contested issue of whether devalued people would choose the same "good things in life" as people in more privileged circumstances.

While there are certainly differences in what is valued by people in different cultures and subcultures, and at different points in history, there is also a tremendous amount of agreement or convergence among people as to what they desire. This convergence on what people consider the good things of life is also brought out by some of the work (e.g., Maslow, 1959) on universal needs that people share, such as for security, belongingness, and self-actualization. Too often these days, the differences between people are highlighted, and the similarities or shared universals are played down, ignored, or even denied. But when we look at human history broadly, we find that there has been much *de facto* consensus as to what constitutes "the good life." While some differences must be expected, due to such things as people's highest-order world views and religions, and specificities of culture and time, we still find that for the vast majority of human beings, the good life is intertwined with at least 17 things, some of which could actually be yet further broken down into separate points. The following is a list of those things, not necessarily in order of importance:

1   Family, or an equivalent small intimate group for those who have no family. Most of the latter would prefer a real family to a substitute intimate group.
2   For most people, a place they can call home. This is often where one has family, but not necessarily so.
3   Belonging to an intermediate but still relatively small-scale social body. In many societies, or for many people, families are too small – and sometimes

too far away – to provide the broader and yet intimate sense of belonging that is so important to the good life. Nations are too large and abstract. Somewhere closer to what humans need and desire are tribes or clans, small local communities ..., or communalities (such as a worship community, an intentional community with a common goal or purpose ..., perhaps people with whom one works closely over a long period of time, etc.), even if these are not local bodies.

4   Friends. Even if one has a family, most people still desire the acceptance and companionship of others who are like-minded, who are not duty-bound by obligations of kinship to accept and relate to them, but who do so voluntarily out of affinity with, or affection for, them. ...

5   A transcendent belief system that gives the human being spiritual anchors. Such a belief system has the greatest appeal when it reflects the human wisdom traditions and insights that have a great deal in common even when they evolved relatively independently in different locales and cultures over the course of history. Since many of these share a large number of insights and moral principles, one can conclude that each has grasped some portion of universal truth, or at least of universal human higher aspirations. Such a belief system not only gives a person a sense of belonging and continuity with the larger human community, but also helps a person to cope with the mysteries and tragedies of life.

6   Work, and especially work that can be invested with meaning other than, and usually in addition to, merely a way to gain money or comparable material gain. For many people, this is likely to be work that is of the nature of primary or secondary production, or that is life-enhancing to others or the environment, that hopefully has readily visible results, and that is recognized as valuable by others.

7   Absence of imminent threats of extreme privation (e.g., via penury, starvation, homelessness) and of violent death. One might call this a sense of reasonable safety and security, and perhaps some kind of "insurance" against awful things happening.

8   Opportunities and expectancies that enable one to discover and develop one's abilities, skills, gifts, and talents. In most societies today, this would also include schooling. Probably no one ever develops all their abilities to the fullest, and we are not talking about getting to "actualize" oneself in every way and in every aspect of life. But most people do want to be able to contribute at least something, to be good at one or more things.

9   To be viewed as human and treated with at least a basic level of respect, and by more than just a very few people.

10   To be dealt with honestly.

11   A reasonable assurance that one will not be a victim of gross injustice, even if perfect justice is not to be had. ...

12   Being treated as an individual.

13   Having a say in important decisions affecting one's own life.

14   Access to at least many of the sites of conduct of everyday life; not to be excluded from such places of normal human intercourse.
15   Access to at least many of the ordinary activities of human social life, including their associated opportunities.
16   Being able to contribute, and have one's contributions recognized as valuable.
17   Good health. Though most people would agree that one can lead "*a* good life" even with illness, still most people would count good health as one element of "*the* good life."

It seems self-evident that people who fill valued roles in society are vastly more likely to attain the things that society values (or to have others accord these to them) than people who do not fill valued roles. However, we are, of course, speaking only in probabilistic terms. After all, the good things in life are not accorded or attained only by people in valued roles; ... some people will accord others at least some of the "good things in life" out of moral imperatives rather than because of the roles those people hold; and yet other people will have other good and bad motives for according some people some of the time the good things in life. ... Nonetheless, on an overall and societal basis, we can say that whether people are accorded the good things of life by others depends heavily on their social roles: how many valued roles they hold, how valued these roles are, how narrow or broad (i.e., how life-defining) these roles are, and to what degree people's valued roles are balanced off by their incumbency of devalued roles.

Therefore, while SRV does indeed have dimensions that are culturally relative (because it is tied to what is valued by a particular society in a particular time), we can still say that people who fill roles that are valued in whatever society at whatever time are apt to have access to many good things, including a great many – such as the 17 listed above – that are likely to be valued in any culture. Further, we can say with confidence that almost everyone would agree that the 17 goods listed above are a big part of the good things in life that everyone would like for him- or herself.

Chapter 4

Advocacy

Introduction

The previous two chapters have noted the international acclaim given to Wolfensberger through his formulation of, and attempts to implement, normalization and SRV. It is the editor's opinion, already noted in the introduction, that another of his ideas, arising from experiences in Nebraska and elsewhere, is at least as well-known, and certainly in terms of practical projects, as large a legacy of Wolfensberger's original concepts. Still more so perhaps, in terms of a developed and developing international movement. This is advocacy, and in particular Citizen Advocacy. The main aim of this chapter is therefore to reflect, through two key extracts, Wolfensberger's concept of Citizen Advocacy and its place in the overall range of advocacy possibilities. This was outlined at length in publications in 1973, including an international presentation, but our first key extract is taken from an attempt by Wolfensberger to provide a comprehensive description of what he described as a 'multi-component advocacy schema'. The details of that attempt had a number of contemporary considerations that have been succeeded by events, and so have been left out in an attempt to get to the essence of Citizen Advocacy as it was then proposed, revealing how little the core ideas have changed up to the point of the celebratory conference in 2000 from which the second extract of this chapter is taken.

16 From: *A Balanced Multi-component Advocacy/ Protection Schema*, 1977, (Law and Mental Retardation monograph series) Toronto: Canadian Association for the Mentally Retarded.

For the first extract then, Wolfensberger's overview, taken from the mid-1970s, of advocacy as a whole is given. After examining some of the current issues of social systems, human services organizations, and increasing demands for change that had given rise to the advocacy movement, Wolfensberger goes on to analyze its historical and conceptual roots.

...

A clearly conceptualized advocacy construct in the human service context is relatively new. While advocacy itself has always taken place, the clear formulation of advocacy as a schema or system has a much more recent history. Indeed, the novelty of a clearly conceptualized advocacy approach and component in the human services context is such that the very term "advocacy" can scarcely be found in the human services literature prior to approximately 1970. ...

   As is often the case, various circumstances, including the needs of the times, can propel a concept to wide public attention in a remarkably short period. So it has been with the advocacy concept. However, when this sort of thing happens, there is almost invariably a great deal of confusion and distortion. People may be exposed to a new word, may incorporate the word into their vocabulary, but may not as yet have internalized a clear concept as to what the word is all about, or what it stands for. ... As we proceed to delineate a global advocacy system, it is useful to review at least three ideological-historical roots of the recent advocacy movement, and then proceed to various definition issues.

   One major contributor to the advocacy/protection movement has been the Judeo-Christian tradition. The Old Testament is full of admonitions to protect the lowly, the orphaned, the widow, etc. In the New Testament, concern with the weak, sick, handicapped and abandoned became even more central, and is epitomized in the parable of the Good Samaritan, and that of the sheep and the goats ... . Many people, despite their flight from Judeo-Christian denominations, still idealize this altruistic orientation to the disadvantaged or cast-off members of society.

   A second major tradition is that which has found its way to us through Hegelian philosophy and its various Marxist interpretations and applications. Often quite unconsciously, the idea of the operation of mutually opposed forces (as in thesis and antithesis) has become widely accepted and adopted in the minds of people, especially in various fields of social science and social change that are concerned with social tensions and conflict resolution. Within this ideological tradition, advocacy is conceptualized as the antithesis of an established power or interest ... which is seen as detrimental to a person or group – and in most instances an assumedly disadvantaged group. Thus, we see many elements of the conflict model in many advocacy approaches, and can often detect its Marxist-Hegelian roots by its (not uncommonly unconscious) vocabulary: class struggle, the people, ... masses, ... oppressors, establishment, ... reactionaries, liberation, power, the cause, coalition, ... etc.

   A third major intellectual tradition that has given rise to the advocacy movement is the growing realization in just the last few years that human organizations are subject to certain laws, and that they operate with certain sets of built-in dynamics which can scarcely be overcome by individual efforts, and then only for short periods of time, or for a limited number of occasions, but not for most organizations most of the time. Thus, through the study of complex social systems ..., we have come to recognize a number of distressing realities:

1   Over the long run, organizations serve themselves more than they serve any other purpose.

2   Excellence in complex social systems contexts is most difficult to attain; and once attained, it is subject to dynamics and stresses which make it extremely unlikely that it will be maintained. In other words, probabilistically, human institutions, social systems, and organizations ... tend toward decay, mediocrity and worse.

3   The entire concept of conflict of interest has received much clearer conceptualization in recent years. Because the above-mentioned organizational dynamics tend to possess organizational members to a degree which was previously unrecognized (largely because of the unconsciousness or counter-intuitiveness of organizational processes), it is now widely acknowledged that the representation by individual actors (and even organizations) of particular interests should not be jeopardized by the co-existence of clashing interests within the same mandate or organization. ...

Recognition and gradual admission of these and related organizational realities has brought more people to at least an intellectual acceptance of the need for independent and powerful representation of impaired citizens, and indeed of any citizens who must deal with powerful organized societal structures. However, it is also essential to recognize the source or sources of the remaining opposition to the advocacy movement. It is quite likely that most of this opposition results from ignorance or denial of the existence and power of various organizational dynamics ... . Such opposition may come from politicians and from human service agency people whom one would often expect to be more sophisticated about organizational realities than ordinary citizens. The opposition may be embodied in the view that good clinical agency service *is* advocacy; that if professionals only practiced sound techniques, no other advocacy would be needed; that efforts should be directed toward service improvement rather than advocacy; ... and/or that ... advocacy structures should be dismantled once they have cleaned up a service area that had lost its (former?) purity and quality. Of course, such a conceptualization – even if well-intentioned rather than merely defensive – simply fails to incorporate the empirical facts of human and especially organizational behavior. Even in human service workers who are intimately familiar with organizational dynamics, the reality that they are a factotum of an organization that has all sorts of purposes and functions other than the officially stated and nobly worded ones may be so threatening to self-concept and self-esteem as to elicit denial. Indeed, the prevalence of this type of self-defensive blindness and even arrogance is, itself, one of the overwhelmingly real, maladaptive and yet universal dynamics of organizations.

...

What is advocacy?

One major problem in the wider dissemination, and at least partial acceptance, of the advocacy concept has been the tremendous confusion surrounding the definition of the term. Today, it is possible to find almost anything labeled advocacy, including some highly traditional and even highly dehumanizing services. Thus, placing a person in an institution might very well be called "institutional advocacy"; providing a person with very traditional case work counseling might be called "case work advocacy" or "counseling advocacy"; submitting a news release regarding a devalued group of people to the media might be called "public advocacy"; etc. In fact, this bandwagon phenomenon has almost the effect of perverting and undermining a genuine advocacy approach, ... people would like to continue doing what they have always done, but add the word advocacy to it.

In order to shed light on this confused scene, it is necessary to first clearly differentiate between advocacy and non-advocacy, and to secondly define various, and strikingly different, types of advocacy.

All definitions are arbitrary. All one can do is offer for wider adoption a definition that has clarity and utility. The current affixation of the advocacy label to just about anything obviously loses both of the desirable attributes of any definition: clarity, and utility; other definitions might possess one but not both of these two desirable criteria.

It is useful to start with the culturally normative meaning of the noun or verb "advocate." As most people know, it comes from the Latin, and means to speak to a matter or issue. In time, it has come to mean speaking on the behalf of a person or issue; and where a person is involved, it almost invariably has come to mean speaking on the behalf of *another* person, rather than oneself. Of course, we often speak of self-advocacy, and that concept is certainly a legitimate one to which we shall return, especially when discussing the balance between the need for self-advocacy and other-advocacy. However, of necessity, we must focus primarily on advocacy on the behalf of others. Even when individuals band together in order to advocate on their own behalf, this type of advocacy becomes as much advocacy on behalf of an issue as on behalf of any one specific individual – indeed, to the degree that each member of a self-advocating group really advocates on behalf of an issue that benefits other members of his/her own group, and perhaps benefits them even more than oneself, this form of self-advocacy may actually be more other-advocacy than self-advocacy.

Further, merely speaking on behalf of a person or group does not seem to be enough. After all, in the narrow and non-vigorous sense of the word "advocacy," almost anyone can lay claim to being an advocate for all sorts of causes and other people. ... Is it not true that in a technical sense, perhaps every human service worker, every human service agency, every public official, every church, etc., could claim to be advocating? Obviously, much more is needed if the concept of advocacy is to hold the special meaning it is intended to convey.

I propose that this "much more" consists of three components. The first one is vigor and vehemence. Speaking for someone in inaudible whispers is conscience-salving at worst and prayer at best. Advocacy implies fervor and depth of feeling in advancing a cause, or the interest of another person; it calls for doing more than what is done routinely, and what would be found routinely acceptable; in this sense, the advocate acts at least as vigorously for another person or group as for him/herself.

Secondly, I propose that even fervent advocacy is cheap advocacy if it costs nothing more significant than a shout here, a little excitement there, or a bit of traditional consideration and thoughtfulness. I propose that the essence of advocacy implies a distinct cost to the advocate. This distinct cost may involve any number of things: time that one would much rather have spent on something else; wear and tear on one's emotions, such as one would ordinarily avoid; investment of one's material substance and possessions; sacrifice of rest, sleep and/or recreation; etc. Indeed, the cost may involve one of the highest prices of advocacy, and that is risk, such as the risk of incurring resentment and hostility from others, of being taunted, or becoming an object of ridicule, of being considered foolish or crazy, of being rejected by one's peers and colleagues, of being in danger of loss of job; the risk may involve that of being hurt in violence, of loss of health – perhaps even loss of life itself. Indeed, without significant cost, an action should not be viewed as advocacy ... even if it is otherwise valuable action, such as described in the next section. In fact, it is fervor and cost that may distinguish all sorts of protection from advocacy, in that protection may often be viewed as being advocacy from which the cost has been removed ... .

Thirdly, ... whenever advocacy is intended to be defined as constituting a social institution (in the form of advocacy agencies, citizen advocacy, ombudsmanship, etc.), it must also be structured so as to be maximally free from conflict of interest. If it is not so structured, then the social institution that is being established should be defined as not an advocacy institution, but as some other service quality safeguard ... . This is not to say that an individual worker in a non-advocacy type of social institution (e.g., agency) could not function as an advocate on some occasions by taking on a cause in a vigorous fashion and at significant personal cost, but the institution itself is not to be viewed as an advocacy institution. In fact, the advocacy action of one of its members constitutes an example of an individual rising up against the strong anti-advocacy dynamics that have been imposed on and by his/her organization, thus constituting an exception to the prevailing forces and probabilities.

So as to further sharpen our image of what advocacy is, we will now also review a number of activities that may be mistaken for, confused with, or called advocacy. Some of these may actually be advocacy under certain conditions, as when they meet the above criteria.

What advocacy is not

Not all change agentry is advocacy

In addition to emphasizing the other-directedness of much of the advocacy concept, I also propose that a major distinction must be made between those activities which are of a general change agentry nature, and those change agentry activities which indeed constitute advocacy. Too often, people equate all change-oriented activities with being advocacy; I do not. I can conceive of various types of developmental efforts, community organization, planning, training, and other change strategies that are most certainly strategies or tactics within the process of change, and that are designed to achieve a certain type of change objective, but that I do not view as constituting advocacy. ...

Most desirable and sound service system quality safeguards are not advocacy

There are numerous sound principles of service development, service operation, evaluation, organizational arrangements, etc., that should be adopted, and that would contribute significantly to service quality. Probably the bulk of these principles are not adopted – indeed, they are often not even studied or known; or if studied, they tend to be rejected or avoided. However, the point here is that most of these adaptive processes and structures are not of an advocacy nature, although it may take advocacy to attain their implementation. ...

However, it might be fit to mention here that "protection" (as in the concept of "advocacy and protection") is often *not* advocacy, even if it does protect. Both advocacy and protection are needed; sometimes they are the same; often they are not the same; and therefore, they certainly are not to be viewed as synonymous. Sometimes, that which is advanced as being protection could actually be termed to be "anti-advocacy" in nature. Even such an anti-advocacy act as putting someone into prison may be defined as "protection", as in "protective custody". ...

Not everything good is advocacy

Some people have become so enchanted with the word advocacy that they bestow it on anything they think is positive or benevolent. When a fraternity runs a fund-raising marathon, they may call it advocacy; when a teacher teaches a child to read, that may be called advocacy; when a passer-by drops a dime into the Salvation Army kettle, he/she may consider that advocacy. Even ordinary professional services (supervising a workshop, giving counseling) may be called advocacy. Good intentions alone, nor even desirable actions, are not necessarily advocacy, as we shall see.

Case work can rarely be advocacy

Some people, and particularly social workers, rehabilitation counselors, and similar personnel, seem particularly tempted to claim that case work-like professional services are, and perhaps always have been, advocacy, and that the more recent advocacy movement is really an unnecessary duplication of long-standing efforts which, at most, need a little cleaning up in consciousness or efficiency.

In my own experience of all types of human service agencies, residential institutions have been the most resistive to advocacy; and among human service professions, social work and medicine (including psychiatry) have been the most resistive. Perhaps the resistance from many professionals can be understood as a derivative of the above view of case work-type services already being advocacy. ...

In-house "advocacy" is not advocacy

In recognition of some of the dynamics briefly discussed in the historical review, many agencies or even service systems have established certain internal safeguards designed to protect the individuality of a consumer, to prevent a client from "getting lost" in the system, or to give consumers an easier internal route for voicing a grievance. Many of these safeguards may be called "ombudsmanship," although they are not at all what is understood to be the Scandinavian social-legal institution of the Ombudsman ... .

The first type consists of an office with paid staff functioning as a sort of "inspector-general" to a whole service system. An example may be a nursing home Ombudsman for a whole state/province, functioning in the executive branch of government, usually the state/provincial office on aging or equivalent.

The second type typically involves a single staff member (or a few members) within a specific agency (e.g., within a single nursing home, or rehabilitation office), who is available to clients in order to check out grievances, bring problems to the director's attention, etc. This type of ombudsmanship is even less independent than the first one.

The third type involves the designation of different staff members within a specific agency as having a special responsibility for facilitating a specific client's progress through the agency. For instance, an attendant in an institution, a psychologist in a workshop, etc., may be charged with an extra-special concern with one or a few clients. Positions of this type are often called client advocate, patient advocate, counselor advocate, staff advocate, in-house ombudsman, etc.

Desirable as all of the above functions are, they are really clinical service provider, regulator, or funder functions, at best a step or two displaced from the service provider to the service regulator or funder. As such, they are not free from conflict of interest, and are therefore not real advocacy, underlining once more that not everything that is good and desirable is advocacy. ... Advocacy may be restricted to handing out "These Are Your Rights" booklets, or may even assume the role of "cooling off" criticism and defending the service provider. The mere fact that genuine advocacy may take place in some such arrangements at some point in time does not mean that the function itself is set up to be advocacy as it ought to be conceptualized and structured.

The monograph then goes on to discuss various approaches to protection and guardianship and their problems, in particular the issue of conflict of interest, and concludes with the following list of eleven characteristics of an 'ideal schema', prefaced by Wolfensberger's reasons for needing such a list.

...

When I was unable to identify a single schema that was a) adequately comprehensive, b) satisfying in conceptualization and ideology, and c) actually adaptively operational somewhere, I tried to identify the characteristics of an ideal schema, and it appeared that such a schema would have eleven characteristics

1   Separation from casework and other direct services
2   Individualization of provisions
3   Potential for long-term continuity of personal relationships
4   Instrumental, expressive, and combined support options
5   Both formal and informal relationship options
6   Forms that are highly flexible, and easily changeable over time
7   A built-in ideological orientation and commitment to the advocacy function
8   Consistency with cultural values
9   Maximally feasible freedom from conflict of interest
10   Practical and feasible in implementation
11   Available as needed

It is out of these considerations, though initially not as systematized as I am presenting here, that starting in 1966 I evolved the citizen advocacy schema ... .

A citizen advocacy overview

The components of citizen advocacy

Citizen advocacy (CA) was evolved in order to maximize as many of the above factors as possible. So citizen advocacy was defined as follows: an unpaid competent citizen volunteer, with the support of an independent citizen advocacy agency, represents – as if they were his/her own – the interests of one or two impaired persons by means of one or several of many advocacy roles, some of which may last for life. In order to make this definition more intelligible, the schema can be conceptualized as having five cornerstones, as depicted in Table 4.1.

The top cornerstone refers to the one-to-one relationship by which a competent citizen volunteer, free from built-in conflicts of interest, advances the welfare and interests of an impaired or limited person, as if that person's interests were the advocate's own. For lack of a better term, I have applied the word protégé to the person who is presumed to be in need of significant unmet instrumental (practical problem-solving) or expressive (affective relationship) supports. The advocate is expected to use primarily culturally normative means that typically are accessible to citizens generally, and that might in fact be widely practiced.

The second cornerstone makes a critically important distinction between two major types of tasks, instrumental (problem-solving) and expressive (emotional-affective), as explained in Table 4.2. The distinction between these tasks helps to

Table 4.1 The five cornerstones of the citizen advocacy schema

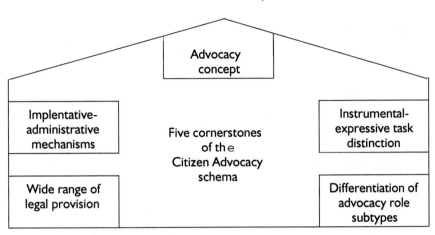

structure relationships so as to provide only the minimally necessary type of supports, and to avoid both excessive as well as inadequate protection, both of which have so often been the hallmark of other guardianship/protective-type schemas – particularly in public guardianship. The principle of minimal protection is implied in the theory of normalization (Wolfensberger, 1972) and its corollary demand for encouraging maximal independence on the part of an impaired person.

Perhaps the most perfect type of advocacy occurs when a citizen chooses to rear as his/her own, and perhaps adopt, a handicapped and neglected child. While few citizens can play such an ideal role, there are many other roles – in relation to adults as well as children – that are less demanding and yet much needed. Among these are the provision of transportation, counsel, or other services for the handicapped child of a family who love and accept the child, but lack the means to solve the child's problems. (N.B. Such actions should not be offered or viewed as a substitute for services that are or should be the responsibility of service agencies, but as either temporary stopgaps, or enrichments. Advocates must resist the temptation to become long-term providers of free services that should be rightfully available, and/or to have their efforts diverted from obtaining for their protégé the services that others should provide.) An advocate can make certain that the child gets the education and training which the community has a responsibility to provide. Advocates can sponsor institutionalized children without (adequate) family ties by visiting them, giving them gifts, or taking them on trips or to entertainments ... even assuming guardianship or at least trying to protect their welfare and rights. Handicapped adults can be assisted in such practical matters as managing money, finding and maintaining living quarters, securing jobs, learning how to use transportation services, and how to vote. Citizen advocates can give friendship and emotional support by offering companionship, and by sharing worship or the observance of holidays and special occasions.

Table 4.2 The distinction between instrumental and expressive tasks

Solving practical and material problems	Meeting needs for communication, relationship, warmth, love and support
"Instrumental" tasks	**"Expressive" tasks**
Advise and assist with day-to-day problems: decision making, transportation, shopping, etc. Administer property and income Represent interests vis-à-vis agencies and the law Insure inclusion in appropriate services: training, work, education, etc.	Provide emotional support during stress and crisis Maintain sympathetic communication and interaction Bring friendship and fellowship to the lonely and abandoned Share emotionally significant activities, trips and events Exchange meaningful tokens (mail, gifts, visits or meals) on special occasions: birthdays, Christmas, Hanukkah, Valentine's Day, Thanksgiving
Meeting relationship needs while also working out practical problems **"Instrumental–expressive" tasks**	
Assume full or partial parental roles for dependent persons Share living quarters with a (young) adult Practical friendship to limited or disadvantaged persons	

A person who is returning from the institution to live in a community group home or apartment needs a wide range of social experiences in the community. A special relationship is desirable for practically all such persons, since group home or other agency personnel must spread their relationships across so many individuals. An advocate for a young handicapped adult can contribute much to the successful adjustment or readjustment of his/her protégé, keeping him/her out of trouble, teaching him/her how to use free time well, and offering advice and support in time of stress and crisis. Young handicapped adults and advocates of the same age can share apartments, with the advocate providing the skills and fellowship that make more independent apartment living possible for the handicapped roommate.

Many parents of impaired children are quite willing and capable of looking after the interests of their child, but have great fears and misgivings about their child's future once their health declines or they pass away. Citizen advocacy can be the means of providing parental successors who would continue to give compassionate, individualized attention to the impaired person, and who would try to preserve the general type and quality of life that the child enjoyed when his/her parents looked after his/her interests.

Advocates are especially needed as "watchdogs" of agencies that serve their protégés, preventing such agencies from "passing the buck," and keeping them relevant, change-oriented, and honest. Particularly in large cities or in large agencies, an individual client may soon lose his/her identity, or may actually be forgotten.

The various advocacy tasks need to be carried out via a wide variety of advocate roles, as indicated by the third cornerstone and Table 4.3. Some of these roles are informal, and it is neither necessary nor desirable that they be recognized by law. Other roles and related aspects do require legal recognition, and this brings us to the fourth cornerstone. While the initiation of citizen advocacy would not require legislation in most countries, the schema could be greatly facilitated if the widest possible range of legal options and supports were available. These include carefully designed guardianship proceedings safeguards; periodic and meaningful review of existing guardianships; a wide range of options for limited guardianships of either the person, the person's property, or a combination thereof; various parental and guardianship successorship options; clearer provisions for guardianship ad litem; and subsidies for the adoption of handicapped children.

There is an inescapable conflict between too much and too little advocacy. In citizen advocacy, the ideal is "minimal advocacy" (just as much help as is needed but no more), in contrast to other services which usually emphasize that more is better. Traditionally, handicapped people have never had enough advocacy, and yet there are people who carry the idea of minimal advocacy to the point where they may deny legal guardianship to people who need it. But if a person is impaired in competency, there must be someone who will make wise and kind decisions for that person, if need be throughout his/her life.

Contrary to much misinterpretation, citizen advocacy was never designed to exclude guardianship. Quite the opposite is true. The need for formal guardianship, or some version thereof, was one of the reasons for the original conceptualization of the citizen advocacy schema. An advocate can be a guardian or a conservator, and not cease being an advocate. Not understanding this, people sometimes speak in terms of a program being *either* citizen advocacy *or* guardianship; the correct phrasing would distinguish between advocates in informal roles in comparison to advocates in formal (i.e., legal) roles. ...

It is also incorrect to assume that those citizen advocates who hold a formal role such as guardianship or conservatorship are somehow unaccountable, therefore apt to misuse their office, and therefore dangerous. Quite to the contrary: a citizen advocate in a formal role is not only in every way as accountable to the courts as

Table 4.3 Examples of the variety of citizen advocacy roles

Instrumental	Expressive
(Legal) conservator Instrumental guardian (i.e., a form of limited guardianship) Informal instrumental guide-advocate	Informal advocate-friend
Both instrumental and expressive	
Adoptive parent (Formal) parental or guardianship successor (Formal) instrumental-expressive guardian (Informal) instrumental-expressive guide-advocate	

is any guardian or conservator, but is doubly monitored, as well as supported, by *additionally* having the citizen advocacy office look over his/her shoulders, offer guidance and referral, etc. Moreover, it is hoped that some of the other safeguards that are desirable in a balanced schema ... would also be operational ... .

The fifth and final cornerstone is a practical implementive administrative mechanism which brings the schema to life on a day-to-day basis. While the efforts of citizen volunteers are noble and desirable, they are not sufficient to sustain a balanced, successful, major and systematic service form unless coordinated and backed-up by staffed local or regional advocacy offices. Such an advocacy office or staff would *not* carry out advocacy functions directly, but instead would attract, select, orient, guide, and reinforce volunteer citizen advocates, and match them with protégés on the basis of criteria such as commitment to the advocacy concept, willingness to undergo orientation and preparation for advocacy tasks, competence in the chosen advocacy area, good character, likely continuity and stability in the community and in a relationship, and possibly, willingness to join a relevant community citizens' action group. The office would assess the needs of a person for advocacy, as well as the ability of a citizen volunteer to contribute through advocacy. It would train advocates, emphasizing commitment to the advocacy concept, understanding of the impaired person and the services of potential use to him/her, and many other areas of action. Finally, advocacy offices would provide emotional and practical assistance, support, and back-up to advocates, and mediate legal and professional services that may be needed by the advocate and his/her protégé. While all the advocates must be unpaid volunteers, it is of critical importance to the success of the schema that the advocacy office have at least one paid staff member who would be available at any time. Without the functions of this office, and without proper matching, citizen advocacy would be equivalent to "ordinary spontaneous everyday moral behavior," but relationships would be less likely to last for long periods, would not reach the numbers of persons that can be reached, and would not make the service of advocates as effective as it might be.

Since an advocate must sometimes represent the interests of his/her protégé *vis-à-vis* a service-rendering agency, an advocacy office ideally should be independently financed and affiliated. Except for initial funding purposes, an advocacy office should never be under the aegis of an agency whose clients might become protégés. Among the desirable alternatives is for voluntary citizen action groups ... to hand over their direct services (if any) to public or quasi-public agencies and to operate advocacy offices instead. Many avenues for funding of such offices suggest themselves. (See Wolfensberger, 1973 [extract 18 – Ed.])

While most advocacy relationships will be informal and have no special status or standing in law, as a volunteer activity citizen advocacy is profoundly different from programs which employ (i.e., hire) people to be advocates, either exclusively (for example, ombudsmen, full-time staff advocates), or as part of their function within an agency. Equally profound is the difference from traditional forms of volunteer activities where individuals perform unpaid work *for a service agency.* Whatever the citizen advocate's role or legal status, in each case, he/she is an independent citizen volunteer whose primary loyalty is to his/her protégé, *not* to an agency. ...

Strengths and limitations of citizen advocacy

Citizen advocacy has the following ... advantages or strengths:

1 It combines the strengths of several other systems while avoiding some of their shortcomings.
2 Reasonable probabilities for continuity and practicality of protection and advocacy exist, due to the back-up of volunteer advocates by paid staff.
3 Conflicts of interest are probably as low as any schema can make them.
4 There is a highly individualized range of advocacy options.
5 Most types of needs can be met via informal relationships.
6 There is a reasonable likelihood that where needed, long-term relationships will exist, whether formal or informal.
7 The cost is relatively low, especially if compared to some other schemas.
8 It has proven success, with almost 200 operational citizen advocacy offices across North America by early 1977.

Like any human endeavor, citizen advocacy also has its shortcomings and built-in limitations. Some are inherent, some are circumstantial. Inherently, 1) citizen advocacy cannot replace all other forms of advocacy/protection; 2) it will probably never be able to meet all of the demand, due to the limited supply of volunteers; and 3) it does not and should not have more than culturally typical social control over the established relationships. Circumstantially, 1) it is very difficult to persuade implementors to preserve and pursue sound ideological as well as practical principles; 2) there is a tendency to over-emphasize informal, reciprocal, and expressive or instrumental-expressive relationships; 3) it is difficult to get funding that is not tainted with conflicts of interest, and 4) sometimes, opposition to citizen advocacy increases as it becomes more successful and effective. Particularly in regard to No. 2, much can be learned from the experience of the nearly 200 citizen advocacy offices to date. There has been a tendency to assign advocates to the more "interesting," more verbal, more affectional and lovable people in need. In consequence, the pool of potential advocates was often drained of advocates who might have taken on the interests of those persons who may have needed advocacy the most: those who are noncommunicative, profoundly impaired, unattractive for some reason, institutionalized, totally abandoned, etc. This issue has been confronted in more recent workshops and discussions in the citizen advocacy movement, and more intensive coverage is more relevant to citizen advocacy personnel and committee workers than to the probably more broadly-oriented reader of this paper. [These and other issues were later to be elaborated at length in Wolfensberger's (1983b) paper *Reflections on the Status of Citizen Advocacy* – Ed.]

Agency response to citizen advocacy can take a wide range of forms, from one extreme of rejection and hostility, to the other extreme of not only support but even maladaptive idealization. In the latter instance, citizen advocacy may be seen as a panacea solution to all the problems of all individuals and all services, and even as a dumping ground onto which are dumped all the clients with whom the agencies cannot cope and with whom they do not know what to do. ...

---

17   From: 'What advocates said', 2001, *Citizen Advocacy Forum*, 11(2), 4–11.

As the first extract shows, therefore, Citizen Advocacy was already firmly established in the USA by the early 1970s. For the next twenty-five years, to the time of writing, it has spread to many countries, and the confusion noted above, between what was and was not advocacy, continued, with further additions, again especially in the UK, of disputes between those who saw self-advocacy as the only 'true' advocacy, and those who sought to continue to emphasise the real need for Citizen Advocacy. Wolfensberger's writings on the subject, apart from the lengthy and detailed analysis in the 1983 monograph mentioned earlier, were less frequent than presentations via the oral teaching culture, and many leaders in the advocacy movement, especially in North America and Australia, continued to develop networks and associations that were only in indirect contact with the Training Institute. Inevitably, disagreements and tensions have arisen over the years, and the issue of 'empowerment,' discussed in relation to SRV in chapter 3, continues to beset the discourse. Despite this, there does exist a large-scale inter-national network in relation to advocacy, and specifically Citizen Advocacy. Such a situation demonstrates, I believe, the validity of the original conceptualization, in that what is revealed by the other extract of this chapter is how relatively unchanged are the basic premises of a voluntary, unpaid, *committed* relationship between an advocate and the 'protégé'.

The extract is taken from an edited version of Wolfensberger's keynote address to the second world congress on Citizen Advocacy, held in Nebraska in October 2000. Space restrictions mean that a number of the illustrations of the key themes have had to be omitted, but it is hoped that the sense of a strong and continuing movement, and Wolfensberger's (and advocates') views on this come across.

Introduction

It was in about 1975, not long after my books on normalization and Citizen Advocacy (Wolfensberger, 1972; Wolfensberger & Zauha, 1973) had come out, that one person mentioned to a second one some other item that I had just published. The second person's jaw dropped, and she said, "You mean he is still alive? I thought he had been dead for ages." As Mark Twain said about himself, the reports of my demise had obviously been greatly exaggerated. Furthermore, we can report instead that even 25 years later, neither Wolfensberger, nor Citizen Advocacy, is dead yet.

This will be one of the most pleasurable speeches about Citizen Advocacy that I have ever given. It is a celebration of 30 years of Citizen Advocacy that is very appropriate to the celebratory context of this congress.

Since the beginning of the Citizen Advocacy movement, I have kept files on issues significant to Citizen Advocacy. With the progress of time, I would add new file topics that seemed to deserve archiving. Among these was one I called "Citizen Advocacy vignettes," i.e., stories about what individual citizen advocates have done. Many of these stories had been told by individual citizen advocates themselves, others by Citizen Advocacy coordinators, or possibly by yet other parties, including some by protégés themselves. A major source of these stories was the newsletters that I received from different Citizen Advocacy offices. Several local offices have had me on their mailing list, so these are naturally the most heavily represented. Later on, many such stories were taken from the *Citizen Advocacy Forum* which itself drew heavily on office newsletters ... while editing the congress speech for publication, I added a few items that had been published after the congress.

When I gave this presentation at the Citizen Advocacy Congress in Omaha, I remarked that advocate stories I drew on turned out to be almost all from Australia, Canada and the United States. It only struck me when I went through my files that I had hardly any vignettes from Britain. After my presentation, Sally Carr from Citizen Advocacy Information and Training in Britain gave me Paul Williams'

1998 monograph *Standing By Me*, which I had not seen before. I discovered that it had many parallels to my own presentation, and I subsequently cited some material from it while preparing my speech for publication.

However, my report to you will not draw exclusively on published material that ended up in my files, but also on what I remember from such vignettes that did not end up in my files ... there is an enormous amount to be learned from accumulating Citizen Advocacy vignettes, and today I will present, for the first time, some important themes that keep emerging over and over in what advocates have said about their Citizen Advocacy engagements. ...

Some of the recurring themes in citizen advocate testimony

Keeping in mind that classifications are arbitrary, it seemed to me that aside from advocates reporting successes and failures, there are five other commonly recurring and overarching themes in advocate testimony, namely: advocate commitment and determination, reciprocity between advocates and protégés, advocates benefiting from the relationship, advocates making various insightful or wise observations, and advocates being grateful for their experience. ...

The single most recurrent of these themes in advocate testimony seemed to be that the advocate had been a major beneficiary of the relationship. And the two benefits that advocates seemed to mention the most are that the advocate learned a lot, and that the advocate has been morally advanced or purified. ...

However, readers should note that I will not dwell on one of the most common themes of Citizen Advocacy stories alluded to above, namely advocacy "war stories," mostly of successes in having averted disasters, saved lives and limbs, given hope, liberated protégés from institutions, the service system, or other bondages, and on and on. There will be some references to these, but such stories are so common, and already so widely disseminated in the Citizen Advocacy culture and literature, that I am making no effort to retell them here. ...

Proclamation of advocate commitment and determination

A certain percentage of advocates expressed deep commitment to either their advocacy role, or to their specific protégé, and stated their determination about one or the other. Some examples follow.

...

"I've got to be there for him, he has no one else who cares" (Rhall, 1997). ...

"I will put my foot in any door that is being closed to her" (Quotes From Citizen Advocates, 1997).

One advocate said about her severely impaired school-age protégé, "I go to all doctor appointments, to all IEP meetings at school, and to all parent-teacher conferences." (The Testimony of Advocates, 1998). Not even many parents could say this. ...

Note how often the expression "being there" recurs verbatim in advocate testimonies. In his compilation of advocacy vignettes, Williams (1998) also noted that the phrase "just being there" was very prominent (pp. 6, 24). ...

Sometimes, the proclamation of commitment takes the form of, or is coupled with, an explicit or implied confession of love for the protégé.

"I have given my heart to this relationship with the belief that the stakes are high" (Grable, 1998). ...

"I think she really knows now that I'm her friend, I'm a real friend, I'm a person that cares about her, really cares. She tried to run me away a couple of times. But I hung in there. Lots of people she knew before took advantage of her. Now she realizes that I care, that someone cares" (Elks, 1999).

Some advocate testimony emphasizes the commitment to the long haul.

One advocate told how she found out that her bodily disfigured protégé of nearly eight years was dying of stomach cancer. She got permission to have her protégé leave the hospital for a few hours to visit with her, and when the protégé felt weak, the advocate put her into her own bed to rest. This was noted by the protégé, who giggled, "I'm in your bed!" The advocate walked the rest of the painful way with her protégé, sat by her deathbed, arranged a church service, gave the eulogy, and attended to the burial. None of the relatives attended, deeming it a waste of time (Joan, 1997).

An advocate in England said about his protégé, "I realised people were always coming and going in his life – I had to decide not to be one of those" (Tyne, 1998). ...

Mind-benighted modernists obsessed with radical autonomy even by severely mentally impaired people keep saying that advocates should only and always do what advocatees tell them. If they did, many would cease being advocates because so many wounded persons will initially distrust an advocate, and/or test the advocate by episodes of rejection. The mainstream of the Citizen Advocacy culture has always taught that this will often happen, and that advocates should persist and reiterate their loyalty, and many advocate testimonies demonstrate this.

One advocate broke the wall of initial rejection by her protégé by telling her, "You might be mad at me right now, but I will never abandon you" (Costa, 2001). ...

In the Citizen Advocacy movement, we tend to consider it an ideal to recruit an advocate for a needy person for as long as that person is needy, which with retarded people is commonly for life. And because of their multiple vulnerabilities, the life expectancy of mentally retarded people is still much briefer than that of the general population, which is why we generally assume that advocates will outlive their protégés. We are therefore often taken aback when a long-standing relationship ends not with the protégé's death, but with the death of the advocate. For instance, in January 2000, a man passed away in Grand Island, Nebraska, who had been another man's advocate for 25 years. His protégé by that time was 77 (Ayoub, 2000). ...

Even though people do not always live up to what they say, some do, and some do at least part of the time. And those who make proclamations of commitment and determination are more apt to live up to them. ...

Advocates express a sense of reciprocity with protégés

One common theme found in advocate testimony is that advocates experience their relationship with their protégé as a reciprocal one, often of a friendship nature, as also noted by Williams (1998, p. 6). Over and over, too often to document here, advocates say, "we have become good friends." ...

A Georgia advocate (Mayes, 1999) said about his protégé Amanda, "We are now friends and extended family to each other. When she needs me, I am there for her, forsaking all other business ... and forsaking everything else." In turn, "Amanda has come to my side. She has been there for me ..." ...

As Williams (1998, p. 6) noted, "friendship can exist without advocacy, and advocacy without friendship, but many ... stories illustrate that the two are closely linked". ...

Advocates claim great benefits to themselves, and sometimes their families, from their advocacy engagement

Even though Citizen Advocacy was not set up to benefit advocates, but advocatees, from the beginning of the Citizen Advocacy movement, I asserted that advocates would benefit greatly from their advocacy engagements .... The Citizen Advocacy culture and literature keeps pouring out a virtual flood of testimonials from individual citizen advocates all over the world to the effect that advocates – and sometimes their entire families – benefited greatly, or even more than their protégés, from their relationship. In fact, this is one of the most persistent themes that keeps coming out of such testimony. ...

Unspecified or general benefits

Some advocates will only say that they have benefited, without going into details how, perhaps because no one asked them to elaborate.

"In a world which values the perfect, the healthy, and the beautiful, we as advocates can make a difference in the lives of people with disabilities. In return, a wonderful difference is made in the life of an advocate by being involved in the life of someone who has a disability" (The Testimony of Advocates, 1998). ...

One way that advocates often speak about how they have benefited from their advocacy engagement is by saying, in almost identical words, "My protégé has given me infinitely more than I have given him/her," or "he/she has given me (or done for me) vastly more than the other way around.". ...

The phrases "rewarding," "getting more than one gives," "enriching," "enjoy," "fun," "being privileged," "fortunate," and "blessed" or "blessing" are heard over and over in advocate testimony... .

Many advocates express regret that they did not discover earlier what being an advocate could give to them. They say things like "if I only had known then what I know now" (Cook, 1997) ... .

The stated benefit of a gift of friendship, love or concern from the protégé

Some advocates are deeply touched by the way their protégé comes to love them and care for them, and see this as a great gift, especially when a protégé had experienced many wounds that might ordinarily have predisposed him/her to never again entrust another person with his/her love.

A Nebraska advocate (Schlueter, 1998) said: "Gary had every reason not to trust me or let me into his life," but "he gave me the gift of love.". ...

"Do you ever wish that you would be accepted for the real you with no strings attached? My friend Kyle can do that for you" (Donna, 1998). ...

Throughout history, observers have noted that mentally retarded persons specifically tend to have a great capacity to love (e.g., Wolfensberger, 1988 [see extract 32 – Ed.]), and will try to please those whom they love. Sometimes, when virtually every other of their capacities is impaired, they still retain the capacity to love, and to try to be good to the ones they love. Because Citizen Advocacy has made more matches with retarded people than with other needy classes, we hear more testimony along these lines. ...

Advocates report that they find enjoyment and fun in their relationships

One thing many advocates have said in some way or other is that they and their protégés have fun together. As one advocate put it (Rozell, 1998), "we ... share many laughs."

One of the early citizen advocates (Julie Meyerson) in Lincoln, Nebraska, was a human service professional who knew that advocates should generally not be sought in such professions, but something surprising happened to her: a 32-year-old man who had spent 16 years in the institution, upon meeting her accidentally, chose her (Meyerson, in Wolfensberger & Zauha, 1973, p. 246). She reported that she and Ray faced serious problems together, but "Some of the things I have been through with Ray have been funny and we do a lot of laughing together." "We have great times together." ...

The fun and joy aspect of Citizen Advocacy tells us many important things, such as the following: being an advocate is not all work; at least within the Citizen Advocacy form of social advocacy, the context of advocating does not have to be – and rarely is – all objectivity and a serious goal-orientedness; and it is the expressive relationship element that in most cases carries the instrumental advocacy along, and sustains it.

The stated benefit of learning important things from one's advocacy, or from one's protégé

One of the most common benefits to themselves that advocates specifically mention is that they learned very important things from their engagement, or from their protégé. A common phrasing is to the effect, "I have been so fortunate to have so-and-so as part of my life. He/she has taught me so much," or "I learned things from my protégé that he/she would not even know he/she taught me.". ...

While some advocates report in a general way that they have learned something, ... others will specify what it is that they have learned. This can range across a very wide spectrum, from the mundane to the cosmic ... I have divided the reported learnings into one distinct sub-theme, and a miscellaneous category.

Advocates learn about the darker side of life, society, social devaluation and human services.

From the beginning of Citizen Advocacy, I asserted that advocates would learn a lot about the bad things that happened to, and get done to, impaired and lowly people. Not only that, but I also asserted that this is one of the benefits of Citizen Advocacy to advocates, and thereby to society This assertion has proven to be correct. It is obvious that Citizen Advocacy is a fast and nearly certain way to learn about the darker side of life about which many advocates had been ignorant, and they do this by finding out what happens to societally devalued people through their protégé. As a result, advocates grow in knowledge, wisdom, compassion, justice, competency and citizenship. While this is very much to their own practical and moral betterment, it contributes in turn to making the world a little less worse than it otherwise would have been.

More specifically, what one hears in advocate testimonies are stories of what we have called the wounds of devalued people. [**See extract 5 – Ed.**] In our teaching (e.g., Wolfensberger, 1998), we speak about 18 common such wounding experiences of devalued people, but these are abstract categories. In real life, these wounds are struck in a virtual infinity of ways, and there is a never-ending novelty in the way an advocate discovers one or more of these many wounds in the life of his/her protégé. At any rate, because human lives are so distinct despite the recurring patterns, I have never gotten bored or weary reading vignettes in which citizen advocates told of learning about these wounds.

One lawyer who had become an advocate said that every time she went to a training session about impaired people and societal attitudes, a light bulb came on in her mind, and "... all of a sudden, I'm saying, 'Oh! Wow! Of course!'" (O'Berry, 1999). ...

In this sub-theme, I also identified three sub-sub-themes.

1   ... that the advocate confesses to having been sheltered from contact with devalued people and the bad things that get done to them, and that the advocacy experience shattered this cocoon.

As one privileged citizen advocate (Lowenthal, 1999) said about himself and his mentally retarded protégé William: "We had come from different worlds. ... My childhood ... was spent within the loving embrace of a large family. ... Opportunities were presented to me throughout my life, while obstacles were present throughout William's. ... Bouncing from foster home to foster home and finally to an institution had filled William with distrust." "We have touched each other's lives in ways that make us better. ..." ...

2   ... many people start out assuming that the human service system is benign, facilitative and helpful. What they experience is so often the opposite. A common type of statement along these lines would be something like, "I had no idea how difficult it would be to ...", and then, we commonly get a thumbnail sketch of some horror story, where the advocate was trying to pursue a reasonable – and often even minor – benefit for the protégé, but had innumerable obstacles thrown into his/her way, usually by human service workers. ...

"What I found out about my protégé and the 'system' was shocking. The unjustice got under my skin" (Jones, 1997). ...

What many advocates say about their family members benefiting or learning is exemplified by what an advocate's daughter said upon getting to know her mother's protégé. "Just about every assumption I made about Pam and her relationship with my mother turned out to be wrong." Then she recited a long list of her mistaken, and sometimes prejudiced, assumptions and said, "For all these things I am sorry ..." She also said, "What I didn't understand then and am only beginning to realize now is that people like Pam need people like my mom and me or they may end up dying ... These 'types' of people are in real danger. Without citizen advocates to protect them, handicapped people are often used and hurt by the system that I had assumed helped them."... (Minis, 1998).

3   ... one way that advocates learn about the realities of social devaluation and wound-striking is that sometimes they come upon a scene where an arm has been raised to strike a devalued person – but the moment the striker perceives that the wounded person is not alone and defenseless, but has an ally from the valued world, the menacing arm withdraws.

Advocates keep telling us how often they are surprised that sometimes, merely being with a protégé will open doors ..., even if the advocate says and does nothing. What this teaches advocates about advocacy is the importance of "just being there" for a protégé, quite aside from whatever benefits an advocate may be able to extract by additional actions for a protégé from other parties in the world.

In turn, there is a lesson in this (though not exactly a new one) for citizen advocacy offices. Namely, while we certainly want advocates to advocate, we should not dismiss as being of little advocacy value the mere but visible presence of an ally from the valued world by the side of a devalued person.

Of course, the entire theme that everyone can learn from Citizen Advocacy had already been brought out in 1987 by O'Brien's *Learning From Citizen Advocacy* materials set, in which he specifically emphasized learning about oneself, the community, the service system and the possibilities for people with handicaps.

Miscellaneous other lessons that advocates claim to learn

Some advocate learnings I have put into a miscellaneous category. Here is an example. "I have learned so many things from Theresa." ... (Abbot, 1999). "Being a citizen advocate has been a profound learning experience for me." She then mentions some of the things she learned. "Helping someone is never just a benign act; help can have an element of harm in it." "It takes patience and courage to be dependent upon others." "Accepting others' control over you does not have to be the same as giving in." ...

However, even many miscellaneous learnings reported by advocates fall into certain sub-themes. ...

1　Aside from learning about social devaluation and the realities associated with it, one sub-theme is that advocates voice other things that they learn about human afflictions and impairments. ... "I have learned so much from someone I never thought I could learn anything from." "People with disabilities want the same thing that I want: a home, real work, friends" (Quotes From Citizen Advocates, 1997). "Michelle's disability is not the most important part of who she is."...

2　Another sub-theme is that advocates learn about themselves. ... "I never thought I could do this, and I have been pleasantly surprised to find out what I can accomplish if I set my mind to it." ...

3　Another sub-theme is learning something about what constitutes the good life. "It has helped me see that there is much more to life than professional success." "It has put things in perspective for me, and shown me what is really important."

4　From looking at the lives of their protégés, advocates learn to no longer take some of the positive things in their own lives for granted.

　　For instance, one advocate said (Rozell, 1998), "She helps me to look at the freedoms that so many of us take for granted in everyday life – the right to have a driver's license, to have a good job and money to buy a car. She must depend on the (paid service worker). I have no staff of people on whom I must depend for the times I need to shop or need to see a doctor. There is no one who is trying to develop an Individual Service Plan for me. ..."

5   Some protégés teach their advocates to be "gooder ."...
    A Nebraska advocate (Schlueter, 1998) said, "[Gary] taught me about patience and acceptance and about appreciation of family."...

One learning theme drawn to my attention by Barbara Fischer after I had given the presentation ... was that advocates often point out that their protégé has taught them important truths about being. This in essence makes a protégé a model for his/her advocate, at least in respect to certain issues of being. Examples could be a protégé modeling forbearance, forgiveness, fortitude, etc.

Miscellaneous other stated advocate benefits

Aside from the benefit themes already mentioned, advocates will also mention specific benefits that do not summate into distinct clusters.

For instance, Carol Rap, the ... world's first citizen advocate, observed that as a result of her family's involvement in advocacy for two young men coming out of the state institution, her whole family benefited, in that they began to do more things together than they previously had ever wished to do, and all this as part of being involved in their relationship to the two young men (in Wolfensberger & Zauha, 1973, p. 248). ...

An English advocate said, "It has been very rewarding. It's about trying to redress the imbalance/inequality I see in others: to level the playing field a bit" (Metiuk, 1998).

Advocates making insightful or wise observations

Some of the things that some citizen advocates have said fall into the category of deeply insightful or wise observations, perhaps about a protégé's experience, and it is not clear whether the advocates were thusly wise to begin with, or learned wisdoms from their advocacy engagement.

An example is what one of the earliest advocates in Lincoln, Nebraska – namely Ruth Hall, herself a parent of a retarded son – said about her protégé, Barbara Jones (in Wolfensberger & Zauha, 1973, p. 244). She noted that as an orphan, Barbara had been put into the institution at age two with a doll on her arm – and 38 years later, this is how she came out, "just as she had gone in."

Observations such as these seem to be vastly more likely to come from a decent, wise, observant, ordinary citizen than from a human service worker whose mind has been turned upside down by his/her professional training and culture.

Advocates express gratitude for their advocacy experience to the Citizen Advocacy office or their protégé

Not only do advocates keep saying that they benefited from being advocates, but they also often express their gratitude – sometimes to their protégé, and often to a

Citizen Advocacy coordinator or office – for having been asked to be a citizen advocate, or for having been matched to their particular protégé. ...

In some cultures, there has existed an imperative to help at least members of one's own clan or tribe. Where Western cultural traditions are still strong, people sense a strong imperative to help anyone in need. In turn, many people have realized that it is by being in an individual Citizen Advocacy relationship that they can live out this imperative in a way that is very harmonious with their ideals. This was expressed by Gayle Johnston, one of the earliest Canadian citizen advocates who advocated for a mentally limited married woman, and often met both with her and her equally limited husband. She said this (in Wolfensberger & Zauha, 1973, p. 254): "They visit me at the office, or we meet downtown at a restaurant in Kingston and have coffee and talk. We've discussed a lot of problems and are becoming good friends. I've been able to help them in some ways and they've helped me. I would like to thank them for letting me help somebody because this is important to me and I'm glad there is somebody who will accept anything I can do for them." Thus, we have here both the themes of reciprocity and gratitude. ...

Multiple themes in advocate testimonies

Some advocates voice not merely one but several of the above themes, and sometimes they manage to do this with great economy of words. We have many examples of such theme bundles. [The paper goes on to give examples of most combinations of themes – two only are presented here – Ed.]

"Jenny was in a living situation that was not only unclean and unhealthy, but also very unsafe – it was, in fact, life-threatening. ... As long as I am Jenny's advocate, she (or her children) will never live in a life-threatening situation again ... the benefits of our relationship do not stop there. I started out ... thinking that I was the one that was going to be helping her, but in essence, I found that I received a blessing far greater than I could ever give" (Kubik, 1997). The themes here are determination and benefiting. ...

Some ... testimonies are virtual grand slams or dense packs of theme combinations. ...

What a Massachusetts advocate said almost sounds as if she had read this article or heard the speech version of it. At first reluctant to become an advocate, upon meeting her 13-year-old protégé Jennifer, "You had me from hello" (citing a song). "Building a friendship together has become an experience full of learning, growth, and commitment. ... My fondness and commitment to Jennifer continues to grow. ... I am sincerely honored to have become a part of a program filled with such integrity, hope, dedication and compassion as the North Quabbin Citizen Advocacy stands for. ... As for Jennifer and I, we anticipate that our friendship will continue to grow and blossom and that in the future, we will continue to share the many up and down phases of both her life and mine" ("Pat and Jennifer," 2001).

Overall comments and conclusion

...

There are a number of things I did not do, or lay no claim to.

1   The sources that I cited are not to be considered the only ones to support my claims. To some degree, I also drew on my memory of advocacy stories that I heard.
2   ... I am not asserting that my classification of themes of advocate testimony is the only, or the best one.
3   I also repeat that most of the themes I brought out are not new. For instance, even in the early 1970s, I used a teaching overhead that listed "satisfaction in serving others," "increased self-awareness," and "knowledge of societal processes and needs" as advocate benefits. "Increased acceptance or tolerance of differentness," often mentioned by advocates, I had listed as a societal benefit. Later, several other benefits were added, and in recent years, A. J. Hildebrand has used a set of teaching overheads listing most or all of the themes mentioned here as benefits either to advocates or to society .
4   I make no claim to an exhaustive delineation of themes ... Paul Williams' monograph (1998) ... brought out advocate themes in a different way, some ... overlapping with my arrangement here. The more vignettes one reads, the more themes are likely to become apparent. However, the delineation of certain themes may require more focused interviewing of advocates. For instance, one often hears advocates say that their protégé is "an important part of my life." This could refer to reciprocity, friendship, or commitment, but could also mean something distinctly different about which one might have to interrogate the advocate.
5   Though reading advocate stories can become addictive, after some time, one discovers that so many advocates keep saying the same things that time to document them all becomes a bottomless pit. ... Thus, at a certain point I gave up documenting further vignettes that merely buttressed the delineation of the above themes. For instance, I already mentioned that I decided not to dwell on the most common theme of all, which ... I call ... "war stories of success." I also did not make a point of bringing out a common theme of advocates saying that at first, "I didn't know what to expect," and "I was rather nervous about our first meeting."

I want to pay tribute to Paul Williams for his collection of 38 advocacy stories (1998). While many of the stories were not first-person accounts, and many of the advocates had not been advocates for long, and a number were human service workers, there was nevertheless a gratifying overlap in the themes he identified with those here, as already noted. For instance, he named the themes of "mutual benefit to both advocate and partner," "partner being enabled to give to advocate," "sticking with it over the long term," "surprise at uncaring systems," and "just being there (existence of advocate is helpful even without action)." Williams also included two pages of advice on collecting and using advocacy stories. ...

I hope that one of the services I have rendered is to illustrate the variety of ways advocates may express a theme, so that from now on, when you hear advocates telling stories, these themes will more readily spring out at you from their background.

Among other uses of this material, I also see the possibility that Citizen Advocacy offices may want to draw on it in service of their fund-raising efforts. Vignettes of what people in Citizen Advocacy do and say are, in my opinion, extremely powerful in convincing people of the merits of this undertaking ... in the Citizen Advocacy literature (and my files), one will also find ... many stories told by Citizen Advocacy personnel, and by protégés, and someone may some day want to take a systematic look at these. ...

Now I want to say some things about reading hundreds of advocate testimonies slowly and thoughtfully in a concentrated fashion over a period of several days, instead of reading a vignette here and there over a period of years or even decades ... this makes a very different impact on one and will affect one differently, and enables one to learn – or at least explicate – certain things ... .

One such thing is that in most cases, advocate testimony does not come as professional technical discourse, but as ordinary people-talk. It does not come with punctuation marks and perfect spelling, and is often not well-organized. It also tends to be laconic, i.e., it commonly tells a great deal in just a few terse words, as many of my citations have already illustrated. ...

Another thing I noticed is that there was a shift in emphasis over the years, from a lot of expressive involvement with instrumental "doing for" and direct helping, to a greater emphasis on the instrumental "advocating for," but apparently without any loss of the expressive element. As late as 1983 (Wolfensberger, 1983b) I had lamented that Citizen Advocacy offices were recruiting too much with an appeal to the expressive element in the relationship, and that this was pushing the instrumental advocacy and representational element to the edge. While in later vignettes, we find that the expressive element is as strong as ever, we also find that the instrumental functions performed by advocates had shifted significantly from helping and doing-for to representing and advocating. I ascribe this difference in part to more resources being available that one can advocate for rather than having to provide them, in part to the spirit of the times, and in part to the evolving maturity of the Citizen Advocacy culture and the offices, in that office personnel have learned to ask more searching questions about the needs of devalued persons, and have in turn brought these needs more clearly to the consciousness of advocates. In fact, many Citizen Advocacy offices now approach potential advocates with a much more explicated description of the plight and needs of a potential protégé.

While the early advocacies may have been overbalanced with expressive elements in relation to the advocative one, reading hundreds of advocate testimonies brings out how important the expressive element is in *supporting* the instrumental and advocative ones. I have always believed that purely instrumental advocacy can be effective; but it is difficult to sustain if the advocate does not develop an affective bond with the protégé, and without that affective bond, many advocates would have difficulty even discerning what is right and best for the protégé. The affection enables them to increase in empathy, and thereby to develop important insights into their protégé.

That many advocates grow in such a way into their relationship with their protégé – even if they do not say it – is one of the more obvious facts about Citizen Advocacy. One only needs to read advocacy stories such as the one in Stephenson's (1983) book, *Roxene.*

While I did not endeavor to dwell on advocate success stories, I briefly want to mention two benefits to protégés that become apparent not only from advocacy vignettes and advocate testimony, but also from observation of Citizen Advocacy relationships.

One is that research study after research study has shown that regardless of how favorable the living situation of handicapped people in the community may be, the one thing that is lacking – and almost invariably so for mentally retarded people – is genuine social integration. However, as far as I know, none of these studies have compared people who have citizen advocates with those who do not, yet judging from the vast informal literature on Citizen Advocacy, it seems virtually self-evident that it is retarded persons with citizen advocates who, in fact, are more likely to experience various degrees of integration. A great deal of this integration results from protégés so often being first included in the family life and events of advocates, and derivatively in the activities of the advocate and the advocate's family in the community. Since in most cases, the advocate is from a valued sector of the population, the protégé then generally also gets drawn into valued physical and social contexts, and into valued activities. We hear this expressed when advocates tell us that their protégé is often with them when they do this or that in open society, and in contact with colleagues or others. As one advocate said, "My family included him … it was just natural to include him in my daily life and also with my family and friends" (Schlueter, 1998).

Further, advocates commonly mediate yet other contacts between their protégé and the members and activities of society. For example, the advocate just mentioned effected a reunion of her protégé with his family in his former hometown, and a visit to his boyhood farm.

Another thing that struck me … was just how creative advocates have been in seeking benefits for their protégé. Often, they would notice a problem or need – even a subtle one – and then come up with things to try that would never have occurred to me, but that usually were commonsensical and often very simple, drawing on resources that one might not think of even though they are readily available. For instance, if one's protégé was a child whose speech was minimal because of numerous ear infections, one might think of all sorts of recourses to pursue, but would one have thought of going with the child to the public library when story-telling times were being offered there (Ott,1996)? Some of us would not even have known that there was such a thing as story- telling in public libraries.

As mentioned at the beginning: two of the most common themes of citizen advocate testimony are that advocates benefit as much or more than their protégés, and that they are glad and grateful that they somehow got involved either as a citizen advocate generally, or in the relationship to their particular protégé. Along these lines, one thing that struck me was that while all sorts of benefits to advocates had been predicted even before the first advocate was ever recruited, I had discoursed about such benefits in the abstract, and had failed to anticipate that advocates themselves would spell out all the benefits they received from their advocacy engagements. For instance, I do not recall it ever occurring to me that any advocate – let alone hundreds of them – would actually say a thing such as, "I received vastly more from my protégé than I ever gave him/her."

One of the reasons for this was, of course, lack of experience, but another was probably that the earliest roots of Citizen Advocacy were in 1967, which was still in an age of paternalism, and where there was an expectation that many advocates would function in a parent-like role to their protégés after the protégé's own parents had passed away. Unlike the modernists of today, I have never thought that paternalism was a bad thing, only that it needed to take into proper account the capabilities and age of a protégé. However, the point is that from a paternalistic perspective, one thinks first and foremost of the benefits for the protégé, not of those for the protector. I must say that even though the theme of advocates feeling benefited was thoroughly familiar to me, I was deeply moved to see this expressed over and over, in some way or other, in story after story.

One obvious benefit of Citizen Advocacy is that it has a way of bringing out the very best in so many people who have undertaken to be citizen advocates, even if they themselves do not say it. About how many human enterprises can one say this? Not about commerce, not about science, not about becoming educated, not about all sorts of enterprises, and not even about most positions in paid human services. It is thus amazing how much good Citizen Advocacy can bring out of so many people.

Particularly in regard to the benefits to themselves explicitly claimed by advocates, when one hears these mentioned by them the first few times, one may be surprised and/or gratified, and perhaps say to oneself that real life has validated what theory had predicted, such as that volunteers would indeed step forward, that they would act in the interests of their protégé as they perceived these, that not only protégés but also the advocates would benefit, etc. But when one hears so many advocates in so many different places from all over the world saying some of the same things about how they have benefited, and say it over and over quite independently of each other, one cannot help but be deeply moved about something very important going on and being said. After all, as far as I know, no one has been coaching the citizen advocates from all over the world to keep saying the same things, nor am I aware that there is a conspiracy among advocates to do this of which the leadership of the Citizen Advocacy movement has not been aware. Thus, we can conclude that we are seeing a universal phenomenon that has the capacity to exert a powerful transformative impact on advocates in a world where people and everything else are falling apart. One could almost say (tongue in cheek, of course), "forget about the benefits of Citizen Advocacy to protégés, because the benefits accrued by advocates alone are worth the whole enterprise."

Now I have a very important point to make about one specific benefit to advocates. Many of you have heard me say that I believe that one's soul comes into serious jeopardy if one does not walk closely with some of the least of society. There are many ways through which such a closer walk can be achieved, and Citizen Advocacy is one of several means for mediating such closeness.

Closeness to a lowly person can upset one's worldview, and most of all so if one acts as that person's protector or advocate. One begins to see the world from the bottom up instead of from the top down (e.g., Wolfensberger, 1989 [see extract 27 – Ed .]).

Many of us have seen politically conservative and/or wealthy people become radicalized in most marvelous ways through their close relationship with a lowly person. Only through this relationship did they come to understand, bit-by-bit and step-by-step, and sometimes with incredulity and amazement, that bad things do not merely happen to lowly people, or are brought upon them by their own behavior, but get systematically *done to* them as part of a process of oppression that they did nothing to deserve. This can be a very radicalizing experience, and to observe a privileged person getting thusly educated and radicalized can be very amusing. ...

In this connection it struck me that one class of people who seemed to have been among the best learners and benefitters along these lines were lawyers who became citizen advocates – or at least, they were more likely to tell their stories. At any rate, how fortunate they were! ...

The soul-saving potential of engaging oneself as an advocate for a lowly and oppressed person has an implication to Citizen Advocacy offices that I have to explain in a bit round-about fashion. Namely, there is one remarkable fact about Citizen Advocacy that is rarely underlined in the Citizen Advocacy literature. It is that citizen advocates do, in fact, come from virtually every sector of society: male and female; from every race and from a vast number of national origins; and perhaps most important of all, from rich to poor, and everywhere along the political spectrum, from liberal to conservative. When one recruits privileged advocates, one often finds that they are very effective because of the esteem in which they are held by many people, and because they hold, or have access to, avenues and positions of influence and power which they can exercise on behalf of their protégé.

However, in a certain transcendent sense, such privileged people need their protégé more than the protégés need them, because it is their protégés who lead their souls to personal compassion and morality. While Citizen Advocacy does not exist in order to bridge the chasms within society, nor in order to save the souls of people of the privileged classes who are suffering from a hardening of their hearts, the fact that Citizen Advocacy *does* contribute to these outcomes is one of its great benefits. Thus, I certainly believe that advocates are right when they say in so many different ways that becoming a citizen advocate has been of great benefit to them – especially moral benefit, and that they should be grateful for it. In fact, the benefit to the advocate may be even bigger than the advocate him/herself realized, especially in the case of citizen advocates who had led a life of privilege, and had previously been cut off from contacts with the lowly and suffering, so that their protégés may indeed have become the instruments for saving their very souls.

Here, I want to chide some of our friends in Britain a bit. Tending to be left-of-center, they sometimes have seemed to imply that they did not want to recruit scum such as conservatives and privileged people as advocates, as if these were either incapable, or undeserving, of such an exalted mission ... it bears saying that an advocate's initial motivation seems to be relatively unimportant as long as it is not dishonorable. Many advocates have started out with all sorts of strange notions and misconceptions, but have nevertheless become good advocates and learned a lot. As one advocate and board member (Catanzarite, 1997) put it, "... If you're sometimes whiny, sometimes selfish, and sometimes hypocritical, well then, you just might make an excellent Citizen Advocate!"

I also want to comment on one very important thing we all know advocates do a lot of, but do not say much about, and about which there has not been much written. Namely, they cry a lot – and not only they, but a lot of other people do who are associated with Citizen Advocacy. That there is a lot of crying going on I have observed when advocates told their stories in person rather than in print, and when Citizen Advocacy coordinators told their stories and those of their advocates. There often are also tears simply from hearing or reading a Citizen Advocacy vignette. On the one hand, the tearfulness of Citizen Advocacy does not really surprise us, but on the other hand, no one in the early Citizen Advocacy literature predicted it.

This crying has to be understood as a wonderful thing, because it is about realities that call for tears, but that so often fail to bring forth tears from a world that in part is unknowing, in part self-centered, uncaring and hardened of heart, and in part just plain too busy. Relatedly, when one hears of all the things that advocates have done for people in terrible straits, one almost cannot bear to think of the life situations of the vast armies of people in equal straits who never had the benefit of a benign human presence, such as that of a citizen advocate, entering their lives.

Tears, grief and sorrow *are* the appropriate responses to all that. But with so many advocates telling us about all the joy and laughter they shared with their protégés, it is easy to overlook the many tears.

Relatedly, it struck me that you can hardly afford to tell potential advocates the full and whole truth up front. First of all, it would overwhelm them and scare them off; and secondly, it is something they need to learn in a very personal way by a combination of discovery and growth, each advocate in his or her own way and time.

Reading advocate vignettes slowly and thoughtfully for several days on end is like going on a retreat, because it will bring one to ask some very deep questions, and to look at oneself. People who describe themselves as agnostics or atheists should try this sometime; it should give them much food for thought. There is a persistent undertone – or even overtone – of religious faith in so many vignettes. Even the prominent theme in advocate testimony that one's good deeds come back manifold to one's own benefit – often referred to as a "blessing" by advocates – is really a spiritual one that would not accord well with a materialistic world view. I could well imagine that Citizen Advocacy might not be very viable in a culture that is thoroughly materialized in its worldview. It is thus ironic that so many people believe strongly that a culture in which people can no longer be motivated to assume unpaid voluntary Citizen Advocacy-like roles is superior to one that they view as riddled with religious superstitions but where these "superstitions" motivate people to act altruistically and unselfishly.

In the light of the many wonderful things that Citizen Advocacy accomplishes, it has long been a mystery to me why anyone who has worked for any length of time in a Citizen Advocacy office, and has had reasonable success making and supporting good matches, would ever want to do any other kind of work instead, and particularly work in formal service agencies, unless one were to do a similar kind of work with volunteers, or were driven by genuine and severe financial hardship.

Chapter 5

Possibilities, limitations, and ethical issues raised by Human Services

Introduction

We have seen, in various chapters, the involvement of Wolf Wolfensberger in voluntary 'Associations for the Mentally Retarded,' specifically at the local and state levels in Nebraska, then at the national level in both the United States and Canada. This produced, as well as academic publications, many committee papers, planning documents, and other efforts to bring some rationality to services in this field, within the overall framework of values and principles associated with normalization. This chapter begins with some reflections from that involvement, but goes on, in subsequent extracts, to mirror Wolfensberger's growing concerns at the limitations of human services to deal with the devaluation of vulnerable people. These stemmed from a more penetrating analysis of the direction Wolfensberger saw society going, and by implication human services and those who ostensibly benefit from them. As we shall see in the next chapter, this analysis had other things to say on threats to vulnerable people, including the very real threat to their lives, but in terms of human services, and human service organisations, it goes beyond simply pointing out their ineffectiveness, and on to their carrying out in practice the values of modern societies. It thus raises some fundamental ethical issues. Wolfensberger's stance on such issues – in fact his very raising of them – then resulted, as discussed in the Introduction and also later in this book, in a degree of distancing of a number of previously supportive groups. One of the earliest to react were the voluntary associations, especially following the address extracted first, and its subsequent publication.

---

18 From: *The Third Stage in the Evolution of Voluntary Associations for the Mentally Retarded, 1973, Toronto: International League of Societies for the Mentally Handicapped, and National Institute on Mental Retardation.*

The extract is taken from a major international conference, where Wolfensberger put forward a controversial view on the role of voluntary associations. As we shall see, it suggests an empirically observable regularity of development of such associations, from small, informally organised responses to a lack of services, through the provision of services, but again in an informal unprofessionalised way and accompanied by campaigning for publicly provided services to replace them, to what Wolfensberger calls the 'second stage', where there is a consistent tendency for the voluntary associations to become major service providers. Along with this stage comes an increase in the size of those organisations, with a concomitant increase in bureaucracy, reduction in the proportion of volunteer members as opposed to paid staff, and many of the other issues that come with organisational dynamics, including the one most often cited in the management literature, the unconscious organisational will for survival and expansion that may totally obliterate the original mission of the association. In pointing out the counter arguments to the long-term operation of services by associations – effectively being stuck at the 'second stage' – and calling for a 'third stage' in his paper, Wolfensberger points to the dangers that being 'stuck' poses to at least an attempt to achieve good quality, comprehensive, values-based services such as he had been advocating in the late 1960s and early 1970s. The counter arguments in this extract are listed after the first two 'stages' have been outlined. Readers three decades later may like to note how many, or how few, voluntary associations have reached the 'third stage' even in countries such as the UK, with its history of public services.

...

Arguments against, or problems associated with, the long-term operation of services by associations

...

At least eleven such counter arguments can be identified.

1 For associations who have had a history of having to initiate services and operate them for some time in the face of a great deal of indifference or actual hostility on the part of the public and/or the government, the thought of ever handing these services over to public offices can be very frightening, and reluctance to seek public operation of services may far outlive its historical justification. The association may have become too strongly identified with the service to give it up even after service operation has outlived its usefulness. Not just occasionally but commonly, operating a service becomes an end in itself ... .

Even where receptivity for public assumption of services has been relatively good, and where associations had at one time made an ideological commitment to this goal, the mere fact of having operated and controlled service empires for some years can set into motion a historical and administrative momentum which can resist ideological pressures for a change. All formal organizations are molded by forces tangential to their rationally ordered structures and stated goals (Selznick, 1949), and day-to-day decisions relevant to the translation of organizational policy into action create precedents, alliances, effective symbols, personal loyalties and other processes which add up into a systematized commitment which eventually assumes sacred status and is no longer perceived as simply a means toward a goal. This is why many organizations are eventually cast aside when new goals are sought, because the old organization, whether public or private, cannot orient itself to the needed goal.

Thus, when service empires are built, when large staffs are hired, and when one begins to identify proudly with buildings, money, power, etc., it becomes increasingly difficult to resist the seduction that these achievements constitute, and it may become too painful to hand these tokens of material success and worldly benefits to someone else. ...

2   Closely associated with the above tendency is the fact that when one has made various commitments to a system, and has become identified with it, one is less capable of seeing its weaknesses, of criticizing it, or of suggesting alternatives. One is even more reluctant to actively seek or accept adaptive criticism or evaluation that comes from outsiders, even though it is well known that change rarely arises from within a system – again, regardless of whether it is public or private. More often than not, changes occur because of external pressures, and it is not unusual for systems to destroy themselves rather than to change. Thus, whenever an association is identified with a service, chances are overwhelming that it is limiting its potential to seek or initiate creative change from within the service. Yet unless an association constantly generates new goals to inspire its present and potential members, the membership is apt to decline, or at least to withdraw from active involvement. The association must have salient issues around which to mobilize and which are apt to attract new members, or it will become stagnant.

In our thinking about the dynamics of voluntary associations in mental retardation, we must be very much aware of the history of other comparable movements, and these include not merely action on behalf of devalued minority groups, but also large political movements such as revolutions or technological and scientific innovations. ... One thing that they virtually all have in common is that once such movements become respectable and successful, they become complacent.

3   It is often difficult for someone intimately identified with a specific service or service system to look at larger problems, larger geographic service areas, and larger potential target groups. For instance, a typical weakness of associations for the mentally retarded has been that they have been constituted to a large extent of parents of the *severely* retarded, and have tended to ignore the problems of the *mildly* retarded.

Also, local associations have not been too adept at dealing with problems which can only be solved on a regional level. It is relatively unusual to see local associations federate into regional bodies that can effectively operate a regional service system; and yet, in the future, it is to regional systems that we must move if we are to achieve the service economy without which we will be denied service comprehensiveness.

Further, too often, a local association is interested in a relatively modest scope of services, such as a single workshop, a single children's centre, a single residence, etc., and often this interest has been additionally restricted by an emphasis on services to one's own child, instead of to all of the retarded in general. Obviously, in the well-developed and comprehensive service systems of the future, the commitment must be to an astonishingly wide range of services, to a regional approach, to a large number of service locations within a region (i.e., to dispersal) and to all of the retarded – not just the more severely impaired ones.

The service commitment must also be to the handicapped as a whole. Public funding sources are increasingly demanding that the boundaries between handicap categories be broken down. ... More and more, we must find ways of representing the retarded when they are included in services not specifically or exclusively aimed at the retarded. An association for the retarded would have a hard time justifying the stand that it should be the operator of such a service.

4   Day-to-day operation of a service requires a great deal of leadership investment. Volunteers must set direction to the executive staff, serve on program committees, etc. Characteristically, this means that the always very limited amount of leadership available must be invested in a demanding process of service governance and administration. However, it is known from the study of organizations that the process of administration is almost inherently opposed to the process of change. Administration is concerned with continuity, harmony, and efficiency, while change brings with it discontinuity and stress.

At any one time, there is only a small amount of capable and dynamic leadership available in an association, and every quantum of leadership which is drained into service operation is a quantum that is withheld from change agentry, while each quantum of leadership invested in change agentry produces many more results than an equal amount of energy invested in service operation. Yet, while *volunteer* leadership is so very precious, and cannot be bought very readily for any amount of money, *administrative* leadership can be. For this work there are professionals who can be trained and hired, but we cannot produce volunteer leaders in this fashion. All this means that service operation will siphon away the efforts of the typically small and unreplaceable number of leaders from change initiation to the perpetuation of what is. ...

5   Where attempts are made to prevent the above problem and to conserve leadership time by giving the executive staff of an association more power, and by involving the volunteer board of directors in only a very distant supervisory capacity, a new dilemma is created. Voluntary associations that

operate services almost invariably drift toward professionalization, and professionalization means what the scientists call formalization, and formalization almost inevitably means at least some bureaucratization. [See later extracts – Ed.] Soon, full-time staff in official offices with paid secretaries can do many things very efficiently that were formerly done inefficiently but with dedication, enthusiasm, flexibility, informality, and often glory, by volunteers. Because of this new staff efficiency, the volunteers rely increasingly on staff, often to such an extent that eventually the staff rather than the board of directors controls the association and sets policy. Unconsciously, and sometimes even consciously, the staff begins to look upon volunteers as a nuisance, and perhaps even attempt to gain or maintain control and prominence over them. The noble words of written constitutions and by-laws notwithstanding, customs and habits often develop which very definitely discourage volunteers from strong leadership or even involvement.

The balance of power between the board of directors and the executive staff is and should be a delicate one, and in a good organization, such a balancing act between these two functions is associated with what theorists have called a "creative tension" from which progress generally springs. If too much power is given to the staff, a danger that is particularly apt to menace a voluntary association is that the staff will replace the volunteer in importance, activism, function, power, and involvement.

There tends to be an interrelationship between professionalization of an association, the power of its executive staff, lack of staff respect for volunteers, subtle displacement by staff of volunteers in committees and other functions, loss of confidence on the part of volunteers *vis-à-vis* technically skilled staff, and loss of volunteer vitality. Members may come to be seen as no more than fund raisers who generate the moneys that pay the salaries for the staff and support their empires. We know that under these conditions, the membership tends to become either complacent or alienated, but in either case, volunteers withdraw from involvement and activism, and eventually, volunteer membership itself declines. Those who have traveled are familiar with associations which have a very small parent and public membership but huge staffs, and where the volunteer membership exists more in order to give a corporate identity and legitimization to an organization which is actually almost completely a professional service agency, and certainly no longer a *movement.* ...

I submit to you that there are some associations which resist a shift from providing to obtaining services only because they have been seduced by power and money, and because they are controlled by their staff who find the idea of any change too threatening to their empire. ... The innocent imagine that when purpose evaporates, function will end – but purpose is among the last and least of bureaucratic needs.

This really is the horn of the dilemma: on one hand, volunteers may end up playing professional and staff roles, and having no time or energy left to work for adaptive change; on the other hand, the association may become so professionalized as to pervert the entire identity, purpose, and spirit of the voluntary association, making it bureaucratic and indistinguishable from public agencies. When this happens, the association loses the spirituality that is its most precious asset and its very heart and gut.

6   In order to operate a service of any consequence, an association must usually depend upon government for subsidies, and therefore becomes indebted and obliged to it. The association may refrain from pressuring the government in other areas, from speaking boldly on controversial issues, and from representing the rights and welfare of all the retarded for fear of stirring up controversy and losing its subsidies. Many of the dynamics discussed here can interrelate and reinforce each other. For example, it appears that in some countries, ... associations providing residential services to the retarded had to design residences so as to meet the requirements of subsidizing agencies rather than the needs of the retarded residents. Had a public body been charged with the operation of residences, the associations could have confronted the issue sharply, which they could not do very well or with great credibility as long as they were involved in the service operation itself.

Instances abound where associations have shrunk from lean, hungry lions with a roar and a bite into fat, complacent, ineffectual, silent or at most yapping lapdogs of their funding sources. ... Fighting for the retarded is a perpetual revolution against both the past and the present, but the rich man is not likely to take to the barricades. Any organization for the downtrodden should seek or possess the charismatic effectiveness that comes from the rightness of a noble cause rather than the righteousness that often comes from wealth. ...

Once a voluntary association loses its autonomy in an effort to obtain or maintain public funding, it loses most of its identity as a voluntary association, and thereby approaches the identity of governmental bodies. In doing so, it may begin to either duplicate functions of existing public bodies (which is wasteful as well as dangerous), or at least perform functions which *could* be performed by such bodies. At the same time, by failing to concentrate on functions that can be performed best, or perhaps only, by voluntary bodies, it will leave a void where there should be a function. And it is unlikely and perhaps even impossible that another group will step into the void, because all the persons and resources capable of filling the void may already have invested themselves into the existing association.

7   Once an association receives substantial public funding for the operation of services, this income becomes one of the major interests it has to protect. It is very common to see associations become dependent upon this income, so that they can no longer differentiate between the benefits to the association and the benefits to the retarded individuals served. For instance, in one jurisdiction, associations receive a certain amount of money from the government for every child they serve ... and the retarded persons served have begun to be looked upon as sort of a milk cow which sustains the flow

of funds into the association coffers and without which the associations could no longer exist. Thus, incredible as it may sound, even as public services have become available, the association has fought very hard to prevent them from serving the mentally retarded. ...

8   A very important asset to an association is an untarnished image – an image of nobility, and of sacrificing dedication in the service to the retarded. As mentioned, when an association operates services of some size that are publicly funded, it accumulates many interests to protect. Its image may shift from that of an independent spokesman for the retarded to that of yet another of so many powerful selfish service agencies and self-perpetuating bureaucracies. The association then loses charisma and credibility in the sight of the public and its decision-makers, and despite its current success as a service agency, it is likely to be less effective on other and perhaps much larger issues. ...

9   A very subtle problem which is less obvious than some of the others is that a service agency must apply, at least to some extent, the principle of the largest good for the largest numbers. This means that upon occasion, compromises must be made in order to run a program which is efficient and equitable in balance, even though it may not be optimal for each individual client. If the association is the service operator, this immediately constitutes yet another source of conflict of interest, in that a vigorous representation of the rights and welfare of each and every individual would interfere with administrative efficiency. Such a demand for individualization cannot be sustained adaptively and over a long run *within* a service operation itself if it has a broad service mandate. If the demand is not institutionalized as an *outside* demand, then it will almost certainly be suppressed, perhaps by compromising away the issue.

10   It is part of the principle of normalization not to be stamped with the stigma of differentness. Being served by an association for the retarded is more stigmatizing than being served by an agency that serves children or adults in general. Even if an association were to operate fully integrated services, its image of being identified with "differentness" would be transferred to the persons it serves.

11   Social (not merely physical) integration of the retarded person into society is also part of normalization and will increasingly demand that the retarded be served close to, or even together with, the non-retarded. For a number of reasons, a service operated by an association for the mentally retarded will generally be limited in its ability to integrate the retarded person intimately with other services or even into the community. ... Resistance to transfer of retarded clients to other agencies can then mean loss of the opportunity to integrate, and yet in the long run, only societal integration will bring the respect that must underlie a service system based on right rather than pity. ...

Action on behalf of the rights of the mentally retarded is the theme of our Congress. Obviously, if services are to be a public right, then any rightful service must be publicly funded. A service which is not publicly funded is not assured, and a service which is not assured is not a right. I doubt that there is anyone in this room who would not agree with this view, but there are many persons in this room who would propose that while rightful services must be publicly funded, they can still be privately operated. Here, I would agree in principle, but I would submit to you that the above practical, administrative, and socio-psychological principles and processes argue strongly against the long-term provision of services by voluntary associations for the mentally retarded. ...

From the foregoing, it follows that it should be one of our keenest concerns that there be *one* body which, at all times, constitutes the ultimate *independent* collective or corporate spokesmanship for those retarded persons who cannot speak for themselves. In many other functions of our societies, interests are represented at multiple levels, and have multiple spokesmen. This is not the case in mental retardation, where public agencies often represent the interests of their departments, of government, or of the public; and where professionals often represent the interests of their professions or their agencies. Only an *independent* voluntary group remains as the final bulwark of protection in front of the mentally retarded. The integrity of this bulwark must not be compromised in any fashion, because behind it, there are no additional lines of defence. If the voluntary association is not free to speak with ultimate honesty and disinterest, for all of the retarded at large, and in the long run; or if it is beholden to a significant degree to anyone; then the retarded person cannot be assured of a full representation of his interests. But if the voluntary association cannot be free and unconditional in its militancy, then who can?

The fact that associations are a last bulwark is particularly relevant to consider when critics point out that resistance to criticism, evaluation, and change on the part of those who are identified with a service operation is universal and not unique to associations for the mentally retarded. Why then should associations for the mentally retarded try to overcome problems which are not overcome by others? The answer, of course, is that in many other comparable endeavors, there do exist built-in systems of checks and balances, while in mental retardation, the association itself must be such a system. ...

Change agentry and the third stage in the growth of voluntary associations for the mentally retarded

Change agentry has to do with bringing about adaptive changes on behalf of the mentally retarded, and might encompass things such as the obtaining of services, which might include demonstration of a service; initial operation of a service to be handed over as soon as possible to other bodies; the promotion of research or personnel training; and exerting pressure to pass laws which authorize or fund services. It also requires pursuit of other types of legislation which define the rights of the retarded, including the right to services.

However, legal assurance of the rights of the retarded is not enough. Unless the law goes hand in hand with public opinion, public readiness, and public acceptance, the law will ultimately fail. Since it cannot be taken for granted that the need for services to the retarded will always be adequately clear to the public or internalized by it, it is necessary that someone continue to hold this need before the eyes of the public even when the need is being met adequately at the moment. Without such continued interpretation, it is entirely possible that the public will one day decide to re-allocate funds to more vociferous groups or more glamorous target populations. ...

Change agentry also and especially includes implementation of certain service quality monitoring and safeguard mechanisms. Herewith, I propose that the shift from obtaining more and new services on the one hand, to the forceful monitoring of services on the other, will be *the third stage* in the evolution of adaptive associations, and will be one of the major manifestations of change agentry particularly in those societies where the quantity of services is substantial. ...

At this point the paper goes into great detail on suggested safeguards and systems by which an association might try to fulfil this third stage, and the likely benefits of so doing. For reasons of space, and also because, with the exception of a brief period in Canada, no association seems to have been able to set up such systems, they are omitted. The results have been as Wolfensberger implies in his conclusion, and the resulting lack of safeguards provided by associations has, in varying degrees, proved a thin defence against other developments in the service system covered later in this chapter.

...

Conclusion

In some countries, an association may never be able to advance beyond the first stage of service provision. Resources may be so scarce, and social attitudes or conditions so adverse as to make large-scale provision of services through any other auspices very unlikely in the foreseeable future. In many other countries, associations are even now highly successful in obtaining new services, in extending the quantity of old services already under public auspices, and in safeguarding and expanding the rights of the retarded. I submit to you that even though the content of these changes is often very different, their process has universality, and an association that is currently in one stage of development can learn a great deal by looking at the processes through which more advanced associations had to go in order to solve their problems successfully. Similarly, associations in earlier stages of development could study the reasons for the decline in relevance and activism of associations which are or were at a more advanced stage, but which have begun to stagnate.

Nor are the trends and issues discussed here specific to mental retardation. In many other fields, voluntary action groups pass through the same processes as we, experience the same problems, and grope for similar solutions. ... Among these other groups, monitoring and watchdog roles are also mentioned increasingly as the most important functions for the future.

Actions are rarely as noble as words. To fit our actions to our noble words, and then to make our actions count, requires a combination of two strong forces: the elemental drive of a deeply-felt movement of the spirit in service of a good cause, and a hard-headed use of knowledge and of the ways of the world. This combination is rarely achieved, and more rarely sustained. Yet, in the world of the future, this is what our associations shall need if they are to succeed – or perhaps even survive.

19   From: "A brief reflection on where we stand and where we are going in human services," 1983, *Institutions, Etc.*, 6(3), 20–3.

As the introduction to this chapter noted, the extract above contains many of the seeds of a more far-reaching critique of the way services, as reflections of societal values, were progressing. One of the earliest and most concise expressions of this thinking forms the next extract, which is an edited version of a presentation given in 1981 to an informal gathering of members of the Quebec Association for the Mentally Retarded, the Quebec Institute on Mental Retardation, and human service workers with the Quebec government. It is reproduced virtually verbatim.

...

Human services have to be viewed in the context of the larger society. We cannot understand human service unless we first understand our society profoundly. If one wishes to be a philosopher of human service, one has to be a philosopher of society and of its history.

My mind is very heavily preoccupied with visions of cataclysm that I think will befall our society – indeed, our world as we know it. I believe that possibly in the lifetime of my generation, and certainly within the lifetime of the children of my generation, we will witness upheavals of global and cataclysmic proportions. And yet, most people live in a dream world, a world of what we might call "modernism" [see later extracts – Ed.] in which they stick their heads into the sand in a hedonistic denial of reality – a reality that they do not want to be true, that they cannot relate to. They deny the reality that a reckoning must come for generations of rape and abuse of the earth and for an idolatrous faith that science and technology can lift the human race above its nature and, indeed, above nature itself.

What I am telling you is the truth; indeed, it is the truth. But relatively few people believe it, and yet fewer are mentally prepared to face the cataclysm when it comes. And if it is true that societal calamities will occur, then it will also be true that human service calamities will take place. The world is full of policy makers, planners, administrators, law makers, and government leaders who are inflicting the same classes of mistakes on human services that they are transacting in the realm of industry and manufacturing, business, raw materials, conservation, energy, and so on. We can see a translation of the same errors, of the same atrocities, of the same denials, of the same blindnesses, from the larger society to the subsystem of human services. Virtually every sound principle of service development gets violated virtually everywhere (at least virtually everywhere in North America, but to a large extent across the world as well), and the same dysfunctional strategies get recapitulated endlessly. In other words, those things which never really work always get promoted, while those things which have the highest likelihood of being fruitful rarely get done or even attempted.

One prime example is that the age of modernism has exalted technology to godhood – yet that very technology is destroying us. We are creating what is destroying us: a moloch, a god that eats its children. In human services, we see this reality reflected in beliefs that it is technologies that will work, that will save, heal and cure people and their afflictions. In consequence, human service workers, like people in general, lust for technologies, and everybody seeks, employs and deploys technologies in a frenetic denial of the overriding fact that it is ideologies that control human services, and ultimately really only ideologies. Yet people chase after, embrace, and fornicate with one technology after another.

The law is an example of a technology, and so everybody today is law-crazy, and thinks that they can solve human service problems by passing more laws: federal laws, state or provincial laws, longer laws, better laws, time-limited laws, etc. They have to pass longer laws because the shorter laws are not working anymore – but the longer laws are not going to work any better, either. And the reason people think that they must pass ever longer, and longer, and longer laws, with more, and more, and more, and more regulations, is because whatever preceded it did not work. Yet people think that more technology heaped on top of earlier dysfunctional technology will solve the problems. Of course it will not, yet everywhere you look, if a human service technology – especially a new or novel-appearing one – is promoted, people will eat it up. If you offer ideologies, values, principles, and sound strategies, people dismiss them as irrelevant, theoretical, speculative, armchair, futuristic, utopian, or what have you – and these are the more positive epithets one is apt to hear.

A second prime example of the breathless pursuit of the dysfunctional, and the rejection of sound approaches, is that of segregation of devalued people, which itself is a result of bad ideology and poor values. Such segregation has been elevated into a social policy that is practically defining of modern human services. If we ask what a handful of the most defining characteristics of our human services are in this age, one surely would have to say that segregation is one of them. Anybody who is afflicted, handicapped, or devalued is apt to end up somehow segregated – if not fully, then partially.

In contrast, the single most important priority in human services is the promotion of positive attitudes toward people who are at risk of being societally devalued. This strategy underlies everything; without it, *nothing else can be expected to work*, especially in a society which devalues almost a third of its population. (... North America has one of the highest rates of people who are devalued, or at high risk of societal devaluation.)

Concurrently, in a world that is falling apart and where virtually every single social glue that can hold a society together is coming unstuck, and in which we may experience all sorts of physical and social cataclysm, the promotion of communality is another essential and basic priority. We need a communality by means of which people at risk of social rejection and devaluation are included and embedded in communal, supportive, primary and secondary social groups and networks. When the world falls apart, the only security for handicapped persons is their communal support system – which they are not apt to have in segregated settings (or only modestly so), and especially not if the setting is operated by hired staff.

However, consistent with the profound dysfunctionality of our human service system, it is almost impossible to get support for either human service, or informal social, efforts to create communities in which handicapped and non-handicapped people share intimately and informally, and in which they are indeed embedded. Instead, massive funding and other supports are typically available to efforts that destroy community and communality. That is true in the larger society, and it is true in human services. Somebody once said that one of the criteria for whether a policy or development in the larger society is good or bad is to ask the question "Does it build community, or does it destroy community?" There are many policies which may look very desirable on the surface but which are destructive of societal communality. Take any number of agricultural policies that may promote what appear to be increases in productivity, but that do so at the cost of the destruction of the land, of community, of generations of a mutually supportive lifestyle, by displacing people who were rooted in the land and its communities, and alienating them in decadent urban settings. Thus, modernistic economics is destroying communities across the face of every developing nation. In the long run, a day of reckoning will come for destructive policies like that. Lowering the price of food in a wealthy society is not worth the price of wholesale destruction of its communities and of entire societies.

Since our society is destroying communality in general, the same destruction is to be expected in human services, and is actually found there. Massive human service funding goes to patterns of services that destroy community (a good example are institutions), and very little funding may go to patterns that build community, of which an archetypal example is citizen advocacy... [see Chapter 4 – Ed.].

Citizen advocacy is one of the most culturally normative service forms there is, in that it strives to embed people into natural relationships; yet it is the one service form for which it is almost impossible to get support in North America. So it is with many similar measures. It is becoming harder and harder for handicapped and non-handicapped people to live together in community residences, because regulations, wage and hour laws, and other formalisms are hassling the people who are prepared or eager to undertake such life-sharing, to the point where many of them who have strong commitments to this way of serving are opting out of public funding, and even accept voluntary poverty so that they can be free to build community. There are states where it has been impossible to get funding for residential settings in the community that either are (a) family-sized, and/or (b) that attempt to create permanent homes for handicapped people. "Transitional services" may be the only ones that get funded. Everybody must be "transitional"; nobody is accorded the right to have a permanent home, a permanent communal social system.

It is ironic: how to affect people's attitudes is a technology, and it is one that is thoroughly understood, and yet it is also a technology that is almost totally non-understood by people in human services. There, it is a technology that is rarely sought out and pursued in any systematic, long-term, large-scale effort, not even by the voluntary associations on behalf of devalued people, though theoretically, they should make this their highest priority. So where we *do* have workable and adaptive technologies, we make very little use of them. We do not even acknowledge that such technologies exist, or that they ought to be learned and studied, mastered, and massively applied. Similarly, of course, where in North America can we really point to a government that has made public attitudinal change a priority commit-ment, and backed it up with realistic supports and measures?

Though time is very late, my foreboding of cataclysm does not tell me what will happen when. The dysfunctionalities are clearly getting bigger and bigger, more blatant, more destructive, more massive, more "intelligent," and people are widely misled by them – led into a desert. There is an increasing number of people who have glimpses of the gathering storm, but they are in a small minority. Also, many of those who see that things are dysfunctional do not as yet know why or how, but only have a "gut vision" that things are very, very wrong. Yet the time is at hand where we as individuals, in the literal sense of the word "individual," i.e., as separate persons, have to make highly personal and conscious decisions on where we are going to stand in a world that is falling apart, and in a human service system that is very, very dysfunctional and destructive. Will we permit ourselves to be used by the dysfunctionalities? If so, we are often destroyed thereby, and I see people thusly being destroyed left and right. They begin by being used, and they end up by being morally dead. Another choice is to not just be used, but to join and to become the transactors, the leaders, in the dysfunctionalities: to embrace, glorify, promote, implement them, and thereby, in essence, to transact death – because that is what it all really is: a form of deathmaking, the creation of havoc and chaos. Another option is to stand aside quietly, and let things take their course. Finally, we can choose to stand in the door, in the pathway of the juggernaut, the death engine (so to speak), the engine of destruction that is grinding along, and to bear witness to truth, to reality, and to moral principle – though undoubtedly, this can only be done at great personal cost.

---

20   From: "Human services policies – the rhetoric versus the reality," 1989, In L. Barton (ed.) *Disability and Dependency*, 23–41, London: Falmer Press.

Over the next twenty or more years since the above address was made, it would be fair to say that the issues raised therein have formed a major part of the teaching carried out directly by Wolfensberger, usually in conjunction with Susan Thomas, and increasingly with other associates. This has, to some small extent, detracted from his opportunities to write about the issues, especially to the degree of detail that his teaching workshops enter into. Three-, four-, five-, or even, in Australia in 1997, eleven-day workshops do not lend themselves easily to articles in journals or even book chapters. The restrictions of space in a collection of this kind mean even more abbreviation, but we have attempted to address this by covering what seem to be the key points in this and the two final Chapters. The closing extracts in this chapter deal with two of those issues, though the original papers contain elements of both of them and give linkages to the others, which we will note in editorial comment as we go along. They relate to the overall theme of the chapter, in that they consider the effects of societal, even global, trends that affect human services and their organization, and follow on from the previous extract. They are taken from edited versions of keynote speeches made by Wolfensberger at conferences in the UK. One was then edited into a book, the other produced as edited proceedings. The first, from a conference in Bristol, contains further analysis of the difficulties of human services in meeting the needs they purport to meet – not, as might have been Wolfensberger's at least partial view earlier, due to lack of rational planning and comprehensiveness, but through being the inevitable, if often unwitting, agents of societal purposes.

… In many societies, human services are de facto shaped and steered by an overall pattern of policies, structures and practices which are remarkably consistent with each other across local communities, agencies, fields and professions. This pattern is what I call the 'human service supersystem'. It can also be viewed as being a paradigm – at least, a superparadigm. The service system as a whole is thus much like an organisation. The reason this human service supersystem is relatively consistent throughout all of what one might call its 'regions' is relatively obvious: the service supersystem overwhelmingly reflects the larger culture within which it functions, and its control mechanisms. In fact, there has been such a convergence of cultural patterns taking place in recent decades that even the human services of separate nations reflect the same controlling influences.

One thing that all groups and organisations have in common is a tendency to function unconsciously, i.e., they may perform functions, or pursue goals, or have processes, of which the members, and commonly also observers, are unaware. Not only that, but even worse, a language may develop that actually proclaims the opposite of what is going on, which usually deepens the prevailing unconsciousness of the organisational realities. The organisational literature uses two terms to encapture this reality, at least as it pertains to the functions of organisations. Namely, it speaks of 'manifest ' and 'latent' organisational functions.

Manifest functions are the obvious, apparent, and usually stated ones. In human services, these appear to have something to do with meeting the needs of the people served, and to allay all sorts of afflictions and miseries. These goals are also almost universally those that human service organisations, and their function-aries, publicly proclaim. …

In contrast, latent functions are those which are hidden, unannounced, underlying, and implicit rather than stated. Often, members of an organisation or field are not even conscious that their organisation or field has and plays these functions, though they are nonetheless utterly real, and possibly even of overarching proportions. ...

If the real functions and outputs of a social system are contrary to the positive ideals of most of its members, then unconsciousness is virtually guaranteed to be high and deception even more widely prevalent. For instance, if one's highest belief system calls one to be peaceful, to love, to build, etc., but a system with which one is intimately identified is violent or destructive, then persons who remain part of such a system over any length of time are overwhelmingly likely to reinterpret the bad things that their system is and does as reflecting their nobler values and intents, and they are overwhelmingly likely to deny – indeed, to run away from – the unpleasant gruesome truth. ...

Further examples of what is said by services, and what happens in reality are then provided.

This brings us to the crucial question: what are the major latent but real functions played by the human service system in our society today? In order to answer this question, we must do three things:

(a)   We must look at human services in their entirety, or at least at the entirety of major sectors thereof. We must not be distracted by looking only at specific agencies or locales.
(b)   We must look at what an entirety of services actually accomplishes.
(c)   We must not be influenced or distracted by what is said or written by politicians, service organisations, professional organisations, or individual human service workers or leaders, or even in the law.

If we do this, and are not sidetracked by rhetoric, we find an answer that is shocking and unpleasant. Because it is so unpleasant, it is extremely controverted, though is amazingly easy to demonstrate. The answer is that the major function of contemporary human services is to support a post-agricultural and post-industrial, and therefore 'post-primary production', economy. We will now explain what this means.

Largely since the end of World War II, and largely as a result of technological developments, there has been a transformation in the economic structure of Western societies; namely, the economy has changed from one in which the vast majority of the population was engaged in primary production – i.e. farming, fishing, mining, manufacturing, and construction, the things which produce what we need in order to live – into one in which only a very small proportion of the populace is engaged in such labour, and even that small proportion is decreasing. Thus, we have entered a post-primary production economic era, which we abbreviate as PPP, in which human services play a crucial but very hidden/latent function. Figures 5.1 and 5.2 illustrate this.

Until relatively recently, the production of basic goods, mostly needed for relatively short-term survival, absorbed the vast majority of human labor, and supported a small tip of leisure, culture, art, and other non-productive pursuits. Today, the more developed a society is, the more this ancient pattern is turned upside down.

In the United States at least, the PPP phenomenon resulted in a mere 20 per cent of the labor force in 1983 engaged in some form of primary production... Further declines have taken place since then, and the total primary production labor force in the US is predicted to be down to 10 per cent by the year 2000. Similar figures, or at least trends, obtain for other nations in the developed world.

If only 10–20 per cent of the people produce all the wealth – the food we eat, the clothes we wear, the shelter over us, the goods that we can otherwise enjoy – this presents, among others, the following two problems:

(a) If the primary producers of the wealth were permitted to keep the proceeds of all the wealth they produce, then they, and probably only they, would be rich, and everyone else would be poor and dependent, and perhaps 'on welfare'.

(b) If so few people are engaged in producing goods, then how is one going to occupy the rest of the labor force?

Conceivably, one could allow the primary producers to keep the profits of their labors by setting whatever prices they want for them – but, as we all know, that

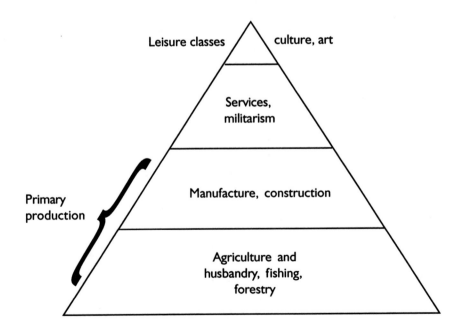

Figure 5.1 The historical patterns of labour

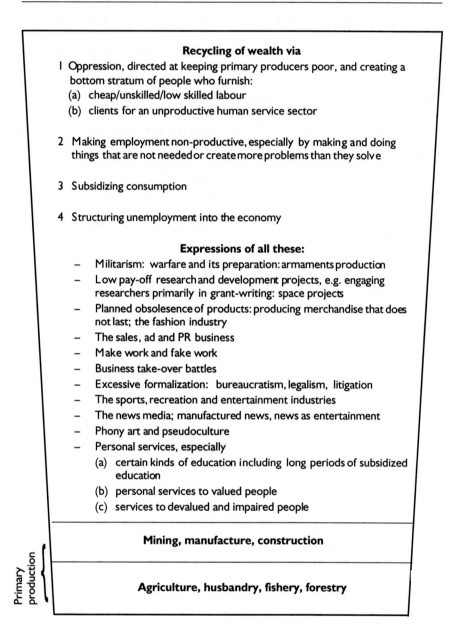

Recycling of wealth via

1 Oppression, directed at keeping primary producers poor, and creating a
   bottom stratum of people who furnish:
   (a) cheap/unskilled/low skilled labour
   (b) clients for an unproductive human service sector

2 Making employment non-productive, especially by making and doing
   things that are not needed or create more problems than they solve

3 Subsidizing consumption

4 Structuring unemployment into the economy

Expressions of all these:
   − Militarism: warfare and its preparation: armaments production
   − Low pay-off research and development projects, e.g. engaging
      researchers primarily in grant-writing: space projects
   − Planned obsolesence of products: producing merchandise that does
      not last; the fashion industry
   − The sales, ad and PR business
   − Make work and fake work
   − Business take-over battles
   − Excessive formalization: bureaucratism, legalism, litigation
   − The sports, recreation and entertainment industries
   − The news media; manufactured news, news as entertainment
   − Phony art and pseudoculture
   − Personal services, especially
      (a) certain kinds of education including long periods of subsidized
           education
      (b) personal services to valued people
      (c) services to devalued and impaired people

Mining, manufacture, construction

Agriculture, husbandry, fishery, forestry

Primary production {

Figure 5.2 Our post-primary production patterns of labour

has not happened. In fact, it is the very primary producers who are being forced by various shenanigans into economic marginality and even outright poverty: for example, witness what is happening to the farmers, the fishers, and to many blue-collar laborers, such as miners.

The strategy that Western society has *de facto* adopted – though largely uncon-sciously – is to oppress the primary producers, keep them poor or nearly so, take away the fruits of their labor at artificially low prices, create unproductive employ-ment for the rest of the population, and create and maintain a large class of the population that is unemployed, and whose reduced identity and oppression provides employment to another whole class of the populace.

All of this is done in such subtle and seemingly legitimate-appearing ways that hardly anyone recognises it for what it is. [A number of examples are then given, of which we include the last – Ed.]

...

Another example is bureaucratisation. The more formal, organised, and bureau-cratised things become, the more people are required in order to manage the complexity, and the more these people strive very hard not to get anything done, and not to let anyone else get anything done. Again, this occupies unimaginable numbers of people, it occupies them in unproductive paid work, and it uses up resources at an unimaginable rate. ... This particular example is also very apparent in human services, because every day, formal organised human services ... are subjected to more and more formalisms, requirements and regulations to the point where hardly anybody can do anything for the clients anymore.

... Of special relevance to us is how human services participate in a PPP economy. By defining ever more human conditions as requiring human service, and especially paid, trained and professional human service, one can create a 'need' for ever more human service workers. Thus, we are witnessing the redefinition of age-old problems of living – growing old, grieving the loss of a loved one, ... inability to control one's eating, ... – as being diseases for which one must receive special treatment by professional paid human services. Also, by defining all these people as human service clients, one keeps many of them out of the labour force, and therefore reduces the number of people that one has to occupy unproductively.

But merely enlarging the human service empire is not sufficient to meet all the requirements that a post-primary production economy poses. In addition, one has to make all the services that do exist as unproductive as possible – indeed, one has to make them counterproductive if at all possible, so that they create dependency, and so that they create impaired people, rather than habilitate them. After all, if more people were habilitated, then they would again present a problem of how to occupy not only them, but also the people who used to be kept occupied serving them. Thus it turns out that, in fact, the net product of the contemporary service system is more dependent people ... .

While most human service workers have no difficulty perceiving some of the other ways we have explained of circulating the wealth and employing people in unproductive work (such as militarism and the inciting of consumerism), they often have difficulty acknowledging the truth of what we have just proposed about organised human services – and for obvious reasons, because to admit this would pose all sorts of moral dilemmas of the most wrenching type to them. ...

Obviously, if human services were truly productive, then clients would be habilitated, would no longer need human services, the service system would collapse, and all the workers who make their living at it would be out of work, and largely unqualified for any other type of employment. ... As one homeless man in Washington, DC noted: 'It would really upset the economy if people were put straight. ... All those policemen, social workers and blood banks – just think how many people would be unemployed if things got better'.

...

The controlling interests of PPP societies have good reason to keep the PPP realities hidden, and thus they engage in various forms of deception. A common one in developed countries, including Britain, is to construct the official unemployment figures so as to grossly (virtually fraudulently) understate the true and high rate of unemployment. For instance, official figures generally exclude anyone who has been defined out of the labour force ... it has been estimated that 58 per cent of European women looking for work were not registered as unemployed. ...

That the human service and welfare system is not really designed to diminish the proportion of afflicted and dependent persons is underlined by the fact that this proportion has actually been increasing in recent decades, and this at the very same time that more and more services have been provided, and even yet more grandiose societal and human service aspirations and accomplishments proclaimed.

The unconsciousness that pervades, and indeed even controls, human service is shown in deinstitutionalisation efforts. Such efforts are seen and purveyed as something positive and glorious, a very progressive step – when in actuality the bulk of the scheme turns out to consist merely of different expressions of society's rejection of devalued people ... what is, in effect, merciless dumping of people without genuine supports into abject poverty, slums and ghettoes, into a violent street culture, into other institutions (such as nursing homes), into other hostile, violent, dissocial, asocial or antisocial environments, and into the prison system, is proclaimed as being a beneficent scheme. ...

All of this is having a devastating impact on everyone involved, but especially on vulnerable classes of people. Rather than benefiting from the bounty of wealth of primary productivity, they are the ones who end up being impressed into clientage, to serve as the unrecognised food on which human service workers, as well as other sectors, enjoy a cannibalistic feast. In a most peculiar fashion, where the labouring child of the English cotton mill was once the food of the economy, an old woman in a nursing home may now be. ...

We can now see that this chapter might have been entitled 'Disability and Dependency: A Creation of Industrial Societies Part II' . ...

21 From: "Major obstacles to rationality and quality of human services in contemporary society," 1997, in R. Adams (ed.) *Crisis in the Human Services: National and International Issues* – Selected papers from a conference held at the University of Cambridge, September 1996, 133–55, Kingston upon Hull: University of Lincolnshire and Humberside.

As can be seen from the reference, the last extract in this chapter comes from the opening address of an international conference entitled 'Crisis in Human Services,' held at Cambridge in 1996. As the note within the extract explains, the address itself covered the full range of issues under the general heading of 'modernism,' but the extracts for this book are specific to the explication of what Wolfensberger sees as the values prevalent in modern societies, and the effects on human services.

...

Societal prerequisites for good service quality

For thousands of years, learned people have debated what a good society would be like and ironically, many awful wars have been fought over this issue. I will propose no grand or utopian answers to this question, but posit only some very modest criteria – one could almost say, minimal criteria – for functionality. I am also only talking about a reasonable degree of societal functionality, not of a utopian arrangement such as the Marxists – among many other utopianists – have been promising. I am not even speaking of a "golden age". ...

The description I will use for this kind of societal functionality is that of a certain degree of comity combining with a certain degree of polity to yield an at least functional comitous polity. Comity refers to things like civility, social harmony, a preparedness to be mutually helpful – something more than merely living indifferently beside each other without being at each other's throat. Polity refers to a set of political and governmental arrangements that manage to unify and order society.

Keep in mind that one can have non-comitous polity. For instance, a bloodthirsty oligarchy may well be able to keep a country together quite efficiently, with great order, but without much comity. I am talking of viable polity with at least viable comity, even if well short of a perfect government ... .

I propose that if a society is to have reasonable comitous polity, then as a minimum, it needs to have large proportions of citizens who function with a fair degree of rationality, self-control and self-direction, altruism, and a moral code on which there is much agreement. The enlightenment philosophers spoke of a "social contract" by which people agree to live with each other – which of course can only exist if there is a sufficient degree of mutual agreement on some of the more important issues and moralities. For instance, one would have to stand on one's head to offer the argument that one can arrive at a viable social contract if one does not first have a reasonable degree of agreement on moral ideals. Again, I am speaking about a population-level and probabilistic presence of these qualities, not that all citizens need to excel at all of them, or that all need all in equal proportion. I am not even saying that having fair amounts of these qualities in a citizenry will assure comitous polity, only that it is a precondition to it.

On the other hand, if we were shown a society in which insanity and delusion were the norm, where people do what they want to, when and how they want to do it, where they put themselves vigorously ahead of all others and cared little what harm their self-will did to others now and in the future, and where each person functioned as his/her own god and could not agree with others on what morality is, and insisted that no one else should tell them what to do – would we not agree that this is a pretty rotten, unhealthy and undesirable society? ... But maybe you have already noticed that this is the kind of society that we see developing more and more in country after country around the world.

Recent and ongoing developments in society that are inimical to service rationality and quality

What is the dynamo that seems to be so widely at work in creating so many disharmonious or non-functional societies in the world today? We believe we can point to five high-level – indeed, overarching – dynamisms that have considerable interrelationship, that contribute to a breakdown in the capacity of societies to have comitous polity, and that in turn disable human service systems in such societies. These are (a) the adoption of a value system that is materialistic, individualistic, hedonistic and utilitarian; (b) the emergence of a post-primary production economy [see extracts 19 and 20 – Ed.]; (c) the "technologisation" of society [see extract 19 – Ed.]; (d) a dramatic increase in the complexity of everything [see extracts 19 and 20 – Ed.]; and (e) formalisation of societal processes [see all previous extracts, this chapter – Ed.]. ...

Of the five 'dynamisms' then listed, all have been covered to a greater or lesser extent in earlier extracts in this or other chapters, as noted against each. This extract will therefore focus on themes a), d) and e), especially the first of these, which is elucidated much more fully in this paper. The order is as in the original paper.

...

Adoption of a value system that is incompatible with human functionality and comitous polity

The first development is a dramatic change of the values of Western societies. This value change consists of a repudiation of one set of values and the adoption of another one instead. What is being repudiated is the value foundation that has undergirded Western societies for as much as 1700 years, and in England for about 1400 years, but that has strands going back much further: to Ancient Greece at least 2400 years back, to Judaism at least 2600 years back, even to Ancient Egypt 3000 and more years back.

What is being embraced instead is a new value system that I call modernism. I have so little time that I can only give the briefest of sketches thereof.

Materialism in three forms

The first element of modernism is materialism which involves most essentially a turning away from things of the spirit and a narrowed focusing on things material. Such a materialism can take three very distinct and yet often related expressions.

1   An obsession with the possession of wealth, objects, goods and their consumption.
2   Even more importantly, an increased preoccupation with the material universe and objects, and especially with technological processes, gadgetry, how things work and how to "fix" them. ...
3   And most impactfully of all, a turning away from metaphysical belief systems and instead, a materialisation of worldview, i.e., a denial of the existence – or at least relevance – of any immaterial, spiritual realm, including a divinity.

Radical individualism

The third kind of materialism quite logically leads to an exaltation of the human and especially of human intellect, human power and therefore also the human will. As such, it might conceivably enthrone collective humanity as the Enlightenment and Marxism have done. But in the presence of other historical factors, it has led instead to the exaltation of the individual human, hence of individual autonomy and power, to an idolatrous degree that makes a godlet of every person. This kind of individualism engenders disregard of other people, of society as a whole and of the interests of other individuals in the future, including even one's own progeny.
...

Merely one example of what this selfish individualism is leading to is that modernistic people have extremely long – and ever growing – lists of what they claim as "rights" but extremely short lists of obligations or duties. The rights are mine, the duties and obligations are someone else's. The trouble is, the "someone elses" also think that they have mostly rights, which of course makes for an adversarial rather than comitous atmosphere. Yet traditionally, rights and responsibilities were always coupled, so that one could not have a right without also incurring a corresponding – and usually equal – responsibility; and vice versa, if one had a responsibility, one also had rights attached to it. ...

Sensualism

The exaltation of the individual, combined with the kind of casting off of external moral codes and constraints that is implied in a materialistic rejection of a metaphysics, quite naturally leads to sensualism, i.e., a preoccupation with comforts and convenience, unbridled pursuit of hedonistic pleasures, exaggerated and uninhibited aspirations for, and indulgences in, sensuality, sexuality, fun, speed, travel, gluttony and "thrills" of all sorts. ...

The fact that our kind of materialism, individualism and sensualism have evolved in the context of material affluence – i.e., a world of material plenty – has strongly contributed to an attitude that one is entitled to all sorts of things much as a god would be. Thus, we see the attitude that one is entitled to freedom from affliction and suffering and even from hardship and inconvenience and that one has a right to material well-being and personal gratification. ...

Externalism

The fourth component is what I call externalism, which is characterised by a deficiency in internal personal identity, strength and mental, moral and emotional substance, to the point that people excessively and pathologically will and must rely on external supports and inputs. These can be physical, chemical, sensory, emotional, social or cognitive in nature. Among the contemporary manifestations of externalism are an inability to be alone, an addiction to noise and therefore a bondage to noise-making gadgets, an excessive reliance on guru figures and cults, an endless involvement in fads and crazes, an almost total reliance on the media and its gadgetry and an inability to live or function without drugs that affect the mind. ...

Externalism can have multiple sources, among which a large role is played these days by an obsession with the object world, a materialistic and mechanistic view of the human and the exaltation of unrestrained sensuality. ...

Here-and-now-ism

Especially where materialism combines with an individualistic pursuit of satisfaction and gratification, it leads to a "here-and-now-ism"... that separates one from time – the past as well as the future. People deny human achievements of the past, lose interest in their history and roots and therefore forget this history, are unable to pass it on to their children, become alienated from the past and are unable to learn anything from it. ...

Memory is deemed and becomes irrelevant. ... As people lose their sense of the continuity of time, they also lose their ability to conceive of a future, to think ahead, to plan rationally, to anticipate the future consequences of any acts and they do not make provision for posterity. Thus, they use up the world's resources without any consideration for what a ravaged world will imply for its future inhabitants ... . What they call planning is really a sketching of fantasies of what they want to happen.

This "here-and-now-ism" is a form of "time-illiteracy", i.e., people are oblivious to the reality of the passage of time, do not grasp the many things that time means (including that all things will eventually come to an end) and are unable to read the signs of their time. ...

Materialism, individualism, sensualism, exernalism and here-and-now-ism feed back on each other in a vicious circle, as when they lead to drug dependence – be it on caffeine, nicotine, alcohol, cannabis, cocaine, heroin, prescription mind drugs, or whatever. Such dependencies are external and material (in this instance, chemical) props, they often also meet the lust for sensory saturation and they are low-level, ad hoc, counterfeit substitutes for enduring values and commitments and for the rich and noble mental, emotional, intellectual and spiritual experiences and engagement of which humans are capable. We should note that enslavement to drugs is rapidly engulfing entire population sectors, has become a major medium of destruction, and yet hardly anyone is giving it truthful high-order explanations, ... or addressing it in the only way that has any chance of working.

I declare to you in strongest terms that the values and lifestyles of modernism are assuredly incapable of sustaining first of all comity, secondly polity and most of all, comitous polity. In fact, contemporary individualism – even by itself alone – would be incompatible with comitous polity. Modernistic people do not bend to each other's will or to an external morality. Relativistic hedonistic individualism divides people, makes each person his/her own god and contains no substance for societal agreement other than to agree on the most extreme moral relativism and thus on moral chaos itself. ...

Of course, value changes do not take place overnight, especially not ones that are so systematic and dramatic as the current one. In fact, this value shift has evolved over several hundred years, receiving several major boosts along the way, one being the ideas of the Enlightenment of ca. 1750–1800 and another the explosive growth in material wealth after WWII. Also, elements of the earlier value system are still around. Nonetheless, it can be stated with confidence that the modernistic values I sketched are now the dominant ones in Western societies, are still gaining momentum ... and are avidly being sought and embraced by the rest of the world. In fact, these values are even being embraced by people who verbally profess a different religion – perhaps even traditional values. ...

The paper then goes on to elaborate the other four dynamics of the value system and state of society that Wolfensberger calls 'modernism,' followed by a brief look at its effects on societies as a whole. We focus, again, on his conclusions as to the effects on human services in a brief examination of the last two dynamics, before moving on to the overall impact of these realities.

...

The complexification of everything to the point of personal and
systemic unmanageability and hence disaster

The fourth overarching development is that everything is becoming more and more complex. The reasons ... include the following.

1   Rising populations increase the size of many things, and increases in size almost always imply some increase in complexity. Today, we see dramatic increases not only in the populations of nations and of cities, but also of specific needy classes ... all of which also adds to complexity.
2   Whenever societies become more heterogeneous, complexity increases; and many Western societies have pursued a deliberate policy of population hetero-genation.
3   Increases in knowledge and the speed of change also tend to increase complexity.
4   Increases in technologisation ... often also increase complexity.
5   So do increases in the formalisation of social processes, because formalisation implies more rules, procedures and regulations and more organisational layers. ...
6   Also, turbulence and strife tend to add complexity and again, we are seeing more of both in virtually every sphere of life, including because of the aforementioned rights and entitlement attitudes.

This increase in complexity has several consequences ... .

First, in complex systems, there are more "parts" and whenever there are more parts, there are more things that can go wrong. Think only of how many more "parts" there are to a jumbo-jet, as compared to a 1920s plane or an oxcart.

A second inherent problem with complexity is that the more complex a system becomes, the less it takes for the system to become destabilised and the more quickly it can become destabilised. A jumbo jet can be disabled by something being wrong with about a pound's worth of small parts, and a continent-wide electric grid can collapse in less than a second ...

Then there is a whole other set of problems with complexity, namely, from the perspective of human beings.

First is that the more complex systems are, the less can humans understand them. Even the people who are experts in computers do not understand well how they work! Societal systems are also very good examples: the social scientists who study them describe them as multi-loop feedback systems that typically behave counter-intuitively and normatively escape the understanding of even those who are enmeshed in and most affected by them.

Because complex systems are so poorly understood, problems can become huge or even irreversible before they are even recognised. It is like a cancer quietly growing in the system and by the time the first symptoms appear, it is beyond remedy. ...

Another problem from the human perspective is that the more complex a system is, the less can humans control or "fix" it. Sometimes, this is because complex systems are so poorly understood, but even systems that are well understood cannot be readily controlled simply because human response capacities are overwhelmed by either the complexity of the task or the speed at which things happen. ...

Even when what is required to fix a system is known or identified, the political, moral, financial or whatever cost of doing so may be so great that people simply cannot muster the will to take relevant action. If they eventually do, it may be too late, because the stability of the system may be past the point of no return. ...

All of this obviously means that complex systems become ever more incomprehensible, unmanageable and even out of control and as everything that is tried seems only to make problems worse. ...

Increasing objectifying formalisation of processes and interactions

Finally, the people of our time are systematically objectifying and formalising the ways in which they deal with the world and each other. Tasks get broken down into component parts and parcelled out to many separate actors who each then carry out only one small part, and all of this is done in a very prescribed, formal fashion as to what should and should not, what may and may not, be done and by whom, that allows very little flexibility and individual discretion. All this also means more and more rules for literally everything. When all this occurs within or by any organisation, it results in what sociologists have called bureaucratism.

The trend toward objectification and formalisation has multiple causes. ...

1   Such objectification is consistent with at least two dominant Western ideologies, namely, the tradition of rationalism and the materialised technologised view of the world ... .

Objectification is consistent with rationalism because objectification seems to impose order on informal, spontaneous and apparently chaotic processes of dealing with people and problems. With objectification, some things become much more predictable and hence – it seems – manageable. And especially since the age of the Enlightenment, human rationality has been exalted and seen as capable of providing the answers for whatever ailed us as long as we were willing to support rationality with sufficient resources and the means of controlling events.

Objectification is also consistent with a materialised worldview and especially materialism in its second and third senses. Materialism in the second sense likes to objectify things so as to deal with them scientifically, technically and via the application of mathematics. Materialism in the third sense implies that this is all one needs to do because there are no such things as gods, souls or spirits that have to be dealt with, only the physical, visible, material world.

2   Another of the major fuels behind the increase in formalisation and objectification in our day is the rights and entitlement culture. Because of its materialistic roots, this culture has very logically turned away from transcendent sources and concepts of rights and toward a purely human formal law ... to spell out what rights people have, what things people in general or in certain classes are entitled to and under what conditions and what recourse there is when a party feels its legal rights have been violated or that it has not gotten all it is entitled to.

But human law, by its very nature, is not informal. It relies on spelling things out, dotting every "i" and crossing every "t", rather than sitting down together over a beer and trying to talk things out in a friendly manner. Also, formal human law is well known to be more concerned with order than with justice. As a result the rights and entitlement culture has managed to generate ever more laws, rules, regulations and conventions governing ever more aspects of life, but often this does not solve problems, or even creates new ones. In fact, this rights culture has never even faced up to the limitations of the law.... .

3   Formalisation and complexification have many mutual feedback loops. For instance, on the one hand, formalisation usually makes things more complex, because it adds parts and layers to a system; on the other hand, people commonly take recourse to formalisation of processes in order to deal with the rising complexity of an enterprise. Thus it is largely in response to some ongoing complexification that people and social institutions make everything more formalised, objectified and bureaucratised in hopes of maintaining control and reducing errors.

Just as the negative consequences of complexification are relatively well understood, so are some of the drawbacks of objectification and formalisation. Here are several of them.

1   Formalisation produces a colder, impersonal human atmosphere.

2   Within organisations, formalisation is transacted as bureaucratism and it is well known that the bureaucratic processes that were supposed to be adaptive means of pursuing a goal end up displacing the goal and become an unacknowledged goal in themselves, so that the former goal is no longer pursued or only secondarily so.

3   Even in those cases where the goals do not get totally displaced, bureaucratisation has the effect of drawing away ever more resources to the transaction of the process.

4   Members of bureaucracies become afraid to make decisions – even those decisions over which they are supposed to have discretion.

5   Members of bureaucracies do not see themselves as responsible for the outcomes to which they contribute and therefore are vastly more easily recruitable to contributing to morally reprehensible outcomes.

6   It is also known that objectification and formalisation make things more complex. Thus, what was done with the intent of bringing rational order to an enterprise ends up making the enterprise more complicated and perhaps even undo-able.

Thus, as problems become ever more urgent, people and systems become ever more tied up in formalisms, legalism and paperwork, to the point where major catastrophes are apt to happen.

We might now contemplate that in developed societies, almost everything is now formalised and complex and/or getting more so. ... We can see this combination of complexity and formalisation all around us in every aspect of our lives, whether it is dealing with a public office, filling out forms, enrolling a child in school, making a long-distance call, trying to get an error in a phone bill or bank statement corrected, getting information about bus or train schedules, or what have you. Even otherwise competent, intelligent and highly-educated people can no longer cope with some of these tasks that used to be so easy. But this complexification has an even bigger negative impact on already vulnerable people. ...

The detrimental impact of the societal realities on human services

It should be obvious that each of the five overarching societal developments, and each of the five clusters of societal consequences that I just listed, create, contribute to or actually are, obstacles to service quality or are just plain bad for service recipients. Often, the same problem is contributed to by several or all of the overarching developments and/or the resultant realities contribute to each other. In this complex web of feedback loops, it is admittedly difficult to disentangle causes from effects.

For our purposes here, I have compiled a list of 15 impacts of the societal realities on human services, but the listing is not meant to be exhaustive nor is the order meant to imply a ranking of some kind.

1   For multiple reasons, the citizenry contributes less to taking care of the needy. Aside from what this does to needy people, it increases demand for formal services even when these do more harm than good.

2   The service system increasingly has to recruit workers who have poor personal and service competency and less and less of a service ethos.

3   Comity declines in all respects in human services, affecting interactions both between and among: recipients, workers, management, families and the public.

4   Services become so complex on both the clinical and systemic levels that they become humanly unmanageable ... we are grinding inexorably toward a state of affairs where it is almost impossible anymore to do anything real and helpful for people in need. After we are done with endless hours of paperwork, liaison and meetings, we may end up with very little service and even that may be of low quality and low effectiveness or outright the wrong

kind of service. The question usually is just which disaster will overwhelm the system first. ...

5   The service system becomes one of several sectors of society that contributes to the creation of the large number of dependent people that a PPP society needs. [See previous extract – Ed.]

6   Since a PPP service system produces a surplus of dependent people, the service system also becomes one of the societal sectors that helps to reduce this surplus by massive transaction of societal deathmaking policies. [The paper goes into some detail here on the topic of 'deathmaking' – this is dealt with at greater length in Chapter 6 of this book, and therefore we proceed here to the next point in the paper – Ed.]

...

7   Just about everybody places expectations on the service system that not even a good service system could meet.

a) Firstly, the service system is expected to have answers to every conceivable personal problem, even though to many such problems there are no service answers. For instance, grief and suffering are the only appropriate responses to the death of a loved one, not mental therapies, mind drugs, support groups of strangers, etc.

b) Secondly, the service system is expected to solve the problems that are created by society in the first place and that may even play hidden societal functions such as PPP dependency-creation and that the service system therefore cannot possibly solve. ... But as if this were not bad enough, the service system has been emitting the message and promise that it can solve society's problems. ...

When one pretends and promises to be able to do what one cannot, then one makes things even worse, for at least three reasons: (a) one will be diverted from doing what one could be doing; (b) one diverts others from doing what really needs to be done because these are not doing what is needed because they are being told that the problem is already being effectively addressed by the service system; (c) one injects craziness into the scene and gets crazified oneself.

8   One of the things that particularly the second and third forms of materialism have quite logically resulted in is that humans have been viewed increasingly as merely physical objects – usually as machines, and handicapped humans specifically as broken machines, or as machines that were poorly "manufactured". Accordingly, human service is seen as body-fixing, i.e., as the application of materialistic technology to material bodies. ... In consequence, humans that cannot be "fixed" ... are to be discarded – at best to be recycled for their parts.

Logically, human service workers too are treated as people-fixing-machines and deployed as if they were objects or as if they were interchangeable with service animals or with gadgets.

9   Materialised mentalities combine with entitlement mentalities, sensualism and here-and-now-ism to produce a service culture that believes in, seeks and promises quick-and-easy solutions. These come in endless waves of service fads and crazes, mostly of a service technology nature. In fact, the service culture has become largely a service craze technology culture where one short-lived super-hyped craze succeeds another.

10 Just as the rest of society gets alienated from its past and culture and oblivious to the future, so does the human service system.

11 Service-related decisions are increasingly made in reference to utilitarian criteria rather than transcendent values. Relatedly, notions of the sacredness of human life are eroding and the value of people – including service recipients – is judged by how much benefit they bring to others, or how much they "cost". As in society, so also in human services, needy people are judged as more or less valuable depending on how pleasant they are to be around and to work with, how responsive they are to servers, how attractive they are, how much they inconvenience the lives of servers, how costly they are, how much they contribute to a worker's status, prestige or career advancement, etc. One can immediately see that such a service environment and mind-set that sees the people served as means towards some end and especially towards the end of the server's own benefits, will be very unfriendly and even outright hostile to all sorts of impaired, devalued and marginal people. Further, one must expect such attitudes to be actualised in hurtful actions towards those recipients who are judged to be "of little use". ...

12 Much as ordinary citizens are cracking left and right, so do service workers. In fact, they are probably even crazier than the rest of the population because the service system realities, on top of everything else, add additional ways of "insanicerating" people [i.e. making people "crazy" – Ed.].

13 Materialism of the third type has separated many people from what they view as "religion", especially in Europe. The problem is that the human being is *homo religiosus,* simply will not live without religion, and there is nothing anybody can do to make it otherwise; it is only a question of which religion people will embrace. And it is particularly in times of stress that people will turn toward some kind of religion, but then often in the form of superstition. ... This also helps explain why there has been such a massive outbreak of superstitions and cults in Western societies lately, and in turn, an intrusion of superstitious and cultish beliefs and practices into human services. ...

14 Contrary to persistent "cut-back" complaints, societal expenditures on welfare and human services have generally been rising but the benefits of these expenditures have been declining, which helps explain the bizarre fact

that dependency rates increase as social spending does – exactly the opposite of what would once have been predicted when we were still in our age of innocence.

In this connection, we may also note that adding layer upon layer of quality safeguards keeps creating human service jobs while having very little impact on service system outcome overall.

15   Amazingly, there is extremely little analysis of, or even consciousness about, any and all of these realities, which is one of the reasons why people will not do much incisive about them, especially in their aggregate.

This is a very depressing list of realities inimical to service quality. One problem with this list and the preceding coverage [even more so in an edited version such as this – Ed.], is that we have vast archives out of which we could give either objective research data or vignette examples to both clarify and document virtually every claim made, and in some of our longer workshops, we do this. This helps people to understand the claims better and secondly, it is more convincing than mere declaratory statements.

On the other hand, the trends that we have sketched are becoming ever more evident by the day and if one fails to perceive them, then soon the point will come when one will no longer perceive anything of importance in larger society or the human service sector. After all, there were people in Germany who would not believe that World War II was lost after it was lost and over .

Some thoughts on action implications

In terms of action implications, the minds of people today have been so shaped by modernism that "doing something" in the face of a problem has to them come to mean almost entirely "fixing it". But for many of the realities I have laid out, and for many of the disfunctionalities that they in turn yield, there is no "fix", no "solution", at least not as modernists understand these words – though there may be any number of relevant and moral stances that can be taken.

At any rate, one overall statement one can make with total assurance is that there is no way in the world that the service problems that we have listed can be boot-strapped into quality from within the service system. In fact, any one of the overarching societal developments by itself could put the jinx on service system quality, even in the absence of the others.

An obvious corollary of the above is that if one wants service quality, one will need a different kind of society. But then the question is whether there is any reasonable sign that society will want, or even be able to reshape itself into one that is healthy enough to allow its human services to have at least reasonable quality, keeping in mind the universal constraints on service quality that we already mentioned. We do not believe that this is the case; in fact, we do not even see much admission that the five overarching trends are problematic. Many people even want them and do whatever they can to promote them.

The analysis that I have presented here explains why, over the years, I and some of my associates have shifted our emphasis away from service system planning and fixing and toward alternative strategies, such as the following.

1 Blowing the trumpet to alert the city that it is about to be vanquished and its inhabitants slain. If the watchman who sees the enemy approach blow not the trumpet, then he is guilty of the blood of the slain. If, however, he blows the trumpet, and the inhabitants heed not the warning, then he is innocent of the blood of the slain, but every man who heard the trumpet but did not heed it is held accountable for his own blood (cf. Ezekiel 3:17–19; 33:2–6,7–9).

2 Raising the consciousness of others about the large-scale and systematic deathmaking of devalued people that is going on [see Chapter 6 – Ed.].

3 Doing what we can to promote schemes that engage as many people as possible on a voluntary and unpaid basis with vulnerable persons, both those who are and are not clients of the human service system [see Chapters 4 and 7 – Ed.].

4 Teaching the importance of extricating vulnerable people from the service system, or at least the system of services for societally devalued people. ...

5 Bringing service workers to the truth. The truths are profoundly unpleasant and their acceptance brings much suffering, but I happen to believe that it is morally better to embrace hard truths than pleasing lies.

6 Helping human service workers specifically to extricate themselves from the lies and deceptions of the service system and to assume personal moral responsibility for doing what is right inside and outside the service system, even if at great cost to themselves. ...

Each individual person has to make up their mind what they believe about our society and where it is headed, and more specifically, to examine whether what I have proposed here is essentially true. ... Most people have not thought about these realities and do not think about them. Instead, they live their daily lives being shaped and socialised by the modernistic mind-set and no more examine it than fish do the water they swim in.

If one agrees even only partly with the picture I have sketched, then another implication is to try to separate oneself as much as possible from the societal dynamics sketched that create all these problems and from living in a way that is dictated by them. Instead, one tries to live in contradiction to them which may take many expressions from among which one may choose some that are concordant with one's readiness, identity and station in life. ...

A number of examples of 'action implications' are then outlined, to end the paper. A number of these, and many others, have figured prominently in Wolfensberger's teaching events, but for this book we would highlight the more general implications at the end of the extract above, in particular the notion of coming to a personal moral judgement on the issues. More on ways to come to such judgements is contained in the final chapter of this book, concerning personal relationships with, and lessons from, vulnerable people. In the next chapter, however, further elucidation is provided on the detail of those moral and ethical issues, as Wolfensberger has developed in his thinking over the years, and as he has revealed more and more about the plight of vulnerable people to the wounding process of extract 5; particularly so in the threats this poses to their very existence.

Chapter 6

Threats to vulnerable people

Introduction

We ended the last chapter with a number of extracts raising deep ethical issues that have figured in Wolfensberger's thinking from at least the early 1970s, though coming more fully to dominate his teaching and publication from the 1980s onwards. As we have also discussed earlier, Wolfensberger's direct involvement in the service system in the 1950s and 1960s generated a number of the shoots of his later thinking. This chapter begins with an extract from that early time that reveals some concerns about vulnerable individuals, in this case the effects of a diagnosis and label of 'mental retardation'. Fairly quickly, however, these particular ethical issues broadened into the full-scale analysis of value trends discussed in the second part of Chapter 5. The resultant threats to vulnerable people are intrinsically bound up with this analysis of ethical issues, and thus formed an equally strong part of Wolfensberger's output at this time, both in teaching events and, more gradually, for reasons discussed below, in terms of publication. The second and third extracts reflect this. The full extension of these threats to the point where people's very lives were at risk was also made at an early point in the process, as the second extract also shows, but was to become what Wolfensberger regarded as the most important of his teaching and writing by the turn of the 1980s, and continues to be so to this day. Thus the remaining extracts examine the issue from a number of perspectives, some being an outright declaration of the dangers, others using particular lessons on the issue to be drawn from the historical experience of both individual lives and the dynamics of the German 'euthanasia' programme. The use of individual cases to make particular points is significant, in view of later criticism of Wolfensberger's 'exclusiveness' from vulnerable people, and we shall return to it in a more general way in Chapter 7. This chapter, however, concludes with Wolfensberger's view on the key impact of the notion of 'Quality of Life' on the 'deathmaking' threat to vulnerable people.

22 From: "Embarrassments in the diagnostic process," 1965, *Mental Retardation*, 3(3), 29–31.

We begin, then, with an early (and for its time very outspoken) account of the threats to people diagnosed as 'mentally retarded' including, as we shall see, the major threat of the diagnosis itself. As elsewhere in this book, the modern reader may well find much to reflect on, given the talk of 'progress' that abounds in the human service field. Though the names and consequences of 'diagnosis' may be different nearly four decades later (some even more serious, as we shall see later in this chapter), much of the practices have an eerily contemporary ring to them.

I propose that the diagnostic process as currently conducted in mental retardation is ridden with contradictions and inefficiencies, thoughtless clichés and bankrupt practices. Specifically, I wish to identify five problems or practices which I believe to constitute embarrassments to the field.

Embarrassment No. 1: Diagnosis is quite often a dead end for the family. Instead of leading to a meaningful service assignment it frequently results only in a frustrating series of fruitless cross-referrals. A typical case in my experience is that of a mildly retarded, homosexually inclined, moderately disturbed teenager who was referred back and forth between the following agencies: regular and special school programs, a child guidance and residential treatment center, a state hospital, two state institutions for the retarded, and the state vocational rehabilitation service. He was judged to be too retarded for the regular grades, too disturbing in special class, too retarded for the outpatient and too old for the inpatient service of the disturbed children's center, too homosexual for the children's ward of the state hospital and too young for its adult wards, too high functioning for the first state retardation institution, not quite enough of a number of things for the special treatment unit of the second, and too effeminate for the programs vocational rehabilitation offered.

This cross-referring took place within a relatively short time span and three or four agencies ran him through their standard diagnostic mill. In the end, the boy somehow did not quite fit in anywhere and lived at home without any service whatever. On paper, however, he was a great success as far as the agencies were concerned. Since he was referred in each instance to what was considered to be an appropriate service by the agency one step ahead in the referral chain, he constituted at least six successful close-outs and will thus enter our national mental health, mental retardation and education statistics. ...

Embarrassment No. 2: Many diagnostic centers do not provide adequate feedback counseling, considering their duty done the moment the diagnostic process is completed *to their satisfaction*. Once the professional staff involved has reached a conclusion, the case is closed except for one, often hurried, impatient and perhaps patronizing, feedback session with the parents. They are given the facts as seen by the professional and told to "accept" them. ...

It is penny-wise and pound-foolish to invest up to several hundred dollars worth of professional man-hours into the diagnostic process only to begrudge a few additional hours of counseling. ...

Embarrassment No. 3: Diagnostic services are often overdeveloped in comparison to other available resources. Indeed, of the services in the field, diagnosis is probably the most readily available. A large number of retardates undergo repeated and redundant evaluations which parents can obtain at relatively little cost if they are willing to expend time and effort. In the writer's experience, the record was held by a boy who, within five years, was subjected to eight evaluations ... . Obtaining needed services, however, was another matter. ...

Embarrassment No. 4: According to theory and cliché, it is of utmost importance that diagnosis take place as early as possible. In practice, however, early diagnosis can be a disaster. When a child is born into a family it is usually accepted and loved with little reservation. Should the child later turn out to be retarded, the problem may be worked out within the family because of the strong bonds that have been formed. However, a child diagnosed as retarded at or near birth may never find the crucial initial acceptance and may be viewed with conflicted attitudes which prevent the formation of deep parental love. This can lead to early and quite unnecessary institutionalization or other consequences detrimental to the child. ...

Embarrassment No. 5: I contend that we really have no strong empirical basis for claiming even a fraction of the benefits attributed to the team evaluation in mental retardation. ... I have concluded that even the best team evaluation is often wasted either because the presenting question could have been answered without it, because it did not concern itself with the underlying problems of the case, or because the data typically collected are not relevant to the prediction to be made. At this point, it seems time to ask: is it at all possible that we have lost perspective? ...

...

---

23 **From: "Normalization of services for the mentally retarded: a conversation with Wolf Wolfensberger," 1974, interview in the "The now way to know" Series, Education and Training of the Mentally Retarded, 9, 202–8.**

By 1974, when this next extract was written, the key development in Wolfensberger's thinking, concerning developments in wider society, had begun to permeate much of his teaching. In terms of writings, however, it tends to be inserted into a number of items nominally about other matters, rather than being more fully explicated, as in some of the extracts later in this chapter. One reason for this is the highly controversial nature of the claims being made, and the political climate of the time, with many 'political correctness wars' being fought out, sometimes literally, in the campuses and in intellectual circles. The extract below is an example. In an interview in an educational journal, ostensibly about normalization and services, and which does indeed contain questions and responses on those issues, the response to a question about the future reveals the way Wolfensberger's thinking was going at the time, particularly with regard to vulnerable people.

...

With as much segregation and dehumanization as we have going on, and with as much devaluation of weak people, of handicapped people, of wounded people, or marginal people, I think that we have to reorient ourselves much more fundamentally to remoralization rather than merely towards better technology, more money, better gimmickry and so on. If we had the proper value orientation and the proper moral underpinnings, all of the other things would be secondary, but without those underpinnings, no technology will work. Not even valid technologies will work if they are not based on a positive morality and ideology.

I think it is terribly important in all of our educational efforts to teach for universality and principles, instead of teaching specificity, and we have not done this very well. We need to teach sensitivity to the process of devaluation in general. We need to teach about deviancy, what it means to society and what it is, because societal response tends to be very universal. ... I think it is very, very important to teach this constantly and to draw the attention of people to the tendency among the majority of our citizens to devalue a significant proportion of fellow citizens – to devalue and even to persecute them to a good degree. Of course, this is what is happening now with aging. The aged are becoming very rapidly one of the primary and largest devalued groups in society.

We have taught almost no sensitivity to certain weak and wounded groups such as the prisoner, the legal offender. The legal offender is an object of wrath ... we have been grossly inconsistent in either unrealistic liberalistic bleeding heart approaches on the one hand, and on the other hand, a punitive destructive approach. And in between, the people get lost. This is why we have a dehumanizing penal system – a maladaptive counterproductive corrective system. We are dealing with human beings, so we do need much broader training towards this whole issue of devaluation, rejection, and isolation.

I think that the liberalization of abortion is one of the expressions of a lowering of the value of human life, and I do believe that we will soon see legalized euthanasia. We will see it applied to the aged and the retarded first, and I think we'll see it in my lifetime, unfortunately. It will have a brutalizing effect on society. I think it will polarize society to a good degree – a lot of people for and a lot of people against. I think we'll have to see massive abuses before we will come back together. We will have to see that you can't have this part way; that once you break through a qualitative barrier of defining human life and its value, then there's no stopping. ...

---

24 From: "How to exclude mentally retarded children from school," 1975, Guest Editorial, *Mental Retardation*, 13(6), 30–1.

The same insertion of the wider issues into a more specific article comes in this next extract, though it also illustrates an important sub-theme of the threats to vulnerable people, namely the deceptions, the excuses: what in his teaching Wolfensberger often calls 'lies and detoxifications' of services that what they are doing is harmful to vulnerable people – in this case children excluded from school. Again, readers in the new millennium might be surprised at the contemporary sound of many of the issues raised.

As a professor in a university that trains a large number of educators, I am painfully reminded that once our students have become "fully qualified" professionally, and are working in the school system, it is often they who exclude children from school. One wonders where the university has failed in its training when a former student becomes what one must now view as a dehumanizer – in a sense even a persecutor of weak and handicapped children. With puzzlement, one reads articles written by professionals about how dedicated the human service professionals are, and how professionalization advances a person toward such dedication. ... I cannot help wondering where literally millions of professionals are, while 2,000,000 children in the United States are excluded from school today, while mental health services are practically on the verge of a relevancy collapse, while millions of elderly people are being stacked into segregated high-rises and nursing homes, and while there are so many other segregated institutions all over our country.

In order to help us maintain a more realistic perspective of our shortcomings as educators, and of our lack of advocacy, it is salutarious to read what a consumer group that has been driven to desperation thinks and does about our shortcomings. One of the more militant such groups has been the Pennsylvania Association for Retarded Citizens that has won a landmark right to education decision in 1972. In order to help its membership to identify illegal exclusion of retarded children from public schools, it developed a list of 17 defenses typically advanced by educators in support of such exclusion. Educators driven by compulsion to exclude weak, handicapped, marginal, defenseless, deeply wounded, or otherwise deviant children from the schools are advised to carefully study this list, since one or more of these arguments can be utilized with great effect in accomplishing their purpose. The list, published in the *Pennsylvania ARC Newsletter* (1972) [referenced under Pennsylvania ARC – Ed.] and elsewhere is reproduced in condensed form.

> We do not have: classes for retarded children; room in our class to include your retarded child; pre-school classes or kindergarten for retarded children; classes for junior or senior high school age retarded children; enough money to provide any classes for retarded children. We do not accept retarded children: until they are 8 years old; who have not reached a mental age of 5; who are not toilet trained; who are behavior problems; who cannot walk; who have other handicaps (such as hearing loss, cerebral palsy, etc.). We cannot send a teacher to your home to work with your retarded child. We shall put your retarded child on a waiting list. We will stop our programs for other retarded children if you make trouble for us. We will postpone your child's admission and let you know when he can come to school. We are not going to educate or provide a training program for your retarded child. Your child can no longer benefit from any education or training

D. Biklen (1974) has identified 8 similar defensive "ploys" often tried on parents by educational administrators and other human service leaders: (a) I agree with your philosophy, but …; (b) I am not the one to make the decision; (c) We don't have the money; (d) The experts agree with our position; (e) These things take time; you must be more patient; (f) Your child is only one of many; our personnel can't spend all their time on your case; (g) Your child is too severe to be helped; (h) The diagnostic data are not in yet.

There are probably many other such compilations. The last one cited here is *The Way We Go To School* (1970) [referenced under Task Force on Children Out of School – Ed.] which classifies the most promising and aggressively defensive exclusion rationales into 10 categeries: (1) Denial: I deny that children are being excluded from school, or that such things are happening to them. Prove it. (2) Exception: The examples you have given are exceptions. Prove that they are widespread. (3) Demurrer: I admit the facts, but feel that you have not presented a problem which is that important. (4) Confession and avoidance: I admit the facts and feel very concerned. But there are overriding considerations which free me from responsibility for action. (5) Improper jurisdiction: I understand the problem, but feel it is not the school's responsibility, but the family's and other institutions'. (6) Prematurity of request: We knew all along that these things were happening, and have made plans to correct the situation. Our efforts must be given a chance. (7) Generalized guilt: What you say is true, but other school systems have similar problems. We are no worse than they are. (8) Improper forum: The problem is really in the hands of the state and federal government. There is little we can do. (9) Recrimination: I admit that children are out of school, but it is their own fault. It wouldn't happen if they and their parents really cared. There isn't much we can do with some of these children.

Many of them are just slow learners. We don't have inferior schools; we have inferior students. (10) Further study: The problem has been referred to the proper officials for further study. We hope to develop a plan sometime in the future.

In order to uphold the tradition of *Mental Retardation's* editorial column, I feel compelled to conclude with a finely polished metered Latinism: "Ubi sunt qui ante nos excluderunt."

---

25   From: "A call to wake up to the beginning of a new wave of 'euthanasia' of severely impaired people," 1980, Guest Editorial, *Education and Training of the Mentally Retarded*, 15, 171–3 .

It is in another 'Guest Editorial' that we find the next extract, being one of the earliest published expositions entirely devoted to what Wolfensberger has termed 'deathmaking' – something he and his Training Institute had been teaching about for some time before this article appeared, and warning about as early as 1974, as part of publications such as the second extract above. Written for a specialist journal, the focus is obviously on 'severely impaired people,' though as we shall see, this already includes a wider group than 'mental retardation.' In view of the previous extract, and its continued relevance in many countries, the introductory sentence might be considered ironic, though it would appear to have been genuine enough at the time it was made. Again readers should note the timing of this paper, and what has happened since with regard to the issues raised, though this will also be covered in later extracts.

Those who ally themselves with severely handicapped or otherwise deeply rejected people can take satisfaction in the fact that major breakthroughs have been experienced in the extension of public funding to the education of severely handicapped children, and even in their inclusion in the public education system. However, a major new calamity now looms over the current scene which renders such advances less significant: the powerful gathering of forces that would assault the very lives of people who are profoundly, severely, and even moderately afflicted; and the beginnings of systematic and large-scale "death-making" of afflicted people. In the context of a brief editorial, I can only sketch a few aspects of these developments. These include the following:

1   The liberalization of abortion in general has resulted in explicit sanction (often outright encouragement) of the abortion of (potentially) handicapped infants; in turn this has led to the now widespread practice of some forms and stages of infanticide which include (a) the abortion of viable fetuses and of fetuses in the last weeks of pregnancy; (b) efforts to kill living and viable aborted infants; and (c) any number of measures applied after birth to maximize the likelihood that a handicapped newborn will not survive.

2   In hospitals (even those run by religious bodies), mentally retarded people, people with other handicaps, and elderly people are commonly denied relatively elementary life supports such as antibiotics, basic resuscitation, or even the simplest medical procedures. In fact, the likelihood is relatively high that persons afflicted with multiple devalued conditions will not leave a hospital alive – even if their affliction and/or illness is relatively moderate. ... Secretly and without involving relevant relatives, advocates, or the other human service providers responsible for the handicapped individuals, death-dealing decisions about such individuals are commonly made by medical personnel. ...

3   Handicapped people are given massive doses of psychoactive drugs, so that they die from drug effects – even though the death certificate will list only the complications, such as cardiac arrest, pneumonia (caused by paralysis of the throat which lets food into the windpipe), etc.

4   Elderly people are subjected to conditions and abuses which make healthy, elderly people sick and feeble, and sick and feeble elderly people dead. Innumerable human service, nursing home, and institutional practices contribute to this. Many elderly people in the community are too poor to eat appropriately, which once more contributes to all sorts of secondary causes of death; violence against elderly people is rampant; in the nursing homes, not enough eating time may be allowed for feeble residents; etc.

5   Infirm people are precipitously moved around from one place to another, which is known to drastically increase the death rate. The list could go on. ...

We should also be aware that for the first time in about 2500 years, the medical profession is abandoning its radical commitment to life, and is massively participating in death-making, even to the point where in state after state, new capital punishment laws are being enacted under which medical personnel would actively participate in the execution of prisoners by means of poisonous injections. ...

Three dynamics appear to prevent many people from recognizing the new wave of death-making: they have been insulated from the evidence; they have seen the evidence, but it has been so disguised that they could not perceive the truth; even if they saw the evidence, and even if it were not disguised, they simply cannot believe that large-scale "euthanasia" could become a reality in our society.

Disguises of the new "euthanasia" movement have included measures (to mention only some samples) such as the following: (a) the use of all sorts of babble that detoxifies the many forms of homicide. Killing may be interpreted as good science, good medicine ("healing intervention," "therapeutic"), compassion ("helping to die"), good law, and even solid theology, religion, and Christianity (e.g., Whytehead, 1979; Whytehead & Chidwick, 1977). (b) The disfigurement (e.g. injection of dyes) of infants prior to abortion, so that attending personnel will not view the aborted infant as human. (c) A major disguised form of death-making is for handicapped people to be dumped into the community without support systems. There, many are severely victimized in any number of ways (having their income and property taken away, being sexually abused and physically assaulted, etc.); many enter into a violent street culture in which they are weak members; many end up in penury, hunger, and poor health. (d) Few people are able to see the connections between legitimized and medicalized mass psychoactive drugging of people and their resulting secondary incapacitation and death. ...

---

26 From: "Extermination: Disabled People in Nazi Germany," 1980, *Disabled USA*, 4(2), 22–4.

Central to the teaching on 'deathmaking' have been the parallels with the 'euthanasia' programme in Nazi Germany, with many lessons being drawn from the processes, the organizations and participants involved, and the underlying values with regard to attitudes to human life of that programme. The next extract is, again, the earliest published account of that process, in a disability journal. Such was the sensitivity of Wolfensberger's views, in particular his inclusion of abortion as one of the 'deathmaking' processes, that the journal thought it necessary to write an introduction clarifying their own position – a feature of being associated with Wolfensberger that was already familiar to some, and was to become much more common as he continued to raise this particular issue, despite the issue itself later becoming one which generated much public debate. The extract is taken from the main text; an inserted 'panel' describing the varying degrees of 'those who took part' is excluded.

Very few people seem to be aware that there are many ominous parallelisms between the mass extermination of handicapped people in Nazi Germany between 1939 and 1945 and what is happening in the United States today. In part, this lack of consciousness derives from unfamiliarity with the basic facts of the events in Germany.

The groundwork for the killing was laid by a 1920 (!) pre-Nazi book (Binding & Hoche, 1920), by two professors of law and psychiatry respectively. ...

The book argued that "euthanasia" was kind, compassionate, reasonable, moral, and cost-beneficial. This book not only served the Nazi purpose well but convinced so many people – especially intellectuals and academicians – that they later participated in "euthanasia" even if they were not Nazis.

World War II provided the opportunity for which the Nazis had waited, and in October of 1939, Hitler authorized the "euthanasia" program. Initially, those institutionalized people were exterminated who were more severely retarded, mentally disordered, tubercular, chronically ill, cerebral palsied, epileptic, etc.

With the quick and easy success of the early phase of the "program," and the fact that a death-making apparatus had been structured that needed further victims in order to survive, the criteria for "inclusion" broadened rapidly into at least four directions, toward people who were *(a) less severely afflicted, (b) physically atypical but not necessarily impaired (e.g., dwarfs), (c) suspected of genetic or racial taint, and (d) devalued mostly because of social characteristics (e.g., gypsies).*

In time, the above group came to include people who had behavior problems or enuresis, who had odd-shaped ears, or who had eyes, hair, or complexion that was unusually dark.

The logistics and organization of the program were probably superior to any large-scale human service enterprise before or since. It began with the most meticulous preparation and planning, detailed working out of methods, the formation of agencies to conduct different parts of the plan (registration, transportation, etc.), the installation of death-dealing equipment, and finally "the action."

Despite the complexity of involving the whole chain of mental institutions, hospitals, universities, professors, etc., and despite war and shortages, everything went like clockwork.

By 1945, up to one million handicapped people had been put to death, including an estimated 100,000 retarded and 200,000 mentally disordered people. Few retarded adults survived; entire institutions were closed down ("de-institutionalized"). Some institutions became extermination centers to which residents from others were shipped to be gassed.

However, there were also extermination units at other institutions, and much killing (especially of children) took place in a large number of pediatric clinics and other medical settings. The use of gas was first piloted in psychiatric institutions. Then the gas – and the medical personnel who had learned to use it – were shipped east to set up the gas chambers in which millions of Jews were killed.

In addition to (and later, in lieu of) gas, poison was injected or given orally; people were bodily exposed to weather, stress, etc., in order to make them sick; medical help was withheld; and young children, especially, were starved to death.

One of the major lessons to us is the linguistic, symbolic, and operational "detoxification" that took place, and that blinded people into participation or collusion.

For instance, the modern arguments that redefine human life were anticipated by Binding and Hoche in such phrases as: "Life without value for itself or society"; "creatures of no value at all who are quite an obstacle"; "a burden serving no useful purpose"; "a life whose continuation is of no interest to any reasonably thinking person"; "the irretrievably lost"; "weaklings"; "life devoid of value"; and the "mentally dead."

The modern euphemisms for the murder of afflicted individuals were also anticipated by terms such as: "death assistance"; "a blessing for the suffering"; "granting death"; "submitting a person to this healing intervention"; "a pure healing action"; "a formulation born out of deep compassion"; "death with dignity"; "abbreviating life"; and "final release."

Unlike people in human services, the Nazis were superb learners and continued the pre-Nazi tradition of detoxification:

Buses that took handicapped people to extermination centers were operated by the "Patients Transport Corporation"; much of the killing was under the aegis of a "Committee for Research on Hereditary and Constitutional Severe Diseases," and several psychiatric facilities instituted "in-service training" on mass killing techniques.

The events of Nazi Germany are not merely a chapter in the history of violence, but a major chapter in the history of medicine, and especially psychiatry, although the psychiatric profession has not oriented itself to that fact.

Similarly, the German "euthanasia" program was not primarily German, but the logical outcome of a materialistic value system.

In Germany, the moral deterioration of "materialistic medicine" was such that the results of experiments performed on concentration camp prisoners were openly presented at medical meetings even after 1942, much as our medical journals today once more freely report infanticide, and carry demands of all sorts of "euthanasia" – not to mention the accomplished fact of from one to two million abortions a year in the United States alone.

People who refuse to acknowledge that all of the forms of "death-making" are related, and who believe that they can contain a legitimated form of death-making to narrow and specific circumstances, and to a highly restricted range of human life, are deluding themselves; at least, they seem to ignore some important lessons from history.

27   From: "Bill F.: signs of the times read from the life of one mentally retarded man," 1989, *Mental Retardation*, 27 (6), 369–73.

As noted in the above extract, one of the key challenges presented by the teaching of many workshops on the issue of 'deathmaking' was not just an acceptance or otherwise of the analysis, but a reflection on one's own life and experiences, in particular with devalued people. A number of associates of Wolfensberger and his Training Institute were moved by this reflection to make time in their lives, in a variety of ways, to be with such people. Wolfensberger himself was, and still is at the time of writing, involved with a group in Syracuse, known as Unity Kitchen Community of the Catholic Worker. The next extract uses some of that experience to illustrate, in stark form, the real live 'wounding and deathmaking' of vulnerable people. It is an edited and expanded version of a funeral oration for a member of the Unity Kitchen Community, which was then published in the journal *Mental Retardation*, though as he makes clear in the article, the lessons to be learnt go far beyond this particular group of vulnerable people. The first part of the paper traces the history of a person referred to as 'Bill F.' from institutionalization in his teens, through involvement with the street culture, the prison system, further attempts at community living, and finally a relative degree of community involvement, albeit in a segregated apartment block in the impoverished area of the city. So much is in accordance with the 'wounds' identified in Chapter 1. The greater dimension of threats to the lives of vulnerable people is picked up in the second part of the paper, which is the more immediate story of Bill F. in the last year of his life. The fact of his deteriorating health, especially diabetes, and his involvement with Unity Kitchen, had also been noted as this extract begins.

...

About a year before his death, Bill's condition deteriorated even more. He was fortunate to be allowed 4 hours of home aide help per day, and doubly fortunate that in these times of such dysfunctionality in the home aide domain, his aide was very kind and patient, even when Bill had his cranky episodes, during which it was hard to please him.

Not so fortunate was that his Medicaid dentures never did fit well. They often rattled when he talked. Then, about 3 months before his death, one of the teeth on the dentures broke, and he quit wearing them altogether – with the consequences that his personal appearance was badly degraded and he became very limited in what he could eat. Because Bill's diabetic diet was so bland anyway, both things together diminished his interest in food. Bill told a Unity Kitchen volunteer that the dental clinic at Upstate Hospital (a state university teaching hospital) had told him that his new teeth would not be ready for a first try-out until about 7 weeks later. These 2 months without teeth must surely have had something to do with his considerable weight loss during this period.

During his last year, Bill's legs had also been giving out. He began to actually need his cane for walking – and then he got a wheelchair. He could still go out in it if someone pushed him, usually his friend Bob, Then, even in his apartment, he moved around less and finally needed a walker there. Because it might take forever to get one from Medicaid, Unity Kitchen volunteers got one for him. Finally, he had a few painful falls. When he was found on the floor after such a fall, he was taken to Upstate Hospital. There he fell once again trying to go to the bathroom. As seemed to happen every time there, he also got tested and diagnosed to death, only this time, it was more than a figure of speech.

... A volunteer visited Bill on Monday, the day after his admission and was pained to see that he had three tubes running things in and out of him and bloody patches all over his body, especially his arms and hands. He was very alert but in foul spirits. The volunteer noticed that his lunch arrived almost an hour late, which is very bad when one is in a debilitated diabetic state – and on top of that, it was the wrong lunch. There was hardly anything there that he could eat without teeth. Thus, the very same agency that was withholding his teeth was giving him food he could not chew. The volunteer, who had come for a quick visit, ended up spending hours mincing a tough slab of very dry roast beef, cutting string beans into tiny bits, and helping Bill to eat. Bill choked several times, and in several hours only managed to eat about 20 per cent of his lunch before he rejected the rest.

When the volunteer expressed concern to a hospital staff person about Bill's emaciated condition and wrong lunch, he got a characteristically modern high-tech response: not to worry, Bill was on an I-V drip that would provide the needed nourishment. The volunteer caught a registered nurse and said that surely Bill's lack of teeth must be a factor in his weight loss and diet, and why couldn't the dental clinic, being in and of the same hospital, fix his teeth right away while he was there. For once, an ally had been found. She agreed and called the dental clinic; they said they had never heard of Bill and had no record on him. It took another day and two more calls before they found Bill's record, but because he had by now missed his appointment, they would not see him again until a week later, and then it would take at least yet another month to make the dentures.

Another Unity Kitchen volunteer visited Bill at noon the next day, Tuesday. This time, the lunch was properly pureed and on time. Another Kitchen volunteer visited him that evening as well. Bill's friend Bob was also in and out several times throughout these days. On Wednesday, a volunteer visited at noon and found an empty bed with an uneaten lunch tray. Bill's roommates told him that Bill had been taken for yet more X-rays just before the lunch arrived. The volunteer sat down to wait for Bill's return when his inner alarms went off. The volunteer started roaming through the building looking for the radiology clinic and there, in a hallway off to the side, all by himself, sat a little, frail, white-haired old man in a wheelchair, half slumped over the side, semiconscious. The volunteer thought he might be dying right then. When he made contact with two staff people some minutes later (most of them being out for lunch), he let himself be buffaloed by their attitude of "the prescribed diagnostic tests must go on," even though there were still four other delays. First, they had failed to bring Bill on a gurney as they should have in the first place, and it took quite a while to get one. Then, Bill screamed in pain when they moved him onto the gurney and then onto the X-ray table, which slowed things down. Then, after they had taken him off the X-ray table and put him back on the gurney, they decided they needed more X-rays. He was transferred once more onto the X-ray table with more screams, then brought out again. They then had to call for an authorized person to wheel him back to his ward. No sooner had Bill arrived back on the ward than an alert student nurse, after taking one look at him, raised the alarm and about a dozen people converged on him. They brought a giant syringe and injected glucose into him. Because he had not been given his lunch on time, he had gone into an insulin reaction and almost died. But his recovery was rapid and seemed miraculous. When things had calmed down, the volunteer was able to administer almost a whole meal to Bill, and he was in top spirits. Another volunteer came at suppertime, but Bill was still full from his late lunch and ate little.

At noon Thursday, a volunteer came and found that despite Wednesday's close call, Bill's breakfast that day had been 1 hour late, and lunch arrived 2 hours late. Further, there was yet another diet error, because tea had been sent instead of the protein-rich broth on his diet sheet, which makes a big difference. A senior dietitian showed up and evidenced profound displeasure and embarrassment but could not account for all the errors that had been occurring. By this time, Bill was withdrawn and ate little. Another volunteer came for supper. Bill ate very little and suddenly expired quietly. The hospital chaplain came and said the prayers for the dead. Though Bill's friends had known that things were not going well for him, his ability to bounce back on Wednesday, and during previous hospital stays, had misled them to expect at least a temporary comeback.

Some Interpretations and Lessons

Valued people in our society rarely die from broken arms, broken teeth, or hangnails – but as we see over and over all the time, societally devalued people do. For instance, in Bill's case, it seemed that for want of a tooth, the whole denture was lost; for want of the denture, appetite was lost; for want of appetite, nourishment was lost; for want of nourishment, bodily weight and strength were lost; for want of strength, three falls occurred. Because of these falls, Bill had to go to the hospital, and, there, Unity Kitchen volunteers were also told that if he recovered, he would almost certainly have to go to a nursing home, because Medicaid not only did not want to increase the hours of home aide he received each day, but wanted to cut it down to 2. So it might have been that for want of a tooth, Bill's apartment would have been lost had he lived; but as it was, his life itself was lost, at least in the sense that all these things must surely have played a role in abbreviating it. The irony of it all is that there were so many well-meaning, competent, and dedicated health workers involved, but the bankruptcy of the overall system just scrambled their minds, defeated their efforts, and even blinded them to some very overarching truths.

Some may say that Bill's life was atypically bad for retarded persons, but we know better. The kinds of things that happened to him happen to innumerable others, though there are also innumerable variations, and an infinite creativity, in the perpetration of atrocities on societally devalued people. Nor is the issue of mental retardation the crucial one; the same realities apply to a broad spectrum of people at the lower end of societal valuation. What is particularly noteworthy in Bill's case is that unlike many devalued people, he did have several friends from the privileged and competent sectors of society, but the assaults on devalued people are so intense that often even efforts of several such defenders are not sufficient to prevent vast harm from being done. In one extreme case that we have encountered, a moderately retarded young man, dumped out of an institution, had at least a dozen competent associates in the community; and yet his problems, and the attacks on him, were so numerous that the efforts of all of these associates were absorbed to the point where they became stretched to exhaustion, and still he only escaped into, at best, a tenuous marginality.

Why is it that the professional literature in our field almost totally fails to reflect this aspect of the phenomenology of so many retarded people? Has the prevailing cultural insanity established a schizophrenia in which the phenomenology of the professional/scientific sector has little overlap with that of the people from whom it derives its identity and economic existence?

Although I have reservations about various elements of contemporary liberation ideology, one of its tenets clearly has a great deal of validity, at least for most people most of the time, and that is that one's entire epistemology can be constrained, and even become grossly invalid, because of lack of a relevant phenomenological experience base. In the case at hand, we are talking about the phenomenology of oppression that is the lot of a large minority in our culture – roughly a third of it.

In over 30 years in human services, I have known many thousands of people who make their living in it. Of these, a significant minority rarely have personal contact with the kinds of needy people from whose existence they derive their income, position, prestige, etc. Some I have known have not had any such contacts in many a year. Another segment – it seems the great majority – only have such contact as part of their work and its associated roles. Obviously, both of these groups, who include not only a lot of administrators, professors, and researchers but also clinicians, see the lives of the oppressed and suffering from "the top down" instead of "the bottom up,"

There is a third segment of people who live off human services, and among them are those who have the greatest likelihood of seeing things from the bottom up: they are the workers (a small minority, as far as I can tell) who go beyond their duties and engage in what I call "life-sharing".... . Nor is it enough to do this on rare occasions, or early in one's life; one really needs to do this on an ongoing basis in order not to be overwhelmed by the consciousness and imagery of the ruling imperial structures. The imperial imagery, and even language, very effectively nullifies the reality of oppression and thus muffles the cries of the oppressed and their expressions of grief until these are no longer perceived. This is why even ethnographic study, or so-called "participant observation," of devalued people may fail to establish a valid epistemology. Although many people engage in such studies as students or researchers, they so often still do it "from the top down" and thus still "do not see."...

28 From: "Let's hang up 'quality of life' as a hopeless term," 1994, in D. Goode (ed.), *Quality of Life for Persons with Disabilities: International Perspectives and Issues*, 285–321, Cambridge, MA: Brookline Books.

In the final extract of this chapter, taken from a far-ranging and critical chapter in a book entitled *Quality of Life for Persons with Disabilities*, we find perhaps the most analytical exposition of the various threads that have been covered in this and previous chapters, and lead to a powerful conclusion about the threats to the lives of vulnerable people. The use of language, the unconscious philosophies that led to a dramatic change in societal values, the power of social devaluation and its logical conclusion, and the participation in this process by the human service system, in particular the medical system – all come together in the elements of the chapter that have to do with 'quality of life' (referred to by the acronym QOL throughout the chapter and the editor's notes) and 'deathmaking'.

…

The sequence of thinking and argument in invoking QOL on behalf of deathmaking has gone something like this.

1   Right from the first, proponents of a QOL concept in a deathmaking context conveyed the message that the value of living was related to the quality of one's living or life. Even the very grammar of the term "quality of life" facilitated a line of thinking that went via "quality of life" to "quality of living," to the "quality of a life," from there to both "the quality of a person" and the "value of a life."

2   Once people began to equate quality of life with value of life or living, they could easily be recruited into endorsing a belief many people already had been harboring unconsciously anyway, namely, that some people are less valuable than others.

3   In turn, by characterizing different lives, and different phases of single and individual lives, as having more or less quality, the idea was conveyed that the value of lives and of people could and should be judged in a quantitative rather than qualitative fashion, i.e., in terms of continua without clear and unequivocal benchmarks, rather than in terms of qualitative, discrete and indivisible criterion entities. In other words, some lives were to be judged as more valuable than others, and some parts of one's life (e.g., one's youth) were judged as more valuable than other parts (e.g., one's senescence). Thus, the unborn were automatically of little or no value, the newborn and very young were less valuable than adults, and as one progressed from one's mid-years into senescence, one again became less valuable.

4   Once the value of life is defined in terms of its quality, it seems inevitable that people who are judged by society to be valued and productive would also be judged as having more quality of life than others, and would therefore be given preference over societally devalued people in matters such as medical treatment.

The chapter then goes on to note the philosophical roots of the above views being found in Nietzsche, and to some extent in Hobbes and Darwin, especially the rejection of Judeo-Christian values by the first of those. It then makes the connection between Nietzsche and the Nazis, and the language and influence on the 'euthanasia' movement of the 1920 book by Binding and Hoche, all discussed above, linking this to the notion of killing people thought to be of low utility. Also noting the fact that such actions as the 'euthanasia' movement and 'materialized medicine' were about to be actioned in other countries as well, merely 'lying low' immediately after the war, and then reasserting themselves, the chapter goes on to look at what Wolfensberger regards as two key events in shifting people's thinking about individuals as 'humans' to the idea of 'persons'. One was the publication by a theologian named Fletcher (e.g. 1972, 1975) of what he called 'indicators of personhood' – a set of 15 somewhat arbitrary criteria, such as 'self-awareness', 'balance and rationality of feelings' and 'concern for others', which determined one's place on a scale of 'personhood'. The other was a US Supreme Court ruling in 1973 that unborn children were 'not persons'.

...

These two developments sketched above convinced many people (a) that the morality of killing someone should be drawn on the issue of personhood, not humanhood, and (b) that personhood was not a qualitative entity but a quantitative continuum, so that the less personhood someone possessed, the more permissible it was to kill him/her/it. In other words, the construct of "quality of life" came to replace the traditional Judeo-Christian belief in the absolute and intrinsic value of the life of each individual, or what one might call the "quality of the value of the human." The concept of "quality of life" also began to be used to characterize the lives of individuals rather than of societies, ... the three concepts of *quality of life, value of life,* and *value of people* began to merge; and the merits of the lives of certain individuals could now be denied. Some people could be interpreted as having no value whatever. ...

One thing that all of this illustrates is just how difficult it is to think straight or moralize well once one has abandoned moral absolutes, and perhaps even abandoned thought framed in terms of discrete and qualitative criteria. ...

Going on to highlight the development, via the shift of 'quality of life' from a population term to an individual one, of various groups being subject to 'legalized medicalized killing', the chapter continues with retrospective accounts from clinicians of how, before it was seen as legal, various impaired infants were quietly disposed of, through more open advocacy and practice of decisions on which impaired infants should be 'allowed to die'. The observations are then extended, as covered in earlier extracts, to the range of groups at risk of being 'made dead'. We pick up the chapter as it then returns to the direct link between the term 'quality of life' and deathmaking.

... It was particularly since ca. 1980 that the term and construct of QOL has been seized by parties (including materialized medicine) that promote the deathmaking of members of unwanted classes. These parties have used the QOL term and construct in order to promote their goals, often in ways that sow confusion among more naive people, and thereby recruit them into acquiescence to – or even collaboration with – deathmaking. ...

For instance, deathmaking leader Peter Singer (1983) explicitly titled one of his articles, "Sanctity of life or quality of life?" In this article, Singer said that compared to a "severely defective human infant," a healthy dog or pig "will often ... have superior capacities ... for ... anything ... that can plausibly be considered morally significant."

Yet more recently, deathmaking promotion has taken the twist of persuading people to commit suicide, or to help others to commit suicide – and QOL talk has played a big role in this. For example, the notorious suicide assistant Dr. Jack Kevorkian claims that he only helps those people to commit suicide (according to some accounts, he also kills people) whose "life quality has to be nil" (*Time* 31

May 1993), but this is either a blatant lie or a gross misinterpretation of "life quality," since some of his victims had very good life conditions, and only poor *long-term* prognosis. ...

After a few more examples of the link of QOL with suicide, the chapter then goes on to examine a further example of the use of language to 'detoxify' deathmaking, namely the use of the word 'futile' when it comes to medical treatment. After citing a number of sources from the 'futility literature', Wolfensberger concludes that ...

One of the profound errors or deceptions that one encounters over and over again ... is that QOL is associated with medical treatment rather than the affected person. Whatever QOL is or is not, it refers to the life circumstances of a person and ... after medicine has done its thing. To link QOL to the medical measure applied, or not applied, is absurd. A smallpox vaccination has no QOL, but a person who gets one may have something that someone can define as QOL. One cannot even say that it is a medical treatment that determines QOL, except in very constrained ways, e.g., when the treatment itself debilitates someone. Otherwise, treatment can only, and at best, *remove obstacles* to QOL [more examples of the 'futility literature' then follow – Ed.]. ...

...

In May 1993, no less than the editor of the *Journal of the American Medical Association* published an editorial (Lundberg, 1993) calling for 90% of US hospitals to have in place by 1996 what the author called "futile care policies," thereby saving up to scores of billions of dollars. He cited as exemplary the policy of one hospital that included in its definition of "futile care" those treatments that do not have a reasonable possibility of restoring "a quality of life that would be satisfactory to the patient." (Of course, in actual practice, people other than the patient often make the determination of satisfactoriness.) And what about all the lowly afflicted people so familiar to us in our work who never had what modernistic medical people would have considered a satisfactory QOL even prior to any treatment at issue? We can easily see how the earlier linkage of the construct of "futility" to QOL in the same journal was a stalking horse for the ever-expanding juggernaut of deathmaking of medically debilitated people, in part in concert with cost-saving arguments. ...

There is then a brief discussion on the economic motives involved in medicalized deathmaking, and the use of essentially economic indicators of quality of life, and resulting quantitative scales, that a critic referred to as the "rather-be-dead rating." It then returns to the issue of vulnerable people, deathmaking and the construct of quality of life, and the subversion of 'the traditional Judeo-Christian belief that human life was intrinsically sacred.' After giving examples, discussed in many different ways throughout this book, of how groups in society, by being classed as 'less human' or even 'non-human' could therefore be vulnerable even within the Judeo-Christian ethic, the chapter proceeds to develop the argument in terms of the inconsistency with which the QOL concept is applied.

...

Once we perceive the politics and historicity of the QOL term, then we are no longer surprised to note that it (and related terms, such as value of life) have an extremely high likelihood of being encountered whenever efforts are underfoot to deprive an impaired or sick person of life. Yet the same people from whose lips QOL language oozes with ease where it serves deathmaking purposes will seldom be heard to invoke the term in order to decry the gross injustices that are inflicted on certain groups and classes in society by those who are more advantaged and privileged.

One can turn this discovery around, and assert that when people who virtually never invoke QOL language in pursuit of social justice and in confrontation of systematic societal oppression begin to invoke it in reference to a debilitated or devalued person – and especially in medical contexts – then it is likely that a fundamental commitment (even if still unconscious) to death has already been made. This likelihood is further and dramatically increased if QOL language is emitted contiguous with other deathmaking-related terms, such as "death with dignity," "right to die," "brain death," "persistent vegetative state," etc., or when QOL is discussed in explicit connection with whether a person should live or die.

Once people got the idea that life with low quality was not worth living, then people who had been deprived of the good things of life by others, usually via oppression and devaluation, could be said to be "better off dead." This results in a gruesome vicious circle. On the one hand, people *always* oppress. This is a human universal: all societies sooner or later engage in social stratification and oppression of their lower strata, and often also of populations outside their own. Such oppression is normatively onerous, and produces what could be called low QOL. By the above circular logic, this implies that at a certain point, oppressed people develop something that one can call – and that has occasionally been called – a "need to die." ...

After further quotations from Nietzsche that lend support to the 'need to die' construct, a number of examples are quoted of such a construct being measurable, scales to do so, or at least a decision being made by the medical profession on the standard of QOL below which a person could be allowed to die, even if they, or their family, had different standards. Crucially, such indices and decisions make reference to criteria that come from the very fact of devaluation and oppression. The extension of this argument is then made.

We might also contemplate the curious fact that QOL constructs are often so conceptualized or operationalized as to actually reinforce the values that underlie the construct. In our modernistically materialistic society, the good things in life are considered to include youthfulness, beauty, intelligence, education, competence, material possessions, and hedonistic sensualistic enjoyment thereof. Thus, the ugly, old, retarded, poor, suffering, etc., who lack these qualities, or who embody their opposites, will automatically be seen or defined to "have" low quality of life, and therefore be better off dead.

Furthermore, and quite obviously, it will be inevitable that it will be people who possess the attributes perceived to make for a high quality of life who would *decide* the needs, quality of life, and life itself, of people who are deficient in them. However, the people who lack them commonly have been brainwashed into the same value system, and can often be brought to agree that they would, indeed, be better off dead if they cannot be or have what the privileged sector of society is and has. …

Within such a framework, there occurs a radical reduction in any incentive to perceive or comprehend the vicious circle of societal wound-striking, oppression and deathmaking. What is interpreted as low QOL does not get addressed so much by raising consciousness about oppression as by making dead the "incumbents" or "inhabitants" of low QOL … .

Many more examples of the use of QOL in deathmaking are then given, especially the use of a 'formula' produced by Shaw (1977) widely used in Wolfensberger's teaching as an example of the absurdity of attempting to 'measure' QOL. The deconstruction of the formula then follows, with the ironic contrast with the fact of similar such schemas being used in many countries for the legal killing, or lack of treatment, of various vulnerable groups, such as elderly people, people with HIV/AIDS, and so on. Our extract ends with the concluding remarks of the section regarding the link between QOL and deathmaking, beginning with the issue of what the vulnerable people might think.

…

While many afflicted people are getting brainwashed into believing that they ought to be dead, advocates of QOL criteria for deathmaking purposes have commonly not been particularly interested in ascertaining, or acknowledging, what handicapped or otherwise afflicted people themselves think about the value or quality of their lives. Yet every formal (e.g., Diamond, 1977, p.70) or informal inquiry I have heard of has found that the vast majority of handicapped people were glad they were born, wanted to live, and had positive anticipations for the future. (Even some non-handicapped people keep expressing the same sentiments.) That afflicted people are so often not asked these questions should not surprise one, since we noted before that the people perceived to possess QOL will be deciding who does not.

However, even if society did succeed in making the lives of handicapped people so miserable that they say they would rather die or wished that they had never been born, this still could not be used as sufficient moral grounds by others to grant them their wish. ...

Chapter 7

Relationships with, and lessons from, vulnerable people

Introduction

Throughout this book we have emphasized the connectedness of the different aspects of Wolfensberger's teaching and writing, and the make-up of this concluding chapter makes the point very well. On a number of occasions throughout earlier chapters, reference has been made to possible 'action implications' of the ideas Wolfensberger is putting across. They invariably begin with a proviso that it is up to each person to reflect on, and make a personal decision on, the material being presented before getting into such implications – in contrast to what Wolfensberger would see as the 'modernistic' tendency to go straight to such 'solutions' before understanding clearly what they are solutions *to*, and, indeed, Wolfensberger's suggestions are not 'solutions' but merely what a personal set of actions might be.

That being said, the notion of personal relationships with, commitment to, and learning the lessons from, devalued and vulnerable people, is a message that has already been conveyed in various ways. This chapter, therefore, is merely an amplification of that notion, rather than a separate subject in itself. In addition, since the sources of Wolfensberger's thinking on these matters have also been covered in the Introduction to the book and elsewhere, editorial comment will be less than elsewhere.

Finally, though we noted earlier that this book has largely excluded Wolfensberger's specifically religious writings, a collection of which is found in Gaventa & Coulter (2001), and which expand considerably on a number of the themes only touched on in these extracts, the presence of religious ideas, in the normally accepted sense, is inevitably found more readily here, and we end with a short extract from one of the items from the above book.

The extracts for this chapter therefore focus on the two aspects of the title. First, the review dealing with the L'Arche movement, especially from its early phase in the 1970s, raises key issues of life-sharing between vulnerable people and others. The second aspect concerns lessons to be learnt from vulnerable people, in this instance people called 'mentally retarded' in Wolfensberger's country. Both aspects, in essence, highlight what society can *receive* from such people: their contribution – often unrecognized but very real – to the betterment of our humanity. This, readers will note, echoes particularly the final extract of Chapter 4, in which advocates spoke tellingly of the benefits given to them by the advocacy relationship.

29 From: Review of *Enough Room for Joy: Jean Vanier's L'Arche: A Message for our Time*, 1974, *Canadian Welfare*, 50(6), 14–17.

The first extract comes from a review by Wolfensberger of a book on the L'Arche movement, in which he not only highlights the key lessons of the movement, but gives some small clue as to its influence on his thinking, a point taken up in later extracts.

There are some leaders and movements which elicit bi-polar responses. If a person is for one of them, he is very, very for it, and one who is against it thinks it's horrid. So it is to a degree in regard to Jean Vanier and the movement of L'Arche.

The movement of L'Arche is not very old, and I first heard about it in late 1971. One could describe it on several levels. On a relatively low one, one could say that L'Arche is a movement to establish humane commune-like residences for retarded adults, somewhat similar to the Camphill movement. Most of these communities are relatively small, and while they maintain a certain apartness from society, they nevertheless tend to be rather well integrated into the community. Many people come on a voluntary basis to work and live in these communes, because it is a basic tenet of L'Arche that a deeply wounded person's self-esteem cannot be improved much if all those who help him are paid to do so. Somewhere, someone must choose to live with the wounded person – and if this is to be constructive, he must do it gladly, with joy, and in a genuinely sharing fashion.

But on a higher level, L'Arche is much more. It is an intensely spiritual Christian movement which, in many ways, plays a function and meets a need for our time as did the monastic orders and other spiritual movements for another era. While having deep roots in Catholicism, the movement is remarkably ecumenical in that its particular approach to spirituality not only appeals to other Christians, but also to Jews, other non-Christians, and even to non-believers.

In its spiritual domain, the movement emphasizes a number of points: awareness of one's own weaknesses, and the need to openly and honestly acknowledge them; the rejection of the absorbing and nervous pursuit of hedonism and possessions that is prevalent within society today; a commitment to a life of at least inner and spiritual poverty, and in many instances of external poverty as well; a concern for all members of society who have been rejected and devalued; an urgent belief that on the international plane, the pursuit of materialism, the unwillingness to share wealth, and the continued armament race is very apt to bring the world to ruin; and a deep sense that the privileged world has a responsibility to the underprivileged or so-called Third World.

It can be readily seen that the basic tenets of the movement of L'Arche as sketched above point strongly to the creation of world-wide community, and the overcoming of irrational and maladaptive nationalisms. Indeed, L'Arche establishments have not only been initiated in four continents, but persons who identify themselves with the movement of L'Arche (which they might do without necessarily joining one of the establishments) soon develop an intimate feeling of brotherhood and community with all other friends within the movement, and with its establishments across the world. There is great interchange and movement among them, exchange visits with fiestas of joyful celebration, all sorts of letters and publications being circulated, etc.

Within the movement of L'Arche, the mentally retarded are a primary focus of involvement but there is also a high level of concern with the imprisoned, the mentally disordered, the poor, and the homeless such as the homeless and transient men of the streets.

For a person who has taken an entirely professional-technical approach to human services – the way most professionals tend to do it – it usually comes as a major surprise, and quite often as an existential shock, to recognize the intrinsic validity of one of the major tenets of the movement of L'Arche: that the superficially weak member of society may, in fact, be really no weaker and no different than anybody else, in that we all have profound weaknesses, profound immoralities, etc.; that therefore it is only proper that human services not be conceptualized and structured as a one-way street in which the handicapped are always the recipients; and that the apparently non-handicapped person can receive as much from the apparently weak ones as they may receive from him.

What gifts can the apparently strong persons receive from the apparently weak, and especially retarded, ones? Some examples would include a much more honest affectivity which so often is lost in the intellectual and achievement-oriented person; a sense of joy, which is often derived from great appreciation of the simpler things in life as well as from often having worked out profound suffering in a spirit of serenity; a desophistication which helps the strong to perceive that every single human being is weak; and a sense of being accepted for one's personal qualities or in one's peculiar uniqueness, rather than for some function which one may play in the world, but which, at least to a retarded observer, is not too intelligible. Also, only at gatherings of the movement of L'Arche have I witnessed retarded people emanating the most profound spiritual wisdoms – almost prophecy in the technical, theological sense – which one often seeks but rarely finds in the pulpits of our cathedrals.

L'Arche brings yet another crushing surprise for the professional-technical human service worker: if he is perceptive and honest, he will learn from L'Arche that *professional-technical skills are totally inadequate in serving other human beings.* Nor is it sufficient that these skills be coupled with humanism, charity, and good intentions. Beyond these, it is absolutely essential to view the person served as a peer, and to be prepared to adopt service forms and lifestyles which result in significant life-sharing with him. Thus, it is a common phenomenon to see L'Arche workers share their own grief and suffering not only with each other, but with the handicapped persons whom, superficially, they may be perceived as serving, and yet by whom, in turn, they themselves are served and helped. Where in human services do helpers consciously go to the "helpee" for help? In what school of service thought and theory is such reciprocity ever acknowledged as legitimate, or even desirable? Yet a L'Arche worker may cry out his problems and griefs on the bosom of a severely retarded resident, and find profound succor and solid spiritual and perhaps even practical counsel.

To my mind, the futility of professionalism is particularly apparent in the recent developments in the field of mental health and aging. In aging, our human service system has adopted an almost 100% technical-professional route, with virtually all of the available professionalism, almost all of the brainpower, almost all of the available money (and lots of it!) and other resources being devoted to the establishment of a service system which is derived essentially and ultimately from a devaluation of elderly people, and which is aimed almost entirely toward total and mass segregation of the elderly, typically in large establishments which can be described with utter justification as nothing but "cities for the socialization unto death." Yet not one major nationally prominent leader, either in Canada or in the United States ... has risen up publicly in moral indignation against this rapid, huge, and North America-wide development.

In mental health, where by definition we are dealing almost exclusively with psychically wounded people, the establishment service model is built entirely upon a profound devaluation of clients, as evidenced by the tremendous status differential that is erected between clients and staff; and by the fact that virtually nowhere in the contemporary psychiatric literature (except its devalued fringe) is the desirability of helper and client living, eating, worshipping, shopping, and genuinely recreating together acknowledged as either practical – nor even at least as an ideal. A field where there is so much money, education, and brains, and so little insight, is bankrupt.

From a more uniquely Christian viewpoint, it may – but should not be – surprising that a movement of such powerful impact (as L'Arche has proven to be in such a short time) should emanate from retarded and other deeply devalued people, and those who work with them. It is often forgotten that from a purely historical viewpoint, the role of Jesus was not so much that of the calculating revolutionary, the blundering rabbi, or what have you, but that above all, his role in the eyes of his contemporaries was that of a dangerous mad man – an obvious point, and yet one that is little recognized even within Christianity itself. Vanier points out again and again that from one's own weakness can come one's greatest strengths, and the weak of society could evoke, or be, some of its greatest strengths – if society would only take a different and more moral view. ...

The extract ends with a more specific review of the book itself, which we omit, as we proceed from what Wolfensberger saw as an ideal form of life-sharing of valued and devalued people to the lessons to be learnt from vulnerable people.

30 From: "Of human courage and dignity," 1970, *Mental Retardation News* (newsletter of the National Association for Retarded Children), 19(9), 6.

The first of these comes from a contemporary example, in the 1970s, of the exemplification of human courage and dignity by one person in one incident, written in the first person for a newsletter-type publication of a national parents group; the second, an example of Wolfensberger's use of historical characters and trends to illustrate some contemporary issues. The first extract begins with an account of how, at a summer programme of study and visits to services across Nebraska, Wolfensberger and the students he was leading attended a supper-seminar in the town of North Platte. The coordinator of the regional mental retardation services gave a brief address.

...

He read a letter which the director of the local sheltered workshop had just received from a mother whose two sons had perished in a fire which had destroyed their home. One of the sons, already a young adult, had been a worker in the workshop because he was a mongoloid and severely retarded. The letter, with spelling errors and exactly as written, follows:

Dear Mike & all

I was in North Platte on a monday but the shop was close
I wanted to thank all of you for every thing you had done for Robert. He was so proud of his job and the ability to do things on his own.
I am very proud of him as he went to the back room to save his brother. He had Donald from the head of the bed to the foot if he had only a few more minites he would of had Donald out – even tho we know Donald was dead at the time.
I am sending his one check back as they say it would not go thru the machine. put the money in your fund so your books will balance.
To day was my first day back at work. It was a long day but I know I have to keep busy. My two boys was my whole life so now I have to start over. My husband is very under standing – was hurt very bad also.
If I can be of any help at any time please feel free to let me know. I feel I proved to the world a retarded child has a place in the world and can be a use ful person.
Many thanks for every thing,

as ever,

(signature and town of residence)

The check the mother enclosed had been carried by the boy; it was burned at the edges, and that was the reason it would not go through the magnetic check-reading machine. It was for 47 cents.

The workshop director then spoke in an almost tear-choked voice; he stated that he would never relinquish this check, that he would keep it as a symbol of the courage of a retarded boy, and that he did not care if his books remained forever unbalanced because of this action. Our students were deeply moved, and so was I. The incident reminded me of an article entitled "The Dignity of Risk," and written by a friend of mine, Chaplain Perske of the Kansas Neurological Institute [Perske, 1972 – Ed.]. In this article, he pointed out that we so rarely think of the mentally retarded as having certain positive qualities that are basic to humanness, such as courage, even though the ideology of normalization and our perception of the retarded as fully human would tell us that they should generally be expected to share all our human emotions – not merely our negative ones, such as fear. Chaplain Perske also reminded us that there is dignity in risk, and that it is dehumanizing to remove all danger from the lives of the retarded. After all, we take for granted that there is risk and danger in our lives, and the lives of our non-retarded children!

Robert could have led a sheltered existence, perhaps in some residential haven for the retarded where no demands are imposed, and where risks are virtually eliminated. There, he might have lived to an old age; but to me, in his charity-inspired and heroic death in the flames, he had found greater dignity.

---

31 From: "Eulogy for a mentally retarded jester," 1982, *Mental Retardation*, 20(6), 269–70.

In a number of his taught workshops, Wolfensberger has used a wealth of historical material to illustrate trends and issues of contemporary relevance. In the previous chapter we had a short glimpse of this in relation to the lessons for contemporary issues of life and death from the German 'euthanasia' movement. In the next extract, the theme of this chapter is continued, in the account of the positive regard in which people, currently devalued, were held historically by the recognition of certain gifts they possessed. It consists of a modern translation of an old English poetic eulogy, author unknown, to a 'court fool' of Henry VIII, the king of England from 1509–47, and Wolfensberger's reflections thereon. The man, who is described as 'almost certainly retarded', was known by the name Lobe, and the extract begins with its source. Because of the importance of the reference notes, they are included with their original notation.

...

The eulogy was preserved in the Rawlinson manuscript collection at the Bodleian Library of Oxford University. Rawlinson lived from 1690 to 1755. The eulogy has been reprinted in several sources, mostly those dealing with fools (e.g., Swain, 1932; Welsford, 1935) ...

"Epitaph of Lobe, the King's Fool"

O lobbe Lobe,[1] on your soul God have mercy,
For as Peter is princeps apostolorum,[2]
So you too may be declared clearly,
Of all fools that ever were, stultus stultorum.[3]
Surely your soul is in regna polorum,[4]
By reason of reason you had none,
Yet all fools are not dead, Lobe, though you be gone.

The loss of you, Lobe, makes many sad,
Though it be not all for your own sake.
The king and the queen you made so merry,
With the many good pastimes that you did make.
If your life could be bought, I dare undertake,
Gold nor silver there would lack none,
Though fools be enough, and you be gone.

You were a fool without fraud,
Shaped and born of very nature,
Of all good fools to you may be laud,
For every man in you had great pleasure;
For our king and queen you were a treasure.
Alas for them! Where should we have such a one
Though all fools be not dead – but you are gone.

You were neither Erasmus[5] nor Luther,
You meddled no further than your pot!
Against high matters you were no disputer,
Among the innocent elect[6] was your lot!
Glad may you be you had that knot,[7]
For many fools near you think themselves none,
And many of these are alive, Lobe, though you be gone.

Tyt Apgnyllamys,[8] prepare his obsequi!
Nature constrain you to do him good;
Mad Lady Apylton,[9] offer the mass penny,[10]
And appear as chief mourner in your own fool's hood.
Your wits were much alike, though nothing of blood,[11]
Save in him was much goodness and in you is none,
Yet you too be a fool, while Lobe is gone.

Now lobbe Lobe, God have mercy on your merry noole,[12]
And Lobe, God have mercy on your foolish face;

And Lobe, God have mercy on your innocent soul,
Which among the innocent I am sure has a place,
Or else my soul is indeed a heavy case;
You, You, and more fools, many a one,[13]
Such fools are alive, Lobe, though you are gone.

　　Now God have mercy on us all,
For wise and foolish, all will die;
Let us to our minds recall,
That to claim to be wise, our deeds will deny.
So to end, my reason will this apply:
God amend all fools that think themselves none,
For many are alive, though Lobe be gone.

The analysis contained in the reference notes should prove conclusively that Lobe was mentally retarded, and was one of those mentally retarded persons who attained not only renown in his age, but esteem – despite his status as a "fool." Obviously, the eulogizer himself had been very fond of Lobe; his poem bespeaks genuine sadness.

　　The poem also strongly reflects the late medieval literary theme that interpreted the world as being a foolish place (a "ship of fools") in which the worldly wise can be the greatest fools of all because of their lack of spiritual and moral wisdom – a wisdom attributed by the eulogizer to the retarded Lobe who had no malice in his heart, who was one of God's innocent, and who surely must have gone to heaven.

Reference notes

1　A play on words. The root lob, and thus the word lobbe, can itself mean heavy, clumsy, clown, etc. Already, this is strong evidence that Lobe was mentally retarded, because concepts such as "heavy" have been used in several languages to denote mental sluggishness.

2　Latin for prince of apostles, i.e., St. Peter.

3　*Stultus* in Latin could mean fool/foolish, or mentally retarded. *Stultus stultorum* means fool of fools, or of fools the most foolish, or of the stupid the most stupid. This is at least suggestive of mental retardation.

4　Latin: the celestial kingdom, i.e., heaven.

5　Erasmus of Rotterdam (1469–1536), a renowned Renaissance scholar.

6　Those unable to sin were often called innocent. This referred almost entirely to infants and the mentally retarded. These innocents would go to heaven if baptized, to limbo if unbaptized, but never to hell. Thus, an adult being called an innocent can be considered conclusive proof that the adult was mentally retarded.

7 I.e., were blockheaded, not very smart. One more indication Lobe was mentally retarded.

8 I was unable to identify who and what Tyt Apgnyllamys was. Presumably it was a rhymster, probably another (but nonretarded) fool at or close to the royal court.

9 More clearly than in the case of Apgnyllamys, Lady Apylton (Appleton) was an official court or house fool, probably also mentally retarded. Reference to these two names might prove the key to obtaining more definite information about Lobe, or at least when and where he flourished. A search of the records of courts and noble households for these names might be fruitful. One should consider the English court both before, during and after Henry VIII, the Scottish court, and even some of the more prominent baronial families. Insofar as the poem mentions Erasmus of Rotterdam, one can assume that Lobe died after Erasmus had become famous for his wisdom, and well before the initiation of the Rawlinson collection.

10 It probably cost one penny to have a funeral or memorial mass said.

11 Probably meaning "though you were not relatives."

12 Apparently pronounced "nole." Could mean either spirit or noodle. The latter often referred to foolishness, hence also the meaning "macaroni," as in "stuck a feather in his cap and called it macaroni." Here, it may also mean "foolish head," in the way we still refer to a head as a noodle.

13 The speaker seems to be addressing people around him, including possibly the reader.

The final two extracts of the book, especially the next one, expand the notion of learning from vulnerable people. Though both were written in the 1980s, their relevance in today's so-called postmodernist world is clear. In his penetrating and largely critical analyses of service systems and societal trends, both in terms of values and actions, Wolfensberger has been accused of being aloof from 'real people', in particular those people who formed the focus of the early decades of his working life. It is to be hoped that readers who have reached this point in the book will be already disabused of that myth, but these final extracts bring out more strongly still Wolfensberger's much deeper understanding of the things that retarded people have to give to other people and society in general. Not in a superficial egalitarian sense, where just giving people their 'rights' is assumed to somehow recognize and allow their gifts, nor in a sentimental stereotyping of the 'happy fool', but in a recognition of real assets, and ones which not only have value in themselves but very often serve to teach about the real worth of what the world values and prizes, and lead us to some important reflection on where to put our energies.

32 From: "Common assets of mentally retarded people that are commonly not acknowledged," 1988, *Mental Retardation*, 26(2), 63–70.

The next extract therefore elaborates on the 'unrecognized' assets of people called 'mentally retarded'. We pick it up after Wolfensberger has noted the common notion of such people as being 'deficient' in most of the qualities that society values, and how even good things that are said about them tend to be either insincere, generalized clichés, or related to specific individuals with no notion of wider applicability.

...

In the present article, I try to bring together some observations of strengths, virtues, gifts, capacities, prosocial dispositions, and resources, here called "assets," that one can find not only in a few retarded people, but among a goodly proportion. Of course, retarded people who have one or more of these assets will almost certainly not have all of them, and some may have none. Thus, I hope readers will not equate what follows with sentimental overgeneralized stereotypes.

Assets

1   Nature or circumstances have denied retarded persons a fuller intellective development, but not necessarily the growth of beautiful "heart qualities." In fact, with the normative preoccupation with intellectual achievement removed or diminished, many retarded people have continued in the growth of these heart qualities that have become "choked out" in others. This implies that mental energies and other resources are more concentrated on relationships – sometimes for worse, but sometimes also for better.

   Vanier (1985) cited an incident where a nonhandicapped man who had been a member of his L'Arche community 14 years earlier came back to visit: "I had completely forgotten him. It was Alfred (a retarded member) who threw himself into ... (the visitor's) arms: he remembered ... (the visitor's) name and where ... (the visitor) had worked." Vanier commented on the capacity of so many retarded persons to "give life and warmth," to "recognize another person and his or her needs" (p. 143).

2   Where heart qualities have not been choked out – most likely by bad treatment from others – retarded people may preserve a natural and positive spontaneity that gets diminished in most of us as we succumb to social conventions. Where this natural spontaneity is linked with goodness, it often manifests itself in retarded people being physically much more demonstrable in their love without suggesting or inviting sexual behavior. Thereby, they often

meet a need in another person that could not be easily met by a nonretarded person without appearing improper. Too often, this affectional spontaneity is regarded negatively by others, and efforts may be made to normalize it out of them when, in balance, it would really have been better to leave things as they are.

Where natural spontaneity is linked with goodness, it can be a beautiful source of interpersonal enrichment and even *joie de vivre*. Vanier (1985) cited a TV cameraman who was filming a world-wide gathering of 12,000 members of the Faith and Light movement, 4,000 of whom were handicapped (mostly retarded), and who observed wistfully, "I like my job, I have money, but they have something I don't have. They have joy."...

3   Even more than many nonretarded people, retarded people tend to respond quickly, generously, and warmly to kindly human contact, approval, and encouragement. One reason may be the presence of one or both of the qualities previously noted. Another reason could be that so many of these persons have had such a long history of rejection, brutalization, or deprivation of positive affectional relationships that they open up to such relationships like a flower famished for water. This responsiveness is often counted against retarded people as suggestibility and may well work to their disadvantage. At the same time, this very wound or weakness can also often become a source of strength – a phenomenon universal to us all. For instance, one positive consequence is that many retarded people are very enjoyable to have around. Many people remark on the fact that relating to a retarded person involves their emotions more than their intellect and challenges their sensitivities ... .

4   In a similar vein, retarded people have a strong propensity to relate to the "heart qualities" of other people, rather than to their status or societal roles and functions. Thus, retarded people are less likely to be put off by appearances, such as impairments, that might cause nonretarded people to distance themselves. Retarded people may relate positively even to a person who is very poor, disfigured, and devalued, as long as that person "has a good heart," is generous, giving, joyous, etc.

Part of this asset is a characteristic that I have heard many people comment upon, namely, that many retarded people seem to see more readily through appearances, in contrast to nonretarded people who tend to be impressed by other people's status, functions, or roles ... . For instance, most nonretarded people would relate to someone named Ronald Reagan in the role of president, but retarded ones are more likely to relate to him as Ronald Reagan the man, who is either a good or bad person, honest or dishonest, reliable or unreliable, and who has to prove himself to them directly. The public will forget the promises of Reagan, but retarded people are likely to take them seriously, remember them, and to judge him, at least in part, by whether these promises are kept or broken.

At several L'Arche communities, when the local bishop has visited, the nonretarded people were tremendously impressed and deferential; but the retarded people wanted to know what the bishop's name was, called him by that, slapped him on the back, watched to see how he behaved himself, and how sociable he was around the dinner table. On the basis of such attributes they might approve of a bishop – not on the basis that the Pope had appointed him.

This capacity not only enables retarded persons to interact often on a deep level with other people whom they encounter, but also can be very instructive to nonretarded people as to how little importance the external incidentals really have.

5   Many retarded persons have a genuine concern for things being well in the world. For instance, unlike the mighty of the world, many would be struck with horror and aversion about all sorts of evil environmental pollutions once the process and its consequences (even the long-term ones) were pointed out to them. Unlike the supposedly sophisticated student body at my university, for instance, they would readily do their part not to contribute to this problem. Many retarded persons really mean it when they ask, "How are you?" and if you do not look well, may not settle for the superficial cultural reply. When someone is in distress, they may be unable to ignore it. We are apt to step over the body of a street person downtown without blinking an eye or interrupting our conversation with a companion. A retarded person might drop everything else and become preoccupied with the person so obviously in distress. ... This kind of readiness to be relationally giving can occasionally even endure for decades, as a retarded person may step forward to provide assistance, solace, support, or even protection to a friend who previously did not need this help.

6   To the degree that retarded individuals have several of the aforementioned assets, they are also much less likely to be in their love what others would view as conditional. This is because the qualities upon which nonretarded people condition their love may hold little or no importance for a retarded person. ...

This observation is not meant to imply that retarded people do, in fact, exercise unconditional love, only that they appear to be able to come closer to doing so than many nonretarded people do. In order to achieve that same capacity, most nonretarded people have to engage in a long and arduous spiritual struggle.

7   Many retarded people are remarkably trusting, even when their trust is not warranted. This propensity may often derive from the reduced conditionality of love mentioned in the foregoing point. At any rate, even in the face of disappointed trust and abuse over a long period of time, a retarded person may remain loyal to the perpetrator, and by no means for selfish motives. On the one hand, such a trust is apt to be bitterly punished; on the other hand, to those of us who are neither retarded nor overly trusting, witnessing the trusting of retarded persons can be a moving and consciousness-raising experience. ...

The trust that some retarded persons emit can also serve to remind us of *its* mirror image, that is, the notorious untrustworthiness and infidelity of the service system, and most of its paid functionaries, to retarded people.

8   The overwhelming majority of retarded persons are poor and always will be poor. In some, this generates a possessiveness and materialism that can be pathological or a vice, but others are remarkably detached from worldly possessions. They may not worry much about their material securities or what wealth they are going to have 10 minutes or 10 years from now, and they may be extraordinarily generous in sharing or giving things away. For this, there probably are several reasons, including their previous exclusion from society and its materialism. At any rate, this is yet another instance where the very wounds that retarded people commonly suffer can sometimes also become sources of strength. ...

9   Some retarded people have a capacity to call forth gentleness, patience, and tolerance from other people, to dissipate the anger and rage of others, and, thus, to be peacemakers. In other words, they have a gift for not only recognizing and relating to people's "heart qualities," as previously mentioned, but also for drawing those qualities forth from others, even from people who are fairly brash, rough around the edges, or even rude.

For example, I once visited a high school that had instituted a program where some of the nonhandicapped students volunteered their free class periods to work on a one-to-one basis with their severely retarded age peers in a separate class within the school. ... As I was observing, a volunteer came in who was one of the school's champion athletes. He was a big and muscular young man, wearing a tight short-sleeved T-shirt, despite the chilliness of that day, probably because he wanted to show off his physique and strength. Although he was probably one of the most glamorous and valued students in the high school, a hero to the girls, he had volunteered to work with one of the severely retarded and rather unattractive young women. Though many of the girls in school would have been delighted if he had paid attention to them, instead he was coming and working with this handicapped student in his free hour, and she adored him as if he were her big brother. When it was time for the young man to leave, she looked up to him with a face radiant with adulation, patted him ever so lightly, and said, "When are you coming back?" And the young man was visibly melting, trying to be strong, nonchalant, and tough, but not quite managing it. He was being gentled by this severely retarded young woman.

It is quite conceivable to me that experiences such as this might change the outlook on life of a young man who might otherwise be oriented toward the body, physical accomplishment, power, and brute strength. But as a result of his relationship with a weak and very dependent woman who loved him, he may no longer have had to show all of this sort of bravado. This is just one small but striking example of the kind of gentling that I am talking about. ...

10   Some retarded persons have a gift that enables them to engage in unfettered enjoyment of life's gifts and pleasures, including the simple ones. Obviously, this is a direct result of their impaired intellect, in that a more sophisticated, advanced, and abstracting intellect tends to seek and enjoy increasingly more advanced, sophisticated pleasures, often, sadly, at the cost of no longer enjoying the simple ones and perhaps no longer even recognizing them. In order to have fun, many nonretarded people need to move at great speed, go far away…, and have expensive things. In contrast, retarded persons still enjoy such simple things as walking in the fresh air, being with friends, having a little party, eating good-tasting food, or playing a fun sport that stretches the body.

11   At least certain kinds of lying require at least some degree of abstracting capabilities, and, therefore, retarded persons have a strong tendency to be direct and concretely honest and a concomitant low inclination – or even ability – to dissemble. Because they take things for real, many do not assume that other people lie to them, and they do not lie to others. Even many retarded persons who would prefer to deceive (because to reveal the truth may bring some unpleasant consequence) may find it hard – even impossible – to do so. Thus, whenever one asks retarded persons such questions as what happened, and how, and where, and by whom, they are almost always apt to give a true answer, providing they are capable of answering at all and are not given (mis)leading cues. True, the answer may be difficult to understand or decipher, but its content is apt to correspond to reality. … This point should not be taken to mean that retarded persons never lie, only that they appear to be both less inclined and less able to do it than are nonretarded people.

12   Similarly, the very concreteness of retarded people can also yield other assets. One is that retarded people apparently have a remarkable tendency to follow an issue, development, or idea in a rigorous, concrete sequentiality to its "logical" conclusion. … If something is said, retarded people are very apt to take it as real and follow it up, and it may even come back to haunt whoever said it.

13   Some "hyper-normalizing" people would like us to believe that retarded people get as easily bored as do nonretarded people, but that is simply not true and possibly reveals the narrowness of the observers' clinical experience. Many retarded persons have the capacity to engage in a single and/or simple activity for an extended period of time, far beyond when it would become boring and tedious to nonretarded persons. This quality, ordinarily judged as a shortcoming, can actually be an asset for retarded people. For instance, if they did become easily bored doing what they can do, vocational services would be in a big fix trying to find interesting tasks that such persons can do, and many kinds of job opportunities would evaporate. In fact, many unskilled but nonretarded young adults today are unemployed precisely because they refuse to hold all kinds of available jobs that, to them, are too boring or tedious – and retarded workers are often replacing them.

One reason why retarded people may not be as susceptible to experiencing certain tasks as boring could be that relatively minute variations in the activity or its context inject novelty for a concrete person, but not for a more intelligent one who views each task of a class as an equivalent repetition thereof and therefore gets bored more easily. ...

14   Paradoxically, it is the very fact that retarded persons are often conceptually rigid and impaired in their ability to abstract that can also keep some of them from being misled, sidetracked, or otherwise confused by clever but erroneous intellectual arguments, clever phrasings, "detoxifications," and other language disguises and deceptions, things that seduce intelligent people all of the time.

15   Because of their reduced intellective capacities, retarded people have fewer intellectual barriers and, therefore, less resistance to a relationship with the divine. Intellect and its achievements is indeed one of the major sources of human pride and commonly leads to aggrandizement of the self or the human race that is really quite ridiculous when viewed from a cosmic perspective. Many very intelligent people have let their intellectual talents and gifts get in the way of an acknowledgment and acceptance of a divine sovereignty, especially as they become prideful of their capacities. Retarded persons have much less to overcome in acknowledging their (and the universal human) smallness and "creatureliness."

Clarifications

I anticipate that no matter how carefully I qualify my generalizations, there will be misinterpretations thereof, statements that I have overgeneralized, or even that, in my old age, I have fallen for the "holy innocent" mystique.

Nothing I have said is intended to convey that retarded persons are holy innocents, that they all have faith, or that they are all submissive to the divine will. Even retarded persons have, in my opinion, free will, although as indicated ... elsewhere (Wolfensberger, 1982), their capacity to exercise volition is apt to be impaired, not merely their intellects.

Several of my points are certainly not meant to imply that retarded persons as a group are morally superior to other people. Also, as mentioned, I am not proposing that one will find these assets in all retarded persons (indeed, some of these assets are not readily compatible with each other, such as Numbers 3 and 14) but, rather, that the majority of retarded people are apt to have at least some of these assets.

Interestingly, many of these assets of retarded people can be the very result of their weaknesses or deficits and, often, of the bad things that others have done to them. It is indeed true that one's weaknesses can also be a source of special strength (2 Corinthians 12:9). For instance, having been deprived of caring by others makes at least some persons more receptive to others who do approach them with caring. Being poor makes some people greedy but helps others develop an attitude of detachment from objects and possessions that, in turn, makes them generous and sharing. Of course, the fact that this is so should not be used as a justification for inflicting bad things on retarded people ... .

Nor are any of the assets delineated here unique to retarded persons. This needs to be stated only to forestall the kinds of misperceptions and misinterpretations that this kind of article is apt to elicit in some readers. Many of these assets, however, are also found in *other* societally devalued groups. For instance, long-term street people can so often see with virtual x-ray clarity through insincerity and the saccharine interactional demeanor of some servers (volunteers or agency staff members). The long-term lowly poor (in contrast to the merely impecunious) have an almost instinctive insight into the disfunctionalities of the endless stream of social and service schemes that are poured out over them, whereas social planners and human service workers are virtually blind to these realities and put their euphoric hopes in one scheme after another, year after year, for a life-time. ...

I am also under no illusions that among certain parties in our field that consider themselves progressive, some of the opinions expressed here will be considered regressive, primitive, condescending, patronizing, and empirically outright invalid. Thus, although I may be wrong, I am certainly not naive.

Conclusion

The thoughts offered in this article are based on a short life-time in the field of mental retardation. ... It is on these 30 plus years of experience in our field that I will also draw in trying to understand why workers in mental retardation have had a hard time recognizing the assets of retarded persons.

One reason is that most of these assets do not readily manifest themselves in certain contexts: most of all, in dehumanizing and brutalizing ones, such as conditions in many institutions; ... in those that simply are not sufficiently culturally normative in regard to facility features and social contexts, even if they are not very degrading; ... and in those where the growth and broadening of retarded persons is systematically blocked, as can happen even in some very environmentally normative and loving homes. Some of these conditions are more likely to constrict some assets than others.

The article then goes on to point out the influence, noted in various earlier extracts, of the 'eugenic alarm' period, and the 'distancing and brutalizing' that resulted, with deficits rather that assets being the currency of services. The 'preconditions' for people to demonstrate their assets and gifts are then outlined, following a similar pattern to the radical developments in the field that were strongly influenced by normalization (see earlier, especially Chapters 2, 3 and 4). This is followed by a reminder of the difficulties of obtaining these conditions in the mental retardation field (see Chapter 2) and of Wolfensberger's earliest contact with conditions and people that 'liberated' these assets.

...

My first contact that I can recall with people who had worked with relatively liberated retarded persons occurred in England during 1962–1963, but my own insights into many of the assets described here continued to be constrained until 1973–1974, when I began to observe some spectacular manifestations thereof in a L'Arche setting. Thereafter, as more retarded people were afforded the life conditions that are virtual preconditions to the flowering and display of their assets, these observations became more routine both for myself and others.

However, many retarded people today still are not afforded liberating life conditions, and many of the remainder experience them only partially and/or for time-limited periods. Accordingly, a significant proportion of workers in our field (and in others as well) have also not had the opportunity to see the assets of retarded people sufficiently displayed or to act appropriately in light of the many positive and negative realities that such experiences reveal.

There are also people to whom some or all of the above assets of retarded persons *have* been displayed, but who nevertheless fail to acknowledge these assets for what they are or to respond appropriately. Why? One possible answer is that it is hard to acknowledge that a person has certain valued assets and even nobilities when that person belongs to a societally devalued class in whose devaluation one is at least partially participating. Further, no serious student of history, sociology, and political philosophy, and especially of the literature in these areas in the last 20 years or so, can seriously doubt that human service structures are one of the major means for carrying out destructive societal policies towards the poor and marginal classes.

Because social structures are expressions of hidden societal control mechanisms, this probably helps explain why, as a group, human service workers seem to have greater difficulty acknowledging the assets of retarded persons than do either family members or those members of the public who have had life-sharing experiences with retarded persons. But again, in my relatively long sojourn in the field, I believe I have seen another obstacle as well: pure old-fashioned universal human pride. After all, human service workers are supposed to be there to help, to be competent, and/or in a place of authority *vis-à-vis* the competency-impaired person. To discover greater truthfulness, gentleness, forbearance, forgiving, fidelity, etc., in retarded persons may be too big a threat, especially to workers who value independence, intelligence, and learning excessively. Thus, they may block out the evidence of these assets or interpret away the evidence that they cannot block out.

Stratford (1986) also pointed to this, or a similar, phenomenon. He noted that especially the affectional qualities of some retarded people, and their readiness to be forgiving, may not be acknowledged because in our culture we have placed such a value on intellectual qualities and worldly achievements that we not only fail to see the more human qualities in those who are distinctly lacking in these respects, but that in the face of such qualities by those whom we devalue, many of us may feel outright indicted or convicted over that which we do value.

33   From: "The prophetic voice and presence of mentally retarded people in the world today," 2001, in W.C. Gaventa, & D.L. Coulter (eds), 11–48, *The Theological Voice of Wolf Wolfensberger*, Binghamton, NY: The Haworth Pastoral Press.

We end the book with a short extract from one of Wolfensberger's theological writings. It will be obvious to readers, even if they have not read the Introduction to this book, what importance Wolfensberger places on personal reflection and decisions on one's position *vis-à-vis* moral issues. On the particular issue of this final chapter, as we have noted, such decisions are the more crucial. If one even goes along part of the way with Wolfensberger's analysis of wounding, of the place of human services in that, and of the pressures of society to perpetuate such wounding – and yet seeks to involve oneself in human affairs, let alone human services themselves – then a way to address the dilemma of trying to do good in a system that rewards doing harm is required. Some have found that in their religion – for Wolfensberger, in the development of a particular Christian-based analysis, influenced, as we have noted, by the work of Stringfellow, but refined and put to the test in many workshops and writings since the 1970s. 'Tried and tested' might have been a better phrase, because for many people those ideas have put Wolfensberger on trial, and in many places the verdict has been a negative, even hostile one, which has also had its effects on those associated with him. If a true attribute of faith is that one is not deterred by the possible consequences of proclaiming what one sees as the truth, then Wolfensberger can certainly be said to have faith. Its consequences, at least in the narrow aspect of this chapter, are spelled out in the extract. Taken from the latter part of an immensely wide ranging and theologically challenging discourse on the 'prophetic voice and presence of retarded people', this short extract comes within a section headed 'The importance of other genuine sharing with retarded people'.

...

Considering therefore the fallenness of nature and of formal human organizations, I now see much more importance in informal human ties and relationships. As Stringfellow points out, the church is like a flame which flickers up more intensely and informally in some place, and then moves and flickers more intensively elsewhere as formalism takes over. The real Pentecostal church [used here in the Christian sense of being inspired and led by the Holy Spirit – Ed.] is not found in huge, formal organization, but in transitory groups and unexpected phenomena; it is fragile, because it resists organization – yet humans organize by reflex. Therefore, the church of Christ comes, goes, moves; and, of course, finds its expression in different ways in different societies and in different places.

So now, I attach vastly more importance to informal human helping forms and relationships between mentally retarded and non-retarded people, as in non-formalized communal living. Even group homes are almost all formal, incorporated structures, with staff, this and that formal funding, evaluations, reports – fine, but theologically more important than such formal structures are the informal ones: people living together in a house, unincorporated, unfunded, life-sharing, Pentecostal. Remember Acts 5: they shared things in common, and anyone who had any want received from those who possessed more. That I see as of terribly deep importance at this time. I would not go so far as to say that members of informal communities today should not accept generic pensions, such as Social Security; but I would prefer it if community living came about not through formal organizations, but through the informal, prophetic and Pentecostal way. Of course, I do not expect that to be a major secular service system solution; I do not expect this to be a quantitative solution for the need of vast numbers of retarded people, but I see it as a qualitative, way-pointing prophetic manifestation.

Perhaps we need to distinguish between what we believe and what we know we will end up doing that violates our belief; and between the weaknesses of two imperfect, fallen helping forms: the formal organized helping form will almost certainly deteriorate to perversion and/or abuse; the informal human helping is more apt to terminate and be unstable. What drives us to insist that stability is worth more than the benefits of informality, and more worth the risk of deterioration to abuse than the risk of discontinuity? I submit that the issue deserves deep, drawn-out thought rather than easy dismissal. …

As editor, I offer this collection of writings, and the many issues they raise, with the same hope.

David Race
Chelmorton
October 2002

References

Editor's note: Whilst every effort has been made to maintain a consistent format for referencing, the inclusion of extracts from different countries and from non-academic sources such as newspapers and locally produced newsletters has meant that this has not always been possible. We are, however confident that the references can be traced to their source via the listing below.

Abbott, L. (1999) *The Citizen Advocate* (Publication of Chatham-Savannah Citizen Advocacy), April–May, 2.

Adorno, T.W., Frenkel-Brunswik, E., Levinson, D.J. and Sanford, R.N. (1950) *The Authoritarian Personality*, New York: Harper.

Ayoub, G. (2000) 'Dick and Wayne: relationship solid and enduring for 25 years', *The Advocate* (Newsletter of Citizen Advocacy, Grand Island, NE), Summer, 1–2. (Reprinted from *The Grand Island Independent*.)

Berelson, B. and Steiner, G. (1964) *Human Behavior: An Inventory of Scientific Findings*, New York: Harcourt, Brace and World.

Biklen, D. (1974) *Let Our Children Go: An Organizing Manual for Advocates and Parents*, Syracuse, NY: Human Policy Press.

Binding, K. and Hoche, A. (1920) *Die Freigabe der Vernichtung lebensunwerten Lebens: ihr Maß und ihre Form*, Leipzig: Felix Meiner.

Blatt, B. and Kaplan, F. (1966) *Christmas in Purgatory: A Photographic Essay on Mental Retardation*, Boston: Allyn and Bacon.

Branson, J. and Miller, D. (1992) 'Normalization, community care and the politics of difference', *Australian Disability Review*, 4, 17–28.

Brown, H. and Smith, H. (1989) 'Whose "ordinary life" is it anyway?', *Disability, Handicap & Society*, 4, 105–19.

Buck, P.S. (1950) *The Child Who Never Grew*, New York: John Day.

Buddenhagen, R.G. (1971) 'Until electric shocks are legal', *Mental Retardation*, 9(6), 48–50.

Catanzarite, S. (1997) 'Thoughts of a sometimes whiny, sometimes selfish, sometimes hypocritical, excellent citizen advocate', *The Citizen Advocacy Forum*, 7(2), 22.

Chappell, A.L. (1992) 'Towards a sociological critique of the normalization principle', *Disability, Handicap & Society*, 7, 35–51.

Colbert, J.N. (1969) 'Philosophia habilitus: towards a policy of human rehabilitation in the post-institutional phase of disability', *Journal of Rehabilitation*, 35(5), 18–20.

Coll, B.D. (1969) *Perspectives in Public Welfare: A History*, Washington, DC: US Department of Health, Education and Welfare.

Columbus, D. and Fogel, M.L. (1971) 'Survey of disabled persons reveals housing choices', *Journal of Rehabilitation*, 37(2), 26–8.

Cook, S. (1997) 'Getting involved in special relationships' *The Advocate* (Newsletter of Citizen Advocacy, Grand Island, NE), Winter, 2.

Costa, A. (2001) 'Heart of the matter' *Person to Person: Citizen Advocacy Newsletter* (Syracuse, NY), January, 3.

Crookshank, F. G. (1924) *The Mongol in our Midst*, London: Kegan Paul.

Deutsch, A. (1949) *The Mentally Ill in America: A History of Their Care and Treatment from Colonial Times* (2nd edn), New York: Columbia University Press.

Diamond, E.F. (1977) *This Curette for Hire*, Chicago: ACPA Foundation.

Donna (1998) 'Donna and Kyle', *The Citizen Advocacy Forum*, 7(3) March, 17. (Reprinted from a publication of stories by the Pennsylvania Citizen Advocacy Consortium.)

Eaton, J.W. and Weil, R.J. (1955) *Culture and Mental Disorders: A Comparative Study of the Hutterites and Other Populations*, Glencoe, IL: The Free Press.

Edgerton, R.B. (1970) 'Mental retardation in non-Western societies: toward a cross-cultural perspective on incompetence', in H.C. Haywood (ed.), *Social-cultural Aspects of Mental Retardation: Proceedings of the Peabody-NIMH Conference*, New York: Appleton-Century-Crofts.

Elks, M. (1999) 'In their own words', *One to One Citizen Advocacy 1998–99 Annual Report* (Beaver, PA), 2.

English, R.W. (1971) 'Assessment, modification and stability of attitudes towards blindness', *Psychological Aspects of Disability*, 18, 79–85.

Farber, B. (1968) *Mental Retardation: Its Social Context and Social Consequences*, Boston: Houghton Mifflin.

Fletcher, J. (1972) 'Indicators of humanhood: a tentative profile of man', *Hastings Center Report*, 2, 1–4.

Fletcher, J. (1975) 'The "right" to live and the "right" to die', in M. Kohl (ed.) *Beneficent Euthanasia*, Buffalo: Prometheus Books.

Flynn, R.J. (1975) *Assessing Human Service Quality with PASS: An Empirical Analysis of 102 Service Program Evaluations* (NIMR Monograph 5), Toronto: National Institute on Mental Retardation.

Flynn, R. J. (1980) 'Normalization, PASS, and service quality assessment: how normalizing are current human services?', in R.J. Flynn and K.E. Nitsch (eds) *Normalization, Social Integration and Community Services*, Baltimore: University Park Press.

Flynn, R.J. (1994) 'Intégration et évaluation de programmes: comparaisons internationaux', paper presented at the conference 'Twenty-Five Years of Normalization, SRV, and Social Integration: A Retrospective and Prospective View', May 10–13, Ottawa, Canada.

Flynn, R.J. and Lemay, R.A. (eds) (1999) *A Quarter-century of Normalization and Social Role Valorization: Evolution and Impact*, Ottawa: University of Ottawa Press.

Flynn, R.J. and Nitsch, K.E. (eds) (1980) *Normalization, Social Integration and Community Services*, Baltimore: University Park Press.

Flynn, R.J., LaPointe, N., Wolfensberger, W. and Thomas, S. (1991) 'Quality of institutional and community human service programs in Canada and the United States', *Journal of Psychiatric Neuroscience*, 16(3), 146–53.

Foucault, M. (1973). *Madness and Civilization: A History of Insanity in the Age of Reason*, New York: Vintage Books.

Gaventa, W.C. and Coulter, D.L. (eds) (2001) *The Theological Voice of Wolf Wolfensberger*, Binghampton, NY: The Haworth Pastoral Press.

Goffman, E. (1961) *Asylums*, New York: John Day.

Gordon, G.A. (1966) *Roles, Theory and Illness: A Sociological Perspective*, New Haven: College and University Press.

Grable, G. (1998) 'Relationships', *The Citizen Advocacy Forum*, 8(2), 28.

Gruenberg, E.M. (ed.) (1966) *Evaluating the Effectiveness of Community Mental Health Services*, New York: Mental Health Materials Center.

Grunewald, K. (1969) 'A rural county in Sweden: Malmohus County', in R.B. Kugel and W. Wolfensberger (eds), *Changing Patterns in Residential Services for the Mentally Retarded*, Washington, DC: President's Committee on Mental Retardation, US Government Printing Office.

Grunewald, K. (ed.) (1971) *Människohantering på totala vårdinstitutioner: Från dehumanisering til normalisering*, Stockholm: Natur och Kultur.

Grunewald, K. (ed.) (1972). *Menneskemanipulering på totalinstitutioner: Frå dehumanisering til normalisering*, Copenhagen: Thaning and Appels.

Howe, S.G. (1866) in *Ceremonies on Laying the Cornerstone of the New York State Institution for the Blind at Batavia, Genesee County, New York*, Batavia, NY: Henry Todd.

Humphrey, Mrs. H.H., Jones, G. and Kugel, R.B. (1968) 'Special report: programs and trends in Europe for the mentally retarded', *PCMR Message* (President's Committee on Mental Retardation), 12, May, 8–12.

Joan (1997) 'Presence of an advocate', *Citizen Advocacy News* (Newsletter of Citizen Advocacy NSW Association, Australia), January, 15.

Jones, M. (1953) *The Therapeutic Community: A New Treatment Method in Psychiatry*, New York: Basic Books.

Jones, M. (1997) 'My experience as a crisis advocate', *One to One* (Newsletter of Citizen Advocacy Perth West, Australia), 18(2), 2.

Kevles, D.J. (1985) *In the Name of Eugenics: Genetics and the Uses of Human Heredity*, New York: Alfred A. Knopf.

Keyes, D. (1966) *Flowers for Algernon*, New York: Harcourt, Brace and World.

King, R.D. and Raynes, N.V. (1968) 'An operational measure of inmate management in residential institutions', *Social Science and Medicine*, 2, 41–53.

Klein, S.D. and Abrams, S.L. (1971) 'Public housing for handicapped persons?' *Journal of Rehabilitation*, 37(2), 20–1.

Kubik, L. (1997) 'In their own words', *One to One Citizen Advocacy 1996–1997 Annual Report* (Beaver County, PA), 7.

Kugel, R.B. and Wolfensberger, W. (eds) (1969) *Changing Patterns in Residential Services for the Mentally Retarded*, Washington, DC: President's Committee on Mental Retardation, US Government Printing Office.

Kugel, R.B. and Wolfensberger, W. (eds) (1974). *Geistig Behinderte – Eingliederung oder Bewahrung?: Heutige Vorstellungen über die Betreuung geistig behinderte Menschen* (W. Borck, trans. and abbrev.) Stuttgart: Georg Thieme.

Kuhn, T.S. (1962) *The Structure of Scientific Revolutions*, Chicago: The University of Chicago Press.

Lakin, K.C. and Bruininks, R.H. (1985) 'Contemporary services for handicapped children and youth', in R.H. Bruininks and K.C. Lakin (eds) *Living and Learning in the Least Restrictive Environment*, Baltimore: Paul H. Brookes.

Lemay, R.A. (1999) 'Roles, identities and expectancies: positive contributions to normaliza-tion and Social Role Valorization', in R.J. Flynn and R.A. Lemay (eds) *A Quarter-century of Normalization and Social Role Valorization: Evolution and Impact*, Ottawa: University of Ottawa Press.

Lowenthal, B. (1999) *The Citizen Advocate* (publication of Chatham-Savannah Citizen Advocacy, GA), April–May, 2–3.

Lundberg, G.D. (1993) 'American health care system management objectives: the aura of inevitability becomes incarnate' [Editorial], *Journal of the American Medical Association*, 269(19), 2554–5.

Maslow, A. (1959) *New Knowledge in Human Values*, New York: Harper.

Maurin, P. (1997) *Easy Essays*, Rifton, NY: Plough.

Mayes, D. (1999) *The Citizen Advocate* (publication of Chatham-Savannah Citizen Advocacy, GA), 3–4.

Menolascino, F.J. (1974) 'The role of parent associations in obtaining and monitoring normalized services for the mentally retarded', in F.J. Menolascino and P.H. Pearson (eds) *Beyond the Limits: Innovations in Services for the Severely and Profoundly Retarded*, Seattle: Special Child Publications.

Menolascino, F.J., Clark, R.L. and Wolfensberger, W. (eds) (1968) *The Initiation and Development of a Comprehensive, County-wide System of Services for the Mentally Retarded of Douglas County* (2nd edn) Vol. 1, Omaha: Greater Omaha Association for Retarded Children.

Menolascino, F.J., Clark, R.L. and Wolfensberger, W. (eds) (1970) *The Initiation and Development of a Comprehensive, County-wide System of Services for the Mentally Retarded of Douglas County* (2nd edn) Vol. 2, Omaha: Greater Omaha Association for Retarded Children.

Metiuk, O. (1998) 'Advocate: Helen; Partners: Ruth and Derek', in P. Williams (ed) *Standing by Me: Stories of Citizen Advocacy*, London: Citizen Advocacy Information and Training.

Minis, F. (1998) 'Citizen Advocacy: seeing others' *The Citizen Advocacy Forum*, 7(3) March, 18.

Morris, J. (1993) *Encounters with Strangers: Feminism and Disability*, London: The Women's Press.

Mullins, J.B. (1971) 'Integrated classrooms', *Journal of Rehabilitation*, 37(2), 14–16.

Nirje, B. (1969) 'The Normalization principle and its human management implications', in R.B. Kugel and W. Wolfensberger (eds) *Changing Patterns in Residential Services for the Mentally Retarded*, Washington, DC: President's Committee on Mental Retardation, US Government Printing Office.

Nirje, B. (1992) *The Normalization Principle Papers*, Uppsala: Uppsala University, Center for Handicap Research.

O'Berry, E. (1999) 'Spotlight on Judge Susan Tate', *Reflections of Citizen Advocacy in Georgia*, 2(1), 9–10.

O'Brien, J. (1987) *Learning From Citizen Advocacy*, Lithonia, GA: Responsive Systems Associates.

Oliver, M. (1990) *The Politics of Disablement*, Basingstoke: Macmillan.

Ott, L. (1996) 'Blessings', *The Citizen Advocacy Forum*, 6(1), 8. (Reprinted from *Citizen Advocacy News*, Fall 1995.)

Parsons, T. (1951) *The Social System*, Glencoe, IL: The Free Press.

Parsons, T. and Fox, R. (1958) 'Illness, therapy, and the modern urban American family', in E.G. Jaco (ed.) *Patients, Physicians and Illness*, Glencoe, IL: The Free Press.

Pat and Jennifer (2001) 'Pat and Jennifer: learning and growing together', *North Quabbin Citizen Advocacy News* (Orange, MA), Winter/Spring, 1–3.

Pennsylvania ARC (1972) *Pennsylvania Message*, 8(2), 4–5.

Perrin, B. and Nirje, B. (1985) 'Setting the record straight: a critique of some frequent misconceptions of the normalization principle', *Australian and New Zealand Journal of Developmental Disabilities*, 11(2), 69–74.

Perske, R. (1972) 'The dignity of risk and the mentally retarded', *Mental Retardation*, 10(1), 24–6.

President's Panel on Mental Retardation (1962) *A Proposed Program for National Action to Combat Mental Retardation*, Washington, DC: US Government Printing Office.

President's Panel on Mental Retardation (1963a) *Report of the Mission to Denmark and Sweden*, Washington, DC: US Government Printing Office.

President's Panel on Mental Retardation (1963b) *Report of the Mission to the Netherlands*, Washington, DC: US Government Printing Office.

President's Panel on Mental Retardation (1963c) *Report of the Task Force on Coordination*, Washington, DC: US Government Printing Office.

President's Panel on Mental Retardation (1963d) *Report of the Task Force on Education and Rehabilitation*, Washington, DC: US Government Printing Office.

President's Panel on Mental Retardation (1963e) *Report of the Task Force on Law*, Washington, DC: US Government Printing Office.

President's Panel on Mental Retardation (1963f) *Report of the Task Force on Prevention, Clinical Services and Residential Care*, Washington, DC: US Government Printing Office.

President's Panel on Mental Retardation (1964a) *Report of the Mission to the USSR*, Washington, DC: US Government Printing Office.

President's Panel on Mental Retardation (1964b). *Report of the Task Force on Behavioral and Social Research*, Washington, DC: US Government Printing Office.

Proctor, R. (1988) *Racial Hygiene: Medicine under the Nazis*, Cambridge, MA: Harvard University Press.

Quotes from Citizen Advocates (1997) *One to One* (Newsletter of Citizen Advocacy Perth West, Australia), 18(2), 5. (Reprinted from *Citizen Advocacy East Side Newsletter.*)

Race, D.G. (1999) *Social Role Valorization and the English Experience*, London: Whiting and Birch.

Race, D.G. (2002a) 'The historical context', in D.G. Race (ed.) *Learning Disability: A Social Approach*, London: Routledge.

Race, D.G. (2002b) 'The "normalization" debate', in D.G .Race (ed.) *Learning Disability: A Social Approach*, London: Routledge.

Ramcharan, P., Roberts, G., Grant, G. and Borland, J. (eds) (1997) *Empowerment in Everyday Life: Learning Disability*, London: Jessica Kingsley.

Royal Commission on the Care and Control of the Feebleminded (1908) *Report of the Royal Commission on the Care and Control of the Feebleminded*, London: Wyman and Sons.

Rhall, D. (1997) 'Loyalty to protégé', *Citizen Advocacy Forum*, 7(2), 17. (Reprinted from *Citizen Advocate*, (Publication of Ryde-Hunters Hill Citizen Advocacy, Denistone East, NSW, Australia), 1(13) June.)

Rosen, M., Clark, G.R. and Kivitz, M.S. (1977) 'Beyond Normalization', in M. Rosen, G.R. Clark and M.S. Kivitz (eds) *Habilitation of the Handicapped: New Dimensions in Programs for the Developmentally Disabled*, Baltimore: University Park Press.

Rosenthal, R. and Jacobson, L. (1968) *Pygmalion in the Classroom: Teacher Expectation and Pupil's Intellectual Ability*, New York: Holt, Rinehart and Winston.

Rowland, G.T. and Patterson, E.G. (1971) 'Curiosity: an educational key to change', *Education and Training of the Mentally Retarded*, 6, 92–7.

Rozell, M. (1998, December) 'In my words – being a citizen advocate' *One-to-One* (Newsletter of Friends In Deed, Holyoke, MA), December, 3.

Schalock, R.L. (ed.) (2002) *Out of the Darkness and into the Light: Nebraska's Experience with Mental Retardation*, Washington, DC: American Association on Mental Retardation.

Scheerenberger, R.C. (1983) *A History of Mental Retardation*, Baltimore: Paul H. Brookes.

Schlueter, B. (1998) 'Gary and Bonnie: he will always be remembered ... and oh so loved' *The Advocate* (Newsletter of Citizen Advocacy, Grand Island, NE), December, 1–2.

Selznick, P. (1949) *TVA and the Grass Roots*, Berkeley and Los Angeles: University of California Press.

Shatto, G. and Keeler, C. (1971) 'Rehabilitation in San Blas', *Journal of Rehabilitation*, 37(2), 10–13.

Shaw, A. (1977) 'Defining the quality of life', *The Hastings Center Reports*, 7(5), 11.

Singer, P. (1983) 'Sanctity of life or quality of life?', *Paediatrics*, 72(1), 128–9.

Stephenson, W. (1983) *Roxene*, Calgary: Temeron Books.

Stratford, B. (1986) 'The acceptable face of mental handicap', *Values*, September, 8–9.

Stringfellow, W. (1973) *An Ethic for Christians and Other Aliens in a Strange Land*, Waco, TX: World Books.

Swain, B. (1932) *Fools and Folly during the Middle Ages and the Renaissance*, New York: Columbia University Press.

Task Force on Children Out of School (1970) *They Way We Go to School*, Boston: Beacon Press.

Testimony of Advocates in Buffalo County, Kearney, Nebraska (1998) *The Citizen Advocacy Forum*, 8(1), 10–11. (Reprinted from the newsletter of Buffalo County Citizen Advocacy, Kearney, NE), Spring 1998.

Thompson, J.D. and Goldin, G. (1975) *The Hospital: A Social and Architectural History*, New Haven: Yale University Press.

Tiffany, F. (1891) *Life of Dorothea Lynde Dix*, Cambridge, MA: Riverside Press.

Tyne, A. (1998) 'Advocate: Robert; Partner: Geoffrey', in P. Williams, *Standing by Me: Stories of Citizen Advocacy*, London: Citizen Advocacy Information and Training.

Vail, D.J. (1967) *Dehumanization and the Institutional Career*, Springfield, IL: Charles C. Thomas.

Vanier, J. (1971) *Eruption to Hope*, Toronto: Griffin House.

Vanier, J. (1985) *Man and Woman He Made Them*, Mahwah, NJ: Paulist Press.

Welsford, E. (1935) *The Fool: His Social and Literary History*, London: Faber and Faber.

White, W. and Wolfensberger, W. (1969) 'The evolution of dehumanization in our institutions', *Mental Retardation*, 7(3), 5–9.

Whytehead, L. (1979) *Report of the Task Force on Human Life*, Winnipeg: General Synod of the Anglican Church of Canada.

Whytehead, L. and Chidwick, P.F. (1977) *Considerations Concerning the Transit from Life to Death*, Winnipeg: General Synod of the Anglican Church of Canada.

Wilkins, L.T. (1965) *Social Deviance: Social Policy, Action, and Research*, Englewood Cliffs, NJ: Prentice-Hall, Inc.

Williams, P. (1987) *Appendix 1: Data on the Performance of Service Groups on PASS*, London: Community and Mental Handicap Educational and Research Association.

Williams, P. (1998) *Standing by Me: Stories of Citizen Advocacy*, London: Citizen Advocacy Information and Training.

Wolfensberger, W. (1965a) 'Diagnosis diagnosed', *Journal of Mental Subnormality*, 11, 62–70.

Wolfensberger, W. (1965b) 'Embarrassments in the diagnostic process', *Mental Retardation*, 3(3), 29–31.

Wolfensberger, W. (1969) 'The origin and nature of our institutional models', in R.B. Kugel and W. Wolfensberger (eds) *Changing Patterns in Residential Services for the Mentally Retarded*, Washington, DC: President's Committee on Mental Retardation, US Government Printing Office.

Wolfensberger, W. (1970a) 'The principle of normalization and its implications for psychiatric services', *American Journal of Psychiatry*, 127, 291–7.

Wolfensberger, W. (1970b) 'Ideology power', *Nebraska Contributor*, 1(1), 1–6.

Wolfensberger, W. (1972) *Normalization: The Principle of Normalization in Human Services*, Toronto: National Institute on Mental Retardation.

Wolfensberger, W. (1973) *The Third Stage in the Evolution of Voluntary Associations for the Mentally Retarded*, Toronto: International League of Societies for the Mentally Handicapped, and National Institute on Mental Retardation.

Wolfensberger, W. (1975) *The Origin and Nature of our Institutional Models* (rev. and ill. edn), Syracuse, NY: Human Policy Press.

Wolfensberger, W. (1980a) 'The definition of normalization: update, problems, disagreements and misunderstandings', in R.J. Flynn and K.E. Nitsch (eds) *Normalization, Social Integration and Community Services*, Baltimore: University Park Press.

Wolfensberger, W. (1980b) 'Research, empiricism, and the principle of Normalization', in R.J. Flynn and K.E. Nitsch (eds) *Normalization, Social Integration and Community Services*, Baltimore: University Park Press.

Wolfensberger, W. (1982) 'An attempt to gain a better understanding from a Christian perspective of what "mental retardation" is', *National Apostolate with Mentally Retarded Persons Quarterly*, 13(3), 2–7.

Wolfensberger, W. (1983a) 'Social Role Valorization: a proposed new term for the principle of normalization', *Mental Retardation*, 21(6), 234–9.

Wolfensberger, W. (1983b) *Reflections on the Status of Citizen Advocacy*, Toronto: National Institute on Mental Retardation, and Atlanta, GA, Georgia Advocacy Office.

Wolfensberger, W. (1988) 'Common assets of mentally retarded people that are commonly not acknowledged', *Mental Retardation*, 26(2), 63–70.

Wolfensberger, W. (1989) 'Bill F.: signs of the times read from the life of one mentally retarded man' *Mental Retardation*, 27(6), 369–73.

Wolfensberger, W. (1992) *A Brief Introduction to Social Role Valorisation as a High-Order Concept for Structuring Human Services* (2nd rev. edn), Syracuse, NY: Syracuse University, Training Institute for Human Service Planning, Leadership and Change Agentry.

Wolfensberger, W. (1994) 'A personal interpretation of the mental retardation scene in light of the "signs of the times" ', *Mental Retardation*, 32, 19–33.

Wolfensberger, W. (1995) 'An "if this, then that" formulation of decisions related to Social Role Valorization as a better way of interpreting it to people', *Mental Retardation*, 33, 163–9.

Wolfensberger, W. (1998) A *Brief Introduction to Social Role Valorization: A High-Order Concept for Addressing the Plight of Societally Devalued People, and for Structuring Human Services* (3rd rev. edn), Syracuse, NY: Syracuse University, Training Institute for Human Service Planning, Leadership and Change Agentry.

Wolfensberger, W. (1999) 'A contribution to the history of normalization, with primary emphasis on the establishment of normalization in North America between 1967–1975', in R.J. Flynn and R.A. Lemay (eds) *A Quarter-century of Normalization and Social Role Valorization: Evolution and Impact*, Ottawa: University of Ottawa Press.

Wolfensberger, W. (2000) 'A brief overview of Social Role Valorization', *Mental Retardation*, 38, 105–23.

Wolfensberger, W. and Glenn, L. (1969) *Program Analysis of Service Systems (PASS): A Method for the Quantitative Evaluation of Human Services* (1st edn), Omaha: Nebraska Psychiatric Institute.

Wolfensberger, W. and Glenn, L. (1973) *Program Analysis of Service Systems (PASS): A Method for the Quantitative Evaluation of Human Services* (2nd edn), Vol. I: Handbook, Vol. II: Field Manual, Toronto: National Institute on Mental Retardation.

Wolfensberger, W. and Glenn, L. (1975) *Program Analysis of Service Systems (PASS): A Method for the Quantitative Evaluation of Human Services* (3rd edn), Vol. II, Field manual, Toronto: National Institute on Mental Retardation.

Wolfensberger, W. and Menolascino, F. (1970a) 'Reflections on recent mental retardation developments in Nebraska. I: a new plan', *Mental Retardation*, 8(6), 20–5.

Wolfensberger, W. and Menolascino, F. (1970b) 'Reflections on recent mental retardation developments in Nebraska. II: implementation to date', *Mental Retardation*, 8(6), 26–8.

Wolfensberger, W. and Thomas, S. (1983) *PASSING (Program Analysis of Service Systems' Implementation of Normalization Goals): Normalization Criteria and Ratings Manual* (2nd edn), Toronto: National Institute on Mental Retardation.

Wolfensberger, W. and Thomas, S. (1989) *PASSING (Programme d'analyse des systèmes de services: applications des buts de la valorisation des rôles sociaux): Manuel des critères et des mesures de la valorisation des rôles sociaux* (2nd edn), (M. Roberge, trans., J. Pelletier, adap.), Toronto: L'Institut G. Allan Roeher & Les Communications Opell.

Wolfensberger, W. and Tullman, S. (1982) 'A brief outline of the principle of Normalization', *Rehabilitation Psychology*, 27(3), 131–45.

Wolfensberger, W. and Zauha, H. (eds) (1973) *Citizen Advocacy and Protective Services for the Impaired and Handicapped*, Toronto: National Institute on Mental Retardation.

Appendix
Full bibliography of publications of Wolf Wolfensberger

This bibliography is up to date as of October 2002. Publications are grouped into seven sections: A) books and monographs; B) chapters and partial monographs; C) articles of significant scope, and/or in major journals; D) minor articles, published letters, or articles in minor journals; E) reviews; F) poems; G) interviews.

A) Books and monographs

1 Menolascino, R., Clark, R. L. and Wolfensberger, W. (1968) *The Initiation and Development of a Comprehensive, County-wide System of Services for the Mentally Retarded of Douglas County* (2nd edn, Vol.1), Omaha, NE: Greater Omaha Association for Retarded Children.

2 Coauthor of: Governor's Citizens' Committee on Mental Retardation (1968) *The Report of the Nebraska Citizens' Study Committee on Mental Retardation* (Vol. 1), Lincoln, NE: Nebraska State Department of Public Institutions.

3 Coauthor of: Governor's Citizens' Committee on Mental Retardation (1968) *The Report of the Nebraska Citizens' Study Committee on Mental Retardation* (Vol. 2), Lincoln, NE: Nebraska State Department of Public Institutions.

4 Coauthor of: Governor's Citizens' Committee on Mental Retardation (1968) *Into the Light*, Lincoln, NE: Nebraska State Department of Public Institutions.

5 Kugel, R.B. and Wolfensberger, W. (eds) (1969) *Changing Patterns in Residential Services for the Mentally Retarded*, Washington, DC: President's Committee on Mental Retardation.
   Republished, or translated in abbreviated form, as/by:
   a. (1971) *Människohantering på totala vårdinstitutioner: Från dehumanisering till normalisering*, Stockholm: Natur och kultur (Swedish).
   b. (1972) *Menneskemanipulering på totalinstitutioner: Frå dehumanisering til normalisering*, Copenhagen: Thaning & Appels (Danish).
   c. (1974) *Geistig Behinderte – Eingliederung oder Bewahrung?: Heutige Vorstellungen über die Betreuung geistig behinderte Menschen*, Stuttgart: Georg Thieme (German).
   d. (1974, reprinted in whole) Harrisburg, PA: Pennsylvania Department of Public Welfare.

6   Wolfensberger, W. and Glenn, L. (1969) *Program Analysis of Service Systems (PASS): A Proposed Review Mechanism for Funding of Service Project Proposals under Nebraska's Community Mental Retardation Services Act of 1969* (1st edn), Omaha, NE: Nebraska Psychiatric Institute (Limited mimeograph edition).

7   Wolfensberger, W. and Kurtz, R.A. (eds) (1969) *Management of the Family of the Mentally Retarded: A Book of Readings*, Chicago, IL: Follett.

8   Menolascino, P., Clark, R.L. and Wolfensberger, W. (1970) *The Initiation and Development of a Comprehensive, County-wide System of Services for the Mentally Retarded of Douglas County* (2nd edn, Vol. 2), Omaha, NE: Greater Omaha Association for Retarded Children.

9   Fritz, M., Wolfensberger, W. and Knowlton, M. (1971) *An Apartment Living Plan to Promote Integration and Normalization of Mentally Retarded Adults*, Toronto, Canada: National Institute on Mental Retardation.

10 Wolfensberger, W. (1972). *The Principle of Normalization in Human Services*, Toronto: National Institute on Mental Retardation. (According to the Canadian definition of best-sellers, this book was a Canadian best-seller in the non-fiction category.)
    Partial reprints:
    a. Blatt, B., Biklen, D. and Bogdan, R. (eds) (1977) *An Alternative Textbook in Special Education: People, Schools, and Other Institutions* (pp. 305–27), Denver, CO: Love Publishing.
    b. Romot, A. (ed.). (1979) *A Collection of Articles on the Subject of Normalization, Individualization, Integration,* Jerusalem: Ministry of Labor & Social Services, Service to the Retarded, Unit for Programs & Information.
    Translated in whole into Japanese by Shimizu, S. and Nakazono, Y. (1982), Tokyo: Gakuen-Sha/Tuttle-Mori Agency.

11 Wolfensberger, W. (1972) *Citizen Advocacy for the Handicapped, Impaired, and Disadvantaged: An Overview* (DHEW Publication No. (05)72–42), Washington, DC: President's Committee on Mental Retardation.
    Reprinted in revised form as Chapter 1 in Wolfensberger, W. and Zauha, H. (eds) (1973) *Citizen Advocacy and Protective Services for the Impaired and Handicapped* (pp. 7–32), Toronto: National Institute on Mental Retardation.

12 Wolfensberger, W. (1973) *The Third Stage in the Evolution of Voluntary Associations for the Mentally Retarded,* Toronto: International League of Societies for the Mentally Handicapped, and National Institute on Mental Retardation. (Edited and expanded opening plenary address to the Congress of the International League of Societies for the Mentally Handicapped, Montreal, October 1972.)
    Summarized as:
    a. Wolfensberger, W. (1973) 'The three stages in the evolution of voluntary associations for retarded persons', *Mental Retardation News*, 22(1), 2.

b. Wolfensberger, W. (1973) 'The three stages in the evolution of voluntary action groups', *Déficience Mentale/Mental Retardation*, 23(1), 4–5. (Appears in French in the same issue as: 'Trois étages dans l'évolution du benevolat', 27–8.)

Republished and translated as: Wolfensberger, W. (1977) *Die dritte Stufe in der Entwicklung von freien Vereinigungen zugunsten geistig Behinderter*, Marburg: Landesverband Hessen der Lebenshilfe für geistig Behinderte.

Translated (in part) into Hebrew, and reprinted in: Aharoni, C. (1988) *By Right Not by Charity*, Hadera, Israel: AKIM Hader

13 Wolfensberger, W. (ed.) (1973) *A Selective Overview of the work of Jean Vanier and the Movement of L'Arche* (Monograph No. 1), Toronto: National Institute on Mental Retardation.

Partially reprinted as: (1974) 'An outsider looks at L'Arche', *Letters of L'Arche*, 7, 35–9.

14 Wolfensberger, W. (1973) *A Look into the Future for Systems of Services to the Mentally Retarded* (Monograph No. 2), Toronto: National Institute on Mental Retardation. (Edited keynote address to 1970 National Conference of the Canadian Association for the Mentally Retarded, October 1970, Vancouver.)

Summarized as: (1971). 'A look into the future for systems of retardation services', *Déficience Mentale/Mental Retardation*, 21(1), 2–8.

(Appears in French in the same issue as: 'Les services de l'avenir pour débiles mentaux', pp. 36–42.)

15 Wolfensberger, W. and Glenn, L. (1973) *PASS (Program Analysis of Service Systems): A Method for the Quantitative Evaluation of Human Services*, Vol.1: Handbook (2nd edn), Toronto: National Institute on Mental Retardation.

16 Wolfensberger, W. and Glenn, L. (1973) *PASS (Program Analysis of Service Systems): A Method for the Quantitative Evaluation of Human Services*, Vol. 2: Field Manual (2nd edn), Toronto: National Institute on Mental Retardation.

17 Wolfensberger, W. and Zauha, H. (eds) (1973) *Citizen Advocacy and Protective Services for the Impaired and Handicapped*, Toronto: National Institute on Mental Retardation.

Reprinted in part as: Wolfensberger, W. (1996) 'Man is both cruel and tender … ', *Citizen Advocacy Forum*, 6(3), 4.

18 Wolfensberger, W. and Vanier, J. (1974) *Growing Together* (Monograph No. 2), Richmond Hill, Ontario: Daybreak. (From material presented at a L'Arche Federation Conference in Aurora, Ontario, in March, 1974.)

19 Wolfensberger, W. (1974) *The Origin and Nature of Our Institutional Models*, Syracuse, NY: Center on Human Policy. (Partial reprint in monograph form of chapter entitled 'The origin and nature of our institutional models', in R.B. Kugel and W. Wolfensberger (eds) (1969) *Changing Patterns in Residential Services for the Mentally Retarded* (pp. 59–171), Washington, DC: President's Committee on Mental Retardation.)

20 Wolfensberger, W. (1975) *The Origin and Nature of Our Institutional Models* (Revised and Iillustrated), Syracuse, NY: Human Policy Press. (Revised and illustrated reprint of chapter entitled 'The origin and nature of our institutional models', in R.B. Kugel and W. Wolfensberger (eds) (1969) *Changing Patterns in Residential Services for the Mentally Retarded* (pp. 59–171), Washington, DC: President's Committee on Mental Retardation.)
Reprinted as: Wolfensberger, W. (1977) *The Origin and Nature of our Institutional Models*, Chicago: Marquis Who's Who, Inc.

21. Wolfensberger, W. and Glenn, L. (1975) *Program Analysis of Service Systems (PASS): A Method for the Quantitative Evaluation of Human Services* Vol.1: Handbook (3rd edn), Toronto: National Institute on Mental Retardation. (Reprinted 1978.)

22 Wolfensberger, W. and Glenn, L. (1975) *Program Analysis of Service Systems (PASS): A Method for the Quantitative Evaluation of Human Services,* Vol. 2: Field Manual (3rd edn), Toronto: National Institute of Mental Retardation. (Reprinted 1978.)
Translated into Spanish:
a. Wolfensberger, W. and Glenn, L. (1982) *Programa de análisis de sistemas de servicios (PASS): Un método par la evaluactión cuantitativa de los servicios sociales*, Gúia (3rd edn), Vitoria-Gasteiz: SADMA.
b. Wolfensberger, W. and Glenn, L. (1982) *Programa de análisis de sistemas de servicios (PASS): Un método par la evaluactión cuantitativa de los servicios sociales*, Manual (3rd edn), Vitoria-Gasteiz: SADMA.
c. Wolfensberger, W. and Glenn, L. (1997) *Programa de análisis de sistemas de servicios (PASS): Un método para la evaluactión cuantitativa de los servicios sociales*, Manual (3rd edn), Agen, France: CEDIS.
Translated into French:
a. Wolfensberger, W. and Glenn, L. (undated, but referenced to 1975 English edition and published ca. 1980) *PASS 3: Méthode d'évaluation quantitative des services sociaux. Manuel pratique* (3rd edn), (1st revision by André Dionne), Montreal: L'Association du Québec pour les Déficients Mentaux.
b. Wolfensberger, W. and Glenn, L. (undated, but referenced to the 1975 English edition, published ca. 1982) *PASS 3: Programme d'analyse des systèmes de services: méthode d'évaluation quantitative des services humains. Manual pratique* (2nd Quebec edn), Montreal: Institut Québecois de la Déficience Mentale.
c. Institut Régional de Formation des Travailleurs Sociaux et Centre Régional pour 1'Enfance et 1'Adolescence Inadaptées de Lorraine (1985) *La méthode d'évaluation PASS 3 (Programme d'analyse de système de services): Compte-rendu de la journée d'information du 10 Juin 1985*, Nancy: IRFTS Nancy/CREAI Lorraine.
d. Garber, K. (1988) *Manuel PASS: Reécriture par le CREAI de la Réunion.* Le Port, Réunion: Centre Régional pour l'Enfance et l'Adolescence Inadaptées (CREAI).

e. Wolfensberger, W. and Glenn, L. (1989) *PASS 3: Manuel pratique (3ième édition 1975), Analyse de programmes pour les systèmes de services: Méthode d'évaluation quantitative des services humains* (A. Dupont, J. Feragus, C. Gouley, J-P. Nicoletti, M. Rakotoarimanana and L. Vaney, adap.), Geneva: Comité Européen pour le Développement de l'Intégration Sociale (CEDIS).
Translated into Japanese:
a. Unauthorized translation at a date and by a party not known to Wolfensberger.

23 Wolfensberger, W. (1977) *A Balanced Multi-component Advocacy/Protection Schema* (Law and Mental Retardation Monograph Series), Toronto: Canadian Association for the Mentally Retarded.
Reprinted in part as: Wolfensberger, W. (1997) 'The historical-conceptual roots of advocacy', *Citizen Advocacy Forum*, 7(2), 4–5.

24 Wolfensberger, W. (1978) *The Normalization Principle, and Some Major Implications to Architectural-Environmental Design*, Atlanta, GA: Georgia Association for Retarded Citizens. (Previously published as a chapter in M.J. Bednar (ed.) (1977) *Barrier-free Environments* (pp. 135–69), Stroudsburg, PA: Dowden, Hutchinson & Ross.)
Reprinted as: Wolfensberger, W. (1995) *The Normalization Principle, and Some Major Implications to Architectural-Environmental Design*, Syracuse, NY: Training Institute for Human Service Planning, Leadership & Change Agentry (Syracuse University).

25 Wolfensberger, W. (1979) *The Limitations of the Law in Human Services* (Law and Mental Retardation Monograph Series), Toronto: Canadian Association for the Mentally Retarded. (Second printing in the 1980s did not list author's name.)

26 O'Brien, J. and Wolfensberger, W. (1979) *Standards for Citizen Advocacy Program Evaluation (CAPE)*, Toronto: National Institute on Mental Retardation.

27 Wolfensberger, W. and Thomas, S. (1980) *Program Analysis of Service Systems' Implementation of Normalization Goals (PASSING)* (Experimental edition), Syracuse, NY: Training Institute for Human Service Planning, Leadership & Change Agentry (Syracuse University).

28 Wolfensberger, W. and Thomas, S. (1983) *PASSING (Program Analysis of Service Systems' Implementation of Normalization Goals): Normalization Criteria and Ratings Manual* (2nd edn), Toronto: National Institute on Mental Retardation.
Updated and translated into French:
Wolfensberger, W. and Thomas, S. (1989) *PASSING (Programme d'analyse des systèmes de services application des buts de la valorisation des rôles sociaux). Manuel des critères et des mesures de la valorisation des rôles sociaux* (2nd edn) (M. Roberge, trans.; J. Pelletier, adap.), Toronto: L'Institut G. Allan Roeher & Les Communications Opell.

29 Wolfensberger, W. (1983) *Reflections on the Status of Citizen Advocacy*, Toronto: National Institute on Mental Retardation; and Atlanta, GA: Georgia Advocacy Office.

30 Wolfensberger, W. (1983) *Guidelines for Evaluators during a PASS, PASSING or Similar Assessment of Human Service Quality*, Toronto: National Institute on Mental Retardation.

31 Wolfensberger, W. (1983) *Normalization-based Guidance, Education and Supports for Families of Handicapped People*, Toronto: National Institute on Mental Retardation; and Atlanta, GA: Georgia Advocacy Office.

32 Wolfensberger, W. (1984) *Voluntary Associations on Behalf of Societally Devalued and/or Handicapped People*, Toronto: National Institute on Mental Retardation; and Atlanta, GA: Georgia Advocacy Office.
    Reprinted as: Wolfensberger, W. (1998) *Voluntary Associations on Behalf of Societally Devalued and/or Handicapped People*, Syracuse, NY: Training Institute for Human Service Planning, Leadership & Change Agentry (Syracuse University).

33 Wolfensberger, W. (1987) *The New Genocide of Handicapped and Afflicted People*, Syracuse, NY: Training Institute for Human Service Planning, Leadership & Change Agentry (Syracuse University).
    Translated and republished as: Wolfensberger, W. (1991) *Der neue Genozid an den Benachteiligten. Alten und Behinderten* (H. Zscherpe, P. Zscherpe, C. Mityorn and K. Dorner, trans.), Gütersloh, Germany: Verlag Jakob van Hoddis.

34 O'Brien, J. and Wolfensberger, W. (1988) *CAPE: Standards for Citizen Advocacy Program Evaluation* (Syracuse Test Edition), Syracuse, NY: Author.

35 Wolfensberger, W. (1991) *A Brief Introduction to Social Role Valorization as a High-order Concept for Structuring Human Services* (1st edn), Syracuse, NY: Training Institute for Human Service Planning, Leadership & Change Agentry (Syracuse University).
    Translated and republished as:
    a. Wolfensberger, W. (1991) *Die Bewertung der sozialen Rollen: Eine kurze Einführung zur Bewertung der sozialen Rollen als Grundbegriff beim Aufbau von Sozialdiensten* (C. Agad and A. Bianchet, trans.), Geneva: Éditions des Deux Continents.
    b. Wolfensberger, W. (1991) *La Valorisation des Rôles Sociaux: Introduction à un concept de référence pour l'organisation des services* (A. Dupont, V. Keller-Revaz, J.-P. Nicoletti and L. Vaney, trans.), Geneva: Éditions des Deux Continents.
    c. Wolfensberger, W. (1991) *La Valorizzazione del Ruolo Sociale: Una breve introduzione al concetto di valorizzazione del ruolo sociale inteso come concetto prioritario per la strutturazione dei servizi alle persone* (M. Costantino and A. Domina, trans.). Geneva: Éditions des Deux Continents.

36   Wolfensberger, W. (1992) *The New Genocide of Handicapped and Afflicted People* (rev. edn), Syracuse, NY: Training Institute for Human Service Planning, Leadership & Change Agentry (Syracuse University).

37   Wolfensberger, W. (1992) *A Guideline for Protecting Patients in Hospitals, Especially if the Patient is a Member of a Societally Devalued Group*, Syracuse, NY: Training Institute for Human Service Planning, Leadership & Change Agentry (Syracuse University).

38   Wolfensberger, W. (1992) *A Brief Introduction to Social Role Valorization as a High-order Concept for Structuring Human Services* (2nd rev. edn), Syracuse, NY: Training Institute for Human Service Planning, Leadership & Change Agentry (Syracuse University).

39   Vater, A., Scheuing, H.-W. and Wolfensberger, W. (1994) *"Euthanasie": Damals und heute*, Mosbach i. O., Germany: Johannes-Anstalten. (Fachtagung auf dem Schwarzacher Hof der Johannes-Anstalten, Mosbach, 13 June 1994.)

40   Wolfensberger, W. (1995) *A Brief Introduction to Social Role Valorization: A High-order Concept for Addressing the Plight of Societally Devalued people, and for Structuring Human Services* (Japanese trans. by Y. Tomiyasu), Tokyo: K. K. Gakuensha. (Based on a revised and enlarged version of: Wolfensberger, W. (1992) *A Brief Introduction to Social Role Valorization as a High-order Concept for Structuring Human Services* (2nd rev. edn), Syracuse, NY: Training Institute for Human Service Planning, Leadership & Change Agentry (Syracuse University).)

41   Wolfensberger, W. (1998) *A Brief Introduction to Social Role Valorization: A High-order Concept for Addressing the Plight of Societally Devalued People, and for Structuring Human Services* (3rd rev. edn), Syracuse, NY: Training Institute for Human Service Planning, Leadership & Change Agentry (Syracuse University).

42   Gaventa, W.C. and Coulter, D.L. (eds) (2001) *The Theological Voice of Wolf Wolfensberger*, Binghamton, NY: Haworth Pastoral Press. (Co-published simultaneously as *Journal of Religion, Disability & Health*, 2001, 4(2/3).)

B) Chapters and partial monographs

1   Wolfensberger, W. (1967) 'Vocational preparation and occupation', in A.A. Baumeister (ed.) *Mental Retardation: Appraisal, Education and Rehabilitation* (pp. 232–73), Chicago, IL: Aldine.

2   Wolfensberger, W. (1967) 'Counseling the parent of the retarded', in A.A. Baumeister (ed.) *Mental Retardation: Appraisal, Education and Rehabilitation* (pp. 329–400), Chicago, IL: Aldine.

3   Wolfensberger, W. (1969) 'The origin and nature of our institutional models', in R.B. Kugel and W. Wolfensberger (eds) *Changing Patterns in Residential Services for the Mentally Retarded* (pp. 59–171), Washington, DC: President's Committee on Mental Retardation.

Reprinted/translated in full or part:

a. (1969) *Exceptional Child Annual*, New York: Brunner/Mazel

b. International League of Societies for the Mentally Handicapped (1969) *Symposium on Residential Care* (pp. 66–73). Brussels: Author.

c. (1971) 'Rolltilldelning och anstaltsutformningen', in K. Grunewald (ed.) *Människohantering på totala vårdinstitutioner: Från dehumanisering till normalisering* (pp. 19–35) (K. Grunewald, trans.), Stockholm: Natur och kultur (in Swedish).

d. (1972) 'Rollefordeling og anstaltsudformningen', in K. Grunewald (ed.) *Menneskemanipulering på totalinstitutioner: Frå dehumanisering til normalisering* (pp. 26–46) (L. Vind, trans.), Copenhagen: Thaning & Appels (in Danish).

e. (1974) 'Ursprung und Eigenheiten unseres Anstaltswesens', in R.B. Kugel and W. Wolfensberger (eds) *Geistig Behinderte – Eingliederung oder Bewahrung?: Heutige Vorstellungen über die Betreuung geistig behinderte Menschen* (pp. 27–30) (W. Bork, trans.), Stuttgart: Georg Thieme (in German).

Reprinted in slightly revised and abbreviated form in R.B. Kugel and A. Shearer (eds) (1976) *Changing Patterns in Residential Services for the Mentally Retarded* (rev. edn) (pp. 35–82), Washington, DC: President's Committee on Mental Retardation.

Reprinted as a separate monograph:

a. Wolfensberger, W. (1974) *The Origin and Nature of our Institutional Models*, Syracuse, NY: Center on Human Policy.

b. Wolfensberger, W. (1975) *The Origin and Nature of our Institutional Models* (Revised and illustrated), Syracuse, NY: Human Policy Press.

4 Wolfensberger, W. (1969) 'A new approach to decision-making in human management services', in R.B. Kugel and W. Wolfensberger (eds) *Changing Patterns in Residential Services* (pp. 367–81), Washington, DC: President's Committee on Mental Retardation.

Translated and reprinted as: (1974) 'Ein neuer Weg zur Entscheidung über die geeignete Betreuung behinderter Menschen', in R.B. Kugel and W. Wolfensberger (eds) *Geistig Behinderte – Eingliederung oder Bewahrung?: Heutige Vorstellungen über die Betreuung geistig behinderte Menschen* (pp. 132–9) (W. Bork, trans.), Stuttgart: Georg Thieme.

5 Wolfensberger, W. and Menolascino, F.J. (1970) 'Methodological considerations in evaluating intelligence-enhancing properties of drugs' in F. Menolascino (ed.) *Psychiatric Approaches to Mental Retardation* (pp. 399–421), New York: Basic Books.

6 Wolfensberger, W. and Menolascino, F.J. (1970) 'A theoretical framework for the management of parents of the mentally retarded', in F. Menolascino (ed.) *Psychiatric Approaches to Mental Retardation* (pp. 475–93), New York: Basic Books.

7 Wolfensberger, W. (1970) 'Facilitation of psychiatric research in mental retardation', in F. Menolascino (ed.) *Psychiatric Approaches to Mental Retardation* (pp. 663–89), New York: Basic Books.

8 Wolfensberger, W. and Kurtz, R.A. (1971) 'Measurement of parents' perception of their children's development', *Genetic Psychology Monographs*, 83, 3–92.

9 Wolfensberger, W. (1971) 'Some not-so-secret secrets of how to make a community service plan work', in H. Ruvin and B. Ruvin (eds) *Proceedings of Special Study Institute on the Trainable Adolescent and Young Adult in School and Community* (pp. 21–48), Boston: Boston University New England Materials for Instruction Center.

10 Wolfensberger, W. (1972) 'Comprehensive community services of the future', in Saskatchewan Association for the Mentally Retarded & Saskatchewan Coordinating Council on Social Planning, *Comprehensive Community Services* (pp. 1–22), Regina, Saskatchewan: Authors.

11 Wolfensberger, W. (1972) 'Implementation of comprehensive community service systems', in Saskatchewan Association for the Mentally Retarded & Saskatchewan Coordinating Council on Social Planning, *Comprehensive Community Services* (pp. 45–60), Regina, Saskatchewan: Authors.

12 Wolfensberger, W. (1972) 'Alternatives to residential institutions', in *Interaction Workshop on Community Living for the Institutionalized Retarded*, Lincoln, IL: Lincoln State School.

13 Wolfensberger, W. (1973) 'A reflection on the movement of L'Arche', in W. Wolfensberger (ed.) *A Selective Overview of the Work of Jean Vanier and the Movement of L'Arche* (pp. 10–17), Toronto: National Institute on Mental Retardation.

14 Wolfensberger, W. (1973) 'Materials and resources relevant to the movement of L'Arche', in W. Wolfensberger (ed.) *A Selective Overview of the Work of Jean Vanier and the Movement of L'Arche* (pp. 18–22), Toronto: National Institute on Mental Retardation.

15 Wolfensberger, W. (1973) 'Citizen advocacy for the handicapped, impaired, and disadvantaged: an overview', in W. Wolfensberger and H. Zauha (eds) *Citizen Advocacy and Protective Services for the Impaired and Handicapped* (pp. 7–32), Toronto: National Institute on Mental Retardation. (Revised version of a 1972 monograph entitled *Citizen Advocacy for the Handicapped, Impaired, and Disadvantaged: An Overview*, Washington, DC: President's Committee on Mental Retardation.)

16 Wolfensberger, W. amd Moylan Brown, B. (1973) 'Youth advocacy', in W. Wolfensberger and H. Zauha (eds) *Citizen Advocacy and Protective Services for the Impaired and Handicapped* (pp. 95–101), Toronto: National Institute on Mental Retardation.

17 Korn, M. and Wolfensberger, W. (1973) 'Implementation and operation of citizen advocacy services via committee activism', in W. Wolfensberger and H. Zauha (eds) *Citizen Advocacy and Protective Services for the Impaired*

and Handicapped (pp. 195–211), Toronto: National Institute on Mental Retardation.

18 Zauha, H. and Wolfensberger, W. (1973) 'Funding, governance and safeguards of citizen advocacy services', in W. Wolfensberger and H. Zauha (eds) *Citizen Advocacy and Protective Services for the Impaired and Handicapped* (pp. 179–92), Toronto: National Institute on Mental Retardation.

19 Zauha, H. and Wolfensberger, W. (1973) 'Dissemination and training in citizen advocacy: guidelines and resources', in W. Wolfensberger and H. Zauha (eds) *Citizen Advocacy and Protective Services for the Impaired and Handicapped* (pp. 215–32), Toronto: National Institute on Mental Retardation.

20 Wolfensberger, W. (1974) 'Safeguarding the rights and welfare of students in the implementation of recent mandates', in *The Right to an Education Mandate: Implications for Special Education Leadership Personnel* (pp. 49–65), Minneapolis, MN: University of Minnesota (3rd Annual Leadership Conference in Special Education).

21 Wolfensberger, W. (1974) 'Can retarded and non-retarded people live together on an intimate, shared basis? Some implications from the Aurora Conference – Part I', in W. Wolfensberger and J. Vanier, *Growing Together* (pp. 1–6), Richmond Hill, Ontario: Daybreak Publications.
Reprinted in revised version as: Wolfensberger, W. (1975/1978) 'Can retarded and non-retarded people live together on an intimate, shared basis?', in National Institute on Mental Retardation, *Residential Services: Community Housing Options for Handicapped People* (pp. F3–5), Toronto: Author.

22 Wolfensberger, W. (1974) 'Some implications from the Aurora Conference – Part II', in W. Wolfensberger and J. Vanier (eds) *Growing Together* (pp. 37–45), Richmond Hill, Ontario: Daybreak Publications.
Reprinted in revised version as: Wolfensberger, W. (1978) 'Twenty possible solutions to relationship discontinuity from the Aurora Conference', in National Institute on Mental Retardation, *Residential Services: Community Housing Options for Handicapped People* (pp. F6–12), Toronto: Author.

23 Wolfensberger, W. (1975/1978) 'What's the difference between an institution and a community residence?', in National Institute on Mental Retardation, *Residential Services: Community Housing Options for Handicapped People* (p. FF 16), Toronto, Ontario: Author.

24 Wolfensberger, W. (1975) 'Citizen advocacy for the impaired' in D.A. Primrose (ed.) *Proceedings of the Third Congress of the International Association for the Scientific Study of Mental Deficiency*, 4–12 September 1973 (pp. 14–19), Larbert, Scotland: IASSMD, Royal Scottish National Hospital.
Reprinted in: (1994) *Citizen Advocacy Forum*, 4(4), 14–20.

25 Wolfensberger, W. (1975) 'Values in the field of mental health as they bear on policies of research and inhibit adaptive human service strategies', in J.C. Schoolar (ed.) *Research and the Psychiatric Patient* (pp. 104–14), New York: Brunner/Mazel.

26 Wolfensberger, W. (1975) 'The principle of normalization as it applies to services for the severely handicapped', in H. Mallik, S. Yspeh and J. Mueller (eds) *Comprehensive Vocational Rehabilitation for Severely Disabled Persons*, Washington, DC: Job Development Lab., George Washington University. (Summary of a keynote address presented at conference for Comprehensive Vocational Rehabilitation for Severely Disabled Persons, Washington, DC, December 1975.)

27 Wolfensberger, W. (1975) 'Transcribed discussion contribution', in A.J. Pulos (ed.) *Closing the Gap: A Seminar on Designing for Everyone*, Syracuse, NY: Syracuse University Department of Design. (Untitled contributions to sections on 'State of the Art', 'Methodology', and 'Priorities & Actions', scattered across pp. 1–40.)

28 Wolfensberger, W. (1976) 'Reaction comment', in M. Kindred, J. Cohen, D. Penrod and T. Shaffer (eds) *The Mentally Retarded Citizen and the Law* (pp. 618–23), New York: Free Press.

29 Wolfensberger, W. (1976) 'Consumer participation in New York State educational structures', in Schuyler, Chemung & Tioga Counties Board of Cooperative Educational Services, *Proceedings of a Special Studies Institute. "The Commissioner's Committee on the Handicapped"* (pp. 104–33), Elmira, NY: Author.

30 Wolfensberger, W. (1977) 'The normalization principle, and some major implications to architectural-environmental design', in M. J. Bednar (ed.) *Barriers in the Built Environment* (pp. 135–69), Stroudsburg, PA: Dowden, Hutchinson & Ross.
Reprinted as a monograph:
a. Wolfensberger, W. (1978) *The Normalization Principle, and Some Major Implications to Architectural-Environmental Design*, Atlanta, GA: Georgia Association for Retarded Citizens.
b. Wolfensberger, W. (1995) *The Normalization Principle, and Some Major Implications to Architectural-Environmental Design*, Syracuse, NY: Training Institute for Human Service Planning, Leadership & Change Agentry (Syracuse University).

31 Wolfensberger, W. (1977) 'Normalizing activation for the profoundly retarded and/or multiply handicapped', in B. Blatt, D. Biklen and R. Bogdan (eds) *An Alternative Textbook in Special Education: People, Schools and Other Institutions* (pp. 409–34), Denver, CO: Love Publishing.

32 Wolfensberger, W. (1977) 'The principle of normalization', in B. Blatt, D. Biklen and R. Bogdan (eds) *An Alternative Textbook in Special Education: People, Schools and Other Institutions* (pp. 435–67), Denver, CO: Love Publishing.

33 Wolfensberger, W. (1977) 'A model for a balanced multi-component advocacy/protective services schema', in L.E. Kopolow and H. Bloom (eds) *Mental Health Advocacy: An Emerging Force in Consumers' Rights* (pp. 16–35), Washington, DC: US Government Printing Office.

34   Wolfensberger, W. (1977) 'A brief overview of the principle of normaliza-
      tion', in S.A. Grand (ed.) *Severe Disability and Rehabilitation Counselor
      Training* (pp. 90–123), Albany, NY: National Council on Rehabilitation
      Education (State University at Albany).
      Reprinted in: Flynn, R.J. and Nitsch, K.E. (eds) (1980) *Normalization, Social
      Integration, and Community Services* (pp. 7–30), Baltimore: University Park
      Press.

35   Wolfensberger, W. (1978) 'The prophetic voice and presence of mentally
      retarded people in the world today', in International Federation of L'Arche,
      Springs of New Hope (pp. 37–80), Richmond Hill, Ontario: Daybreak
      Publications.
      Reprinted in:
      a. Gaventa, V.C. and Coulter, D.L. (eds) (2001) *The Theological Woice of
          Wolf Wolfensberger* (pp. 11–48), Binghamton, NY: Haworth Pastoral
          Press.
      b. Wolfensberger, W. (2001) 'The prophetic voice and presence of mentally
          retarded people in the world today', *Journal of Religion, Disability &
          Health*, 4(2/3), 11–48.

36   Wolfensberger, W. (1980) 'The definition of normalization: update, problems,
      disagreements, and misunderstandings', in R.J. Flynn and K.E. Nitsch (eds)
      Normalization, Social Integration, and Community Services (pp. 71–115),
      Baltimore: University Park Press.

37   Wolfensberger, W. (1980) 'Research, empiricism, and the principle of
      normalization', in R.J. Flynn and K.E. Nitsch (eds) *Normalization, Social
      Integration, and Community Services* (pp. 117–29), Baltimore: University
      Park Press.
      Reprinted as a 'classic article' in: Wolfensberger, W. (1996) 'Research,
      empiricism, and the principle of normalization', *SRV/VRS: The International
      Social Role Valorization Journal/La Revue Internationale de la Valorisation
      des Rôles Sociaux*, 2(2), 29–35. (Appears in French in the same issue as:
      'Recherche, empirisme et le principe de normalisation' (A. Dionne, trans.),
      22–28.)

38   Wolfensberger, W. (1980) 'Mit den Elternvereinigungen ins dritte Jahrzent'
      in Bundesverband für spastisch Gelähmte und andere Körperbehinderte,
      *Integration – Wunsch oder Wirklichkeit? Neue Wege der Arbeit für und mit
      Menschen mit Behinderungen* (pp. 8–16). (Proceedings of 20th Jubilee
      Conference, Berlin, October 1979.) Düsseldorf: Author.

39   Wolfensberger, W. (1981) 'The primacy of values and ideologies in human
      service evaluation', in R.J. Woolridge (ed.) *Evaluation of Complex Systems:
      New Directions for Program Evaluation: A Quarterly Sourcebook*, No. 10
      (pp. 1–7), San Francisco, CA: Jossey-Bass.

40   Wolfensberger, W. and Thomas, S. (1981) 'The principle of normalisation
      in human services: a brief overview', *Research Highlights: Normalization*.

No. 2 (pp. 10–34), Aberdeen: Dept. of Social Work, University of Aberdeen, King's College.

41 Wolfensberger, W. (1985) 'An overview of Social Role Valorization and some reflections on elderly mentally retarded persons', in M.P. Janicki and H.M. Wisniewski (eds) *Aging and Developmental Disabilities: Issues and Approaches* (pp. 61–76), Baltimore: Paul H. Brookes.

42 Wolfensberger, W. (1986) 'Die Entwicklung des Normalisierungsgedankens in den USA und in Kanada', in Bundesvereinigung Lebenshilfe (ed.) *Normalisierung: Eine Chance für Menschen mit geistiger Behinderung* (pp. 45–62), Marburg/Lahn, Germany: Author. (Edited address, in Bericht des Ersten Europäischen Kongresses der Internationalen Liga von Vereinigungen für Menschen mit geistiger Behinderung, Hamburg, October 1985, Vol. 14, *Grosse Schriftenreihe* of Bundesvereinigung Lebenshilfe.)

43 Wolfensberger, W. (1989) 'Human service policies: the rhetoric versus the reality' in L. Barton (ed.) *Disability and dependency* (pp. 23–41), (Disability, Handicap and Life Chances Series), London: Falmer Press.

44 Wolfensberger, W. (1994) 'Let's hang up "quality of life" as a hopeless term', in D. Goode (ed.) *Quality of Life for Persons with Disabilities: International Perspectives and Issues* (pp. 285–321), Cambridge, MA: Brookline Books.

45 Wolfensberger, W. (1994) 'The "Facilitated Communication" craze as an instance of pathological science: the cold fusion of human services', in H.C. Shane (ed.) *Facilitated Communication: The Clinical and Social Phenomenon* (pp. 57–122), San Diego, CA: Singular Press.

46 Wolfensberger, W. (1994) ' "Totmachen": Der neue Genozid an den Benachteiligten, Alten und Behinderten', in A. Vater, H.-W. Scheuing and W. Wolfensberger, *"Euthanasie": Damals und heute* (pp. 35–72), Mosbach i. O., Germany: Johannes-Anstalten (Fachtagung auf dem Schwarzacher Hof der Johannes-Anstalten Mosbach, 13 June 1994).

47 Wolfensberger, W. (1997) 'Major obstacles to rationality and quality of human services in contemporary society', in R. Adams (ed.) *Crisis in the Human Services – National and International Issues*: Selected Papers from a Conference Held at the University of Cambridge, September 1996 (pp. 133–55), Kingston upon Hull, United Kingdom: University of Lincolnshire and Humberside. (This is the published version of Wolfensberger's keynote and opening address.)

48 Wolfensberger, W. (1997) 'The dynamics of a post-primary production economy and society in relation to work for handicapped adults', in S.K. Chandler (ed.) *Transition '96: Building Futures Together* (pp. 1–10), Tallahassee: Florida Blueprint for School to Community Transition, Center for Policy Studies, Florida State University (Conference proceedings, 23–26 April 1996, Orlando, FL).

49 Wolfensberger, W. (1998) 'Die Lebenswirklichkeit von Menschen mit geistiger Behinderung und die Theorie von der Valorisation der sozialen Rollen', in J. Eisenberger, M.T. Hahn, C. Hall, A. Koepp, C. Krüger and B.

Poch-Lisser (eds) *Menschen mit geistiger Behinderung auf dem Weg in die Gemeinde: Perspektiven aus Wissenschaft und Praxis* (pp. 247–96), Reutlingen: Diakonie. (Vol. 5 of: Martin T. Hahn (ed.) *Berliner Beiträge zur Pädagogik und Andragogik von Menschen mit geistiger Behinderung.*) (The editors are listed erroneously on the cover.)

50   Wolfensberger, W. (1998) 'Prinzipien zur Planung von Wohneinrichtungen', in J. Eisenberger, M.T. Hahn, C. Hall, A. Koepp, C. Krüger and B. Poch-Lisser (eds) *Menschen mit geistiger Behinderung auf dem Weg in die Gemeinde: Perspektiven aus Wissenschaft und Praxis* (pp. 111–27), Reutlingen: Diakonie. (Vol. 5 of: Martin T. Hahn (ed.) *Berliner Beiträge zur Pädagogik und Andragogik von Menschen mit geistiger Behinderung.*) (The editors are listed erroneously on the cover.)

51   Wolfensberger, W. (1999) 'A contribution to the history of normalization, with primary emphasis on the establishment of normalization in North America between 1967–1975', in R.J. Flynn and R.A. Lemay (eds) *A Quarter-century of Normalization and Social Role Valorization: Evolution and Impact* (pp. 51–116), Ottawa: University of Ottawa Press.

52   Thomas, S. and Wolfensberger, W. (1999) 'An overview of Social Role Valorization', in R.J. Flynn, and R.A. Lemay (eds) *A Quarter-century of Normalization and Social Role Valorization: Evolution and Impact* (pp. 125–59), Ottawa: University of Ottawa Press.

53   Wolfensberger, W. (1999) 'Response to Professor Michael Oliver', in R.J. Flynn and R.A. Lemay (eds) *A Quarter-century of Normalization and Social Role Valorization: Evolution and Impact* (pp. 175–9), Ottawa: University of Ottawa Press.

54   Wolfensberger, W. (1999) 'Concluding reflections and a look ahead into the future for normalization and Social Role Valorization', in R.J. Flynn and R.A. Lemay (eds) *A Quarter-century of Normalization and Social Role Valorization: Evolution and Impact* (pp. 489–504), Ottawa: University of Ottawa Press.

55   Wolfensberger, W. (2001) 'An attempt to gain a better understanding from a Christian perspective of what "mental retardation" is', in V.C. Gaventa and D.L. Coulter (eds) *The Theological Voice of Wolf Wolfensberger* (pp. 71–83), Binghamton, NY: Haworth Pastoral Press. (Co-published simultaneously in *Journal of Religion, Disability & Health*, 2001, 4(2/3), 71–83.)

56   Wolfensberger, W. (2001) 'An attempt toward a theology of social integration of devalued/handicapped people', in V.C. Gaventa and D.L. Coulter (eds) *The Theological Voice of Wolf Wolfensberger* (pp. 49–70), Binghamton, NY: Haworth Pastoral Press. (Co-published simultaneously in *Journal of Religion, Disability & Health*, 2001, 4(2/3), 49–70.)

57   Wolfensberger, W. (2001) 'The good life for mentally retarded persons', in V.C. Gaventa and D.L. Coulter (eds) *The Theological Voice of Wolf Wolfensberger* (pp. 103–9), Binghamton, NY: Haworth Pastoral Press. (Co-

published simultaneously in *Journal of Religion, Disability & Health*, 2001, 4(2/3), 103–9.)

58   Wolfensberger, W. (2001) 'How we carry the ministry with handicapped persons to the parish level', in V.C. Gaventa and D.L. Coulter (eds) *The Theological Voice of Wolf Wolfensberger* (pp. 85–90), Binghamton, NY: Haworth Pastoral Press. (Co-published simultaneously in *Journal of Religion, Disability & Health*, 2001, 4(2/3), 85–90.)

59   Wolfensberger, W. (2001) 'The most urgent issues facing us as Christians concerned with handicapped persons today', in V.C. Gaventa and D.L. Coulter (eds) *The Theological Voice of Wolf Wolfensberger* (pp. 91–102), Binghamton, NY: Haworth Pastoral Press. (Co-published simultaneously in *Journal of Religion, Disability & Health*, 2001, 4(2/3), 91–102.)

60   Wolfensberger, W. (2001) 'The normative lack of Christian communality in local congregations as the central obstacle to a proper relationship with needy members', in V.C. Gaventa and D.L. Coulter (eds) *The Theological Voice of Wolf Wolfensberger* (pp. 111–26), Binghamton, NY: Haworth Pastoral Press. (Co-published simultaneously in *Journal of Religion, Disability & Health*, 2001, 4(2/3), 111–26.)

61   Wolfensberger, W. (2001) 'Response to the responders', in V.C. Gaventa and D.L. Coulter (eds) *The Theological Voice of Wolf Wolfensberger* (pp. 149–57), Binghamton, NY: Haworth Pastoral Press. (Co-published simultaneously in *Journal of Religion, Disability & Health*, 2001, 4(2/3), 149–57.)

62   Wolfensberger, W. (2002) 'Why Nebraska?', in R.L. Schalock (ed.) *Out of the Darkness and into the Light: Nebraska's Experience with Mental Retardation* (pp. 23–52), Washington, DC: American Association on Mental Retardation.

In addition to the above items, the following monographs written largely or entirely by Wolfensberger were published without authorship listing:

National Institute on Mental Retardation (1973) *A Proposal for the Establishment of Manpower Development and Training Stations in Mental Retardation and Related Developmental Handicap Fields* (Monograph No. 3), Toronto: Author.

National Institute on Mental Retardation (1974) *A Plan for Comprehensive Community Services for the Developmentally Handicapped (ComServ)*, Toronto: Canadian Association for the Mentally Retarded.

National Institute on Mental Retardation (1974) *Guidelines for the Preparation of Proposals for the Establishment of Comprehensive Community Service (ComServ) Experimental and Demonstration (E&D) Projects for Persons with Developmental Handicaps*, Toronto: Canadian Association for the Mentally Retarded.

National Institute on Mental Retardation (1979; reprinted 1988) *The Limitations of the Law in Human Services*, Toronto: Canadian Association for the Mentally Retarded.

The following item was co-authored by Wolfensberger without authorship listing. Base Community of the Unity Kitchen Community of the Catholic Worker (1995) *Christian Personalism: A Manifesto*, Syracuse, NY: Author.

C) Articles of significant scope and/or in major journals

1   Wolfensberger, W. (1958) 'Construction of a table of the significance of the difference between verbal and performance IQs on the WAIS and the Wechsler-Bellevue', *Journal of Clinical Psychology*, 14, 92.

2   Wolfensberger, W. (1958) 'Attitudes of alcoholics toward mental hospitals', *Quarterly Journal of Studies on Alcohol*, 19, 447–51.

3   Hillson, J.S., Wylie, A.A. and Wolfensberger, W. P. (1959) 'The field trip as a supplement to teaching: an experimental study', *Journal of Educational Research*, 53, 19–22.

4   Wolfensberger, W. (1960) 'Schizophrenia in mental retardates: three hypotheses', *American Journal of Mental Deficiency*, 64, 704–6.

5   Wolfensberger, W. (1960) 'Differential rewards as motivating factors in mental deficiency research', *American Journal of Mental Deficiency*, 64, 902–6.

6   Wolfensberger, W., Miller, M.B., Foshee, J.G. and Cromwell, R.L. (1962) 'Rorschach correlates of activity level in high school children', *Journal of Consulting Psychology*, 26, 269–72.

7   Wolfensberger, W. (1962) 'The correlation between PPVT and achievement scores among retardates: a further study', *American Journal of Mental Deficiency*, 67, 450–1.

8   Wolfensberger, W. (1962) 'Age variations in Vineland SQ scores for the four levels of adaptive behavior of the 1959 AAMD behavioral classification', *American Journal of Mental Deficiency*, 67, 452–4.

9   Wilson, J.M. and Wolfensberger, W. (1963) 'Color-blindness testing as an aid in the etiological diagnosis of mental retardation', *American Journal of Mental Deficiency*, 67, 914–15.

10   Wolfensberger, W. (1963) 'Conceptual satiation: an attempt to verify a construct', *American Journal of Mental Deficiency*, 68, 73–9.

11   Wolfensberger, W., Mein, R. and O'Connor, N. (1963) 'A study of the oral vocabularies of severely subnormal patients: III. Core vocabulary, verbosity, and repetitiousness', *Journal of Mental Deficiency Research*, 7, 38–45.

12   Wolfensberger, W. (1964) 'Some observations on European programs for the mentally retarded', *Mental Retardation*, 2, 280–5.

13   Wolfensberger, W. (1964) 'Teaching and training of the retarded in European countries', *Mental Retardation*, 2, 331–7.

Reprinted in full in: Daniels, L.K. (ed.) (1973) *Vocational Rehabilitation of the Mentally Retarded: A Book of Readings*, Springfield, IL: Charles C. Thomas.

14   Wolfensberger, W. (1965) 'General observations on European programs', *Mental Retardation*, 3(1), 8–11.

The above three articles (Nos. 12, 13 and 14) are reprinted in one of the reports of the Joint Commission on Mental Health of Children: David, H.P. (ed.) (1972) *Child Mental Health in International Perspective* (pp. 211–29), New York: Harper & Row.

15   Wolfensberger, W. and O'Connor, N. (1965) 'Stimulus intensity and duration effects on EEG and GSR responses of normals and retardates', *American Journal of Mental Deficiency*, 70, 21–37.

16   Wolfensberger, W. (1965) 'Embarrassments in the diagnostic process', *Mental Retardation*, 3(3), 29–31. Reprinted in or as:
   a. Dempsey, J.J. (ed.) (1975) *Community Services for Retarded Children: The Consumer–Provider Relationship* (pp. 181–5), Baltimore: University Park Press.
   b. Wolfensberger, W. (1979) 'Posibles desajustes en la formulacion del diagnostico', *Siglo Cera*, (63), 23–6.

17   Wolfensberger, W. (1965) 'Diagnosis diagnosed', *Journal of Mental Subnormality*, 11, 62–70. Reprinted in whole or in part in:
   a. Wolfensberger, W. and Kurtz, R. (1969) *Management of the Family of the Retarded: A Book of Readings* (pp. 131–8), Chicago, IL: Follett (Parkinson Division).
   b. Jones, R.L. (ed.) (1971) *Problems and Issues in the Education of Exceptional Children* (pp. 63–72), Boston: Houghton Mifflin.
   c. Gunzburg, H.C. (ed.) (1973) *Advances in the Care of the Mentally Handicapped* (pp. 61–9), London: Baillière Tindall.

18   Wolfensberger, W. and Committee for Behavioral Research and Training in Retardation (1965) 'Administrative obstacles to behavioral research as perceived by administrators and research psychologists', *Mental Retardation*, 3(6), 7–12.

19   Wolfensberger, W. (1967) 'Ethical issues in research with human subjects', *Science*, 155, 47–51. (Featured in 'Medicine' column of *Newsweek*, 6 March, 1967.)
   Reprinted in full or in part in:
   a. Research and Technical Programs Sub-Committee on Government Operations (1967) *The Use of Social Research and Federal Domestic Programs: IV. Current Issues in the Administration of Federal Social Research* (pp. 442–52), Washington, DC: US Government Printing Office.
   b. Council for International Organizations of Medical Sciences (1967) *Biomedical Science Facing the Dilemma of Human Experimentation* (Information document), Paris: Author.

    c. Beecher, H. (1970) *Research and the Individual: Human Studies* (pp. 301–3), Boston: Little, Brown.

    d. Schultz, D.P. (ed.) (1970) *The Science of Psychology: Critical Reflections* (pp. 319–29), New York: Appleton-Century-Crofts.

    e. Katz, J. (1972) *Experimentation with Human Beings: Cases and Materials on the Authority of the Investigator, Subject, Profession and State in the Human Experimentation Process* (pp. 923–4), New York: Russell Sage Foundation.

    f. Coughlin, S.S. (ed.) (1995) *Ethics in Epidemiology and Clinical Research: Annotated Readings* (pp. 59–63), Newton, MA: Epidemiology Resources Inc.

20   Menolascino, F. and Wolfensberger, W. (1967) 'Evocation of career choices in retardation: a summer work experience and training program', *Mental Retardation*, 5(2), 37–9.

21   Wolfensberger, W. and O'Connor, N. (1967) 'Relative effectiveness of galvanic skin response latency, amplitude and duration scores as measures of arousal and habituation in normal and retarded adults', *Psychophysiology*, 3, 345–50.

22   Wolfensberger, W. (1967) 'Research policies and problems in residential institutions', *Mental Retardation*, 5(5), 12–16.

23   Wolfensberger, W. and Menolascino, F. (1968) 'Basic considerations in evaluating ability of drugs to stimulate cognitive development in retardates', *American Journal of Mental Deficiency*, 73, 414–23.

24   White, W. and Wolfensberger, W. (1969) 'The evolution of dehumanization in our institutions', *Mental Retardation*, 7(3), 5–9.

25   Wolfensberger, W. (1969) 'Dilemmas of research in human management agencies', *Rehabilitation Literature*, 30, 162–9.

26   Halliday, R.A. and Wolfensberger, W. (1969) 'County differences in institutionalization of retardates at Nebraska's Beatrice State Home', *Nebraska State Medical Journal*, 54, 519–21.

27   Kurtz, R.A. and Wolfensberger, W. (1969) 'Cultural deprivation, lower class and mental retardation: certain terminological and conceptual confusions', *Social Science and Medicine*, 3, 229–37.

28   Kurtz, R.A. and Wolfensberger, W. (1969) 'Separation experiences of residents in an institution for the mentally retarded: 1910–1959', *American Journal of Mental Deficiency*, 74, 389–96.

29   Wolfensberger, W. (1969) 'Twenty predictions about the future of residential services in mental retardation', *Mental Retardation,* 7(6), 51–4.

30   Wolfensberger, W. (1969) 'An attempt to reconceptualize functions of services to the mentally retarded', *Journal of Mental Subnormality*, 15, 71–8.

31   Wolfensberger, W. (1970) 'Models of mental retardation', *New Society*, 15(380), 51–3.

Reprinted in: Region V Mental Retardation Services (1977) *Orientation Manual* (pp. 12–16), Lincoln, NE: Author.

32 Wolfensberger, W. (1970). 'The principle of normalization and its implications for psychiatric services', *American Journal of Psychiatry*, 127, 291–7. (Subject of a feature in the 'Behavior' column of *Time*, October 12, 1970.)
Reprinted in: Smrtic, J.D. (1979) *Abnormal Psychology: A Perspectives Approach* (pp. 198–203), Wayne, NJ: Avery Publishing Group. (Also in second (1980) and third (1982) editions.)

33 Wolfensberger, W. and Menolascino, F. (1970) 'Reflections on recent mental retardation developments in Nebraska. I: A new plan', *Mental Retardation*, 8(6), 20–5.
Reprinted in: Anderson, R.M. and Greer, J.C. (1976) *Educating the Severely and Profoundly Retarded* (pp. 383–91), Baltimore: University Park Press.

34 Wolfensberger, W. and Menolascino, F. (1970) 'Reflections on recent mental retardation developments in Nebraska. II: Implementation to date', *Mental Retardation*, 8(6), 26–8.

35 Wolfensberger, W. and Halliday, R. (1970) 'Socio-ecological variables associated with institutionalization of retardates', *Journal of Mental Deficiency Research*, 14, 1–15.

36 Wolfensberger, W. (1971) 'Will there always be an institution? I: The impact of epidemiological trends', *Mental Retardation*, 9(5), 14–20.
Reprinted in:
a. Rosen, M., Clark, G.R. and Kivitz, M.S. (1976) *A History of Mental Retardation* Vol. 2 (pp. 399–414), Baltimore: University Park Press.
b. *Association of Mental Health Administrators Newsletter* (1979, July Supplement), 1–7.

37 Wolfensberger, W. (1971) 'Will there always be an institution? II: The impact of new service models', *Mental Retardation*, 9(6), 31–8.
Reprinted in: Rosen, M., Clark, G.R. and Kivitz, M.S. (1976) *A History of Mental Retardation* Vol. 2 (pp. 415–32), Baltimore: University Park Press.

38 Wolfensberger, W. (1972) 'Voluntary citizen advocacy in the human services', *Canada's Mental Health*, 20, 14–18.

39 Wolfensberger, W. (1973) 'The future of residential services for the mentally retarded', *Journal of Clinical Child Psychology*, 2(1), 19–20.

40 Wolfensberger, W. (1973) 'A reflection on the movement of L'Arche', *Déficience Mentale/Mental Retardation*, 23(2), 10–14. (Appears in French in same issue as: Réflexion sur le mouvement de L'Arche, 50–5.)

41 Wolfensberger, W. and Kurtz, R.A. (1974) 'Use of retardation-related diagnostic and descriptive labels by parents of retarded children', *Journal of Special Education*, 8, 131–41.

42 Wolfensberger, W. (1974) 'Reflections on reading old annual government reports on the lunatic and idiot asylums of the province of Ontario', *Canada's Mental Health*, 22(3), 21–4.

43 Wolfensberger, W. (1974) 'Normalization of services for the mentally retarded: a conversation with Wolf Wolfensberger', interview in the 'The Now Way to Know' series, *Education & Training of the Mentally Retarded*, 9, 202–8.

44 Wolfensberger, W. (1975) 'A reflection on Foucault's insights into the nature of deviancy and our residential institutions', *Canada's Mental Health*, 23(2), 21–2.

Also in French edition *(L'Hygiène Mentale au Canada)* as: 'Anormalité et établissements hospitaliers: réflexions sur l'interpretation de Michel Foucault', 22–3.

45 Wolfensberger, W. (1975) 'How to exclude mentally retarded children from school', *Mental Retardation*, 13(6), 30–1.

Reprinted in: *Reachout*, 10(4), 2.

46 Wolfensberger, W. (1976) 'A brief overview of PASS and FUNDET: purposes, uses, structure, content and meaning', *Rehabilitation Psychology News*, 4(1), 9–13.

47 Wolfensberger, W. (1977) 'A dream: was it bad, good, or both?' *Mental Retardation*, 15(6), 37.

48 Wolfensberger, W. (1977) 'The moral challenge of mentally retarded persons to human services', *Information Services* (Newsletter of the Religion Division of the American Association on Mental Deficiency), 6(3), 6–16.

49 Wolfensberger, W. (1978) 'The ideal human service for a societally devalued group', *Rehabilitation Literature*, 39(1), 15–17.

Reprinted in:

a. Regnier, S.J. and Perkovsek, M. (1986) *Rehabilitation: 25 Years of Concepts, Principles, Perspectives* (pp. 141–5), Chicago, IL: National Easter Seal Society.

b. *Dialect* (1987, August), p. 12 (Publication of Saskatchewan Assoc. for the Mentally Retarded) .

c. *Journal of Leisurability* (1988), 15(3), 8–10.

Listed in: Adams, D.S. (ed.) (1982, 1988, 1992) *Handbook of Humorous Teaching Material*. Washington, DC: American Sociological Society Teaching Resources Center (1992 edn is called *Using Humor in Teaching Sociology: A Handbook*).

50 Wolfensberger, W. (1979) 'An attempt toward a theology of social integration of devalued/handicapped people', *Information Services* (Newsletter of the Religion Division of the American Association on Mental Deficiency), 8(1), 12–26.

Reprinted in:

a. Gaventa, V.C. and Coulter, D.L. (eds) (2001) *The Theological Voice of Wolf Wolfensberger* (pp. 49–70), Binghamton, NY: Haworth Pastoral Press.

b. *Journal of Religion, Disability & Health* (2001), 4(2/3), 49–70.

51 Wolfensberger, W. (1979) 'Some historical and moral reasons why members of the clergy and other religious ministries may join the devaluation of

societally devalued people' *National Apostolate With Mentally Retarded Persons Quarterly*, 9(4), 16–17.

Partially reprinted as or in:

a. (1979) 'The clergy and devalued people', *The C. U. Citizen* (Publication of the College for Living, University of Colorado, Boulder, CO), 40(10), 309.

b. (1983) *Newsletter of Persons with Handicapping Conditions* (Publication of the Upper Room, Methodist Church Health & Welfare Ministries, Nashville, TN), 1(4), 3–5.

52 Wolfensberger, W. (1979) 'The case against the use of the term "disability"', *Rehabilitation Literature*, 40(10), 309.

Reprinted in: Spiegel, A.D., Podair, S. and Fiorito, E. (1981) *Rehabilitating People with Disabilities into the Mainstream of Society* (pp. 27–8), Parkridge, NJ: Noyes Medical Publications.

53 Wolfensberger, W. (1980) 'Elemente der Identität und Perversionen des christlichen Wohlfahrtswesens', *Diakonie*, 6(3), 156–67.

54 Wolfensberger, W. (1980) 'A call to wake up to the beginning of a new wave of "euthanasia" of severely impaired people' (Guest Editorial), *Education & Training of the Mentally Retarded*, 15. 171–3.

Reprinted in:

a. Marozas, D.S. and May, D.C. (1988) *Issues and Practices in Special Education* (pp. 233–5), White Plains, NY: Longman.

b. (1989, March) *Speak Out*, (6), 8–11. (Private publication from England.)

55 Wolfensberger, W. (1980) 'Our moral responsibilities as providers or utilizers of human services', *The Bulletin* (Publication of the Christian Association for Psychological Studies), 6(4), 6–8.

56 Wolfensberger, W. (1980)' The challenge of evaluating religiously-based human service settings', *The Bulletin* (Publication of the Christian Association for Psychological Studies), 6(4), 4–6.

57 Wolfensberger, W. (1981) 'The extermination of handicapped people in World War II Germany', *Mental Retardation*, 19(1), 1–7.

58 Thomas, S. and Wolfensberger, W. (1982) 'The importance of social imagery in interpreting societally devalued people to the public', *Rehabilitation Literature*, 43(11–12), 356–8.

Reprinted in: (1988) *Journal of Insurability*, 15(3), 5–7.

Reprinted as a 'classic article' in: (1994) *SRV/VRS: The International Social Role Valorization Journal/La Revue Internationale de la Valorisation des Rôles Sociaux*, 1(1), 35–7.

(Appears in French in the same issue as: 'L'importance de l'imagerie sociale dans l'interprétation des personnes socialement dévalorisées aux yeux du public' (A. Dionne, trans.), 49–50.)

59 Wolfensberger, W. and Tullman, S. (1982) 'A brief outline of the principle of normalization', *Rehabilitation Psychology*, 27(3), 131–45.

Partially reprinted in: Brechin, A. and Walmsley, J. (eds) (1990) *Making Connections: Reflecting on the Lives and Experiences of People with Learning Difficulties* (pp. 211–19), London: Hodder & Stoughton.

60 Wolfensberger, W. (1982) 'An attempt to gain a better understanding from a Christian perspective of what "mental retardation" is', *National Apostolate with Mentally Retarded Persons Quarterly*, 13(3), 2–7.
Reprinted in:
a. Gaventa, V.C. and Coulter, D.L. (eds) (2001) *The Theological Voice of Wolf Wolfensberger* (pp. 71–83), Binghamton, NY: Haworth Pastoral Press.
b. *Journal of Religion, Disability & Health* (2001) 4(2/3), 71–83.

61 Wolfensberger, W. (1982) 'Eulogy for a mentally retarded jester', *Mental Retardation*, 20(6), 269–70.

62 Wolfensberger, W. (1983) 'The most urgent issues facing us as Christians concerned with handicapped persons today' (abbreviation of a presentation at the 13th annual conference of the National Apostolate With Mentally Retarded Persons, Denver, August 10, 1983. Condensed by Dr. Robert R. Lebel) *National Apostolate with Mentally Retarded Persons Quarterly*, 14(3). 4–9.
Reprinted in:
a. Gaventa, V.C. and Coulter, D.L. (eds) (2001) *The Theological Voice of Wolf Wolfensberger* (pp. 91–102), Binghamton, NY: Haworth Pastoral Press.
b. *Journal of Religion, Disability & Health* (2001), 4(2/3), 91–102.

63 Wolfensberger, W. (1983) 'How we carry the ministry with handicapped persons to the parish level'. (Summary of a presentation at the 13th annual conference of the National Apostolate With Mentally Retarded Persons, Denver, August 10, 1983. Condensed by Rev. Charles L. Hughes.) *National Apostolate with Mentally Retarded Persons Quarterly,* 14(3), 9, 12–13.
Reprinted in:
a. Gaventa, V.C. and Coulter, D.L. (eds) (2001) *The Theological Voice of Wolf Wolfensberger* (pp. 85–90), Binghamton, NY: Haworth Pastoral Press.
b. *Journal of Religion, Disability & Health* (2001), 4(2/3), 85–90.

64 Wolfensberger, W. (1983) 'Précis du principe de "Normalisation" et quelques implications pour les personnes agées', *Gérontologie et Société* (Cahiers de la Fondation Nationale de Gérontologie), Numéro special, 59–62.

65 Wolfensberger, W. (1983) 'A brief reflection on where we stand and where we are going in human services', *Institutions, Etc.* (Publication of the National Center on Institutions and Alternatives), 6(3), 20–3.
Reprinted in: (1994) *Citizen Advocacy Forum*, 4(2), 7–9.

66 Wolfensberger, W. (1983) 'Social Role Valorization: a proposed new term for the principle of normalization', *Mental Retardation*, 21(6), 234–9.

67   Wolfensberger, W. (1984) 'Reflections on Gibson's Article', *Mental Retardation*, 22(4), 166–8.
68   Wolfensberger, W. (1984) 'The good life for mentally retarded persons', *National Apostolate with Mentally Retarded Persons Quarterly*, 15(3). 18–20.
      Reprinted in:
      a. Gaventa, V.C. and Coulter, D.L. (eds) (2001). *The Theological Voice of Wolf Wolfensberger* (pp. 103–9), Binghamton, NY: Haworth Pastoral Press.
      b. *Journal of Religion, Disability & Health* (2001), 4(2/3), 103–9.
69   Wolfensberger, W. (1984) 'A reconceptualization of normalization as social role valorization' *Mental Retardation (Canada)*, 34(7), 22–6.
70   Wolfensberger, W. (1984) 'Holocaust II?', *Journal of Learning Disabilities*, 17(7), 439–40.
      Reprinted in: (1992) *Networks* (Publication of The Special Gathering Ministry, Cocoa, FL), April, 1–2.
71   Wolfensberger, W. (1985) 'Social Role Valorization: a new insight, and a new term, for normalization', *Australian Association for the Mentally Retarded Journal*, 9(1), 4–11.
72   Wolfensberger, W. (1987) 'Response to Drash, Raver, and Murrin: Total habilitation – a meritorious concept requiring judicious application', *Mental Retardation*, 25(2), 79–81.
73   Wolfensberger, W. (1987) 'Which sacrament is appropriate?: The continuing controversy over whether retarded persons should receive communion', *National Apostolate with Mentally Retarded Persons Quarterly*, 18(1), 10–13.
74   Wolfensberger, W. (1987) 'Values in the funding of social services', *American Journal of Mental Deficiency*, 92(2), 141–3.
75   Wolfensberger, W. (1988) 'Common assets of mentally retarded people that are commonly not acknowledged', *Mental Retardation*, 26(2), 63–70.
      Translated and reprinted in Hungarian (E. Szauder, trans).
76   Wolfensberger, W. (1988) 'Reply to "all people have personal assets" ', *Mental Retardation*, 26(2), 75–6.
77   Wolfensberger, W. (1989) 'The killing thought in the eugenic era and today: a commentary on Hollander's essay', *Mental Retardation*, 27(2), 63–5.
78   Wolfensberger, W. (1989) 'Self-injurious behavior, behavioristic responses, and social role valorization: A reply to Mulick and Kedesdy', *Mental Retardation*, 27(3), 181–4.
79   Wolfensberger, W. (1989) 'Bill F.: Signs of the times read from the life of one mentally retarded man', *Mental Retardation*, 27(6), 369–73.
      Reprinted in: Saskatchewan Association for Community Living (1995) *Foundations for Community Living: Putting the Human into Human Services* (pp. 19–23), Saskatoon, Sask.: Author.

80 Wolfensberger, W. (1990) 'A most critical issue: life or death', *Changes: An International Journal of Psychology & Psychotherapy*, 8(1), 63–73. Reprinted in: (1992) *Citizen Advocacy Forum*, 2(2), 19–24.

81 Wolfensberger, W. (1991) 'Reflections on a lifetime in human services and mental retardation', *Mental Retardation*, 29(1), 1–15.

82 Flynn, R.J., LaPointe, N., Wolfensberger, W. and Thomas, S. (1991) 'Quality of institutional and community human service programs in Canada and the United States', *Journal of Psychiatry & Neuro-science,*, 16(3), 146–53.

83 Flynn, R.J., LaPointe, N., Wolfensberger, W. and Thomas, S. (1991) 'Measuring the quality of human service programs', *Journal of Leisurability*, 18(3), 22–8.

84 Wolfensberger, W. (1992) 'Deinstitutionalization policy: how it is made, by whom and why', *Clinical Psychology Forum*, 39, 7–11.

85 Wolfensberger W. (1993) 'A reflection on Alfred Hoche, the ideological godfather of the German "euthanasia" program', *Disability, Handicap & Society*, 8(3), 311–15.

86 Wolfensberger, W. (1994) 'The growing threat to the lives of handicapped people in the context of modernistic values', *Disability & Society*, 9(3), 395–413.

87 Wolfensberger, W. (1994) 'The issue of the moral character of citizen advocates', *Citizen Advocacy Forum*, 4(3), 28–9.

88 Wolfensberger, W. (1994) 'A personal interpretation of the mental retardation scene in light of the "signs of the times"', *Mental Retardation*, 32(1), 19–33.

89 Wolfensberger, W. (1994) 'Social Role Valorization news and reviews', *SRV/VRS: The International Social Role Valorization Journal/La Revue Internationale de la Valorisation des Rôles Sociaux*, 1(2), 57–61. (Also published in French in the same issue as: 'Annotations et nouvelles: la VRS en bref' (A. Dionne, trans.), 62–6.)

90 Wolfensberger, W. (1994) 'Strategies which I employ in order to maintain writing productivity', *Clinical Psychology Forum*, (68), 16–19.

91 Wolfensberger, W. and Thomas, S. (1994) 'An analysis of the client role from a Social Role Valorization perspective', *SRV/VRS: The International Social Role Valorization Journal/La Revue Internationale de la Valorisation des Rôles Sociaux*, 1(1), 3–8.

92 Wolfensberger, W. and Thomas, S. (1994). Constraints and cautions in formulating recommendations to a service, especially in the context of an external PASS or PASSING evaluation, *SRV/VRS: The International Social Valorization Journal/La Revue Internationale de la Valorisation des Rôles Sociaux*, 1(2), 3–6.

93 Wolfensberger, W. and Thomas, S. (1994) 'A critique of a critique of normalisation', *Australian Disability Review*, (1), 15–19.

94 Wolfensberger, W. and Thomas, S. (1994) 'Obstacles in the professional human service culture to implementation of Social Role Valorization and

community integration of clients', *Care in Place: The International Journal of Networks & Community*, 1(1), 53–6.

95   Wolfensberger, W. and Thomas, S. (1995) 'Reply to Newnes' "A commentary on obstacles in the professional human service culture to implementation of Social Role Valorization and community integration of clients"', *Care in Place: The International Journal of Networks & Community*, 2(1), 56–62.

96   Wolfensberger, W. (1995) 'An "if this, then that" formulation of decisions related to Social Role Valorization as a better way of interpreting it to people', *Mental Retardation*, 33, 163–9.

97   Wolfensberger, W. (1995) 'Social Role Valorization is too conservative. No, it is too radical', *Disability & Society*, 10(3), 245–7.

98   Wolfensberger, W. (1995) 'A brief outline of some of the most important concepts and assumptions underlying Citizen Advocacy', *Citizen Advocacy Forum*, 5(1), 16–22.
Reprinted in: (2000) *Citizen Advocacy News* (Citizen Advocacy NSW Association, Australia), June, 4–7.

99   Wolfensberger, W. (1995) 'Problems in the use of the term "partner" for the advocate, protégé, or both in a Citizen Advocacy relationship', *Citizen Advocacy Forum*, 5(3), 15–18.

100   Wolfensberger, W. (1996) 'Reply to John O'Brien's: "Nobody outruns the trickster: a brief note on the meaning of the word 'valorization'"', *SRV/ VRS: The International Social Role Valorization Journal/La Revue Internationale de la Valorisation des Rôles Sociaux*, 2(1), 16–20.

101   Wolfensberger, W. and Thomas, S. (1996) 'The problem of trying to incorporate a model coherency analysis into a PASSING assessment', *SRV/ VRS: The International Social Role Valorization Journal/La Revue Internationale de la Valorisation des Rôles Sociau*, 2(1), 12–15.

102   Wolfensberger, W. (1996) 'Social Role Valorization news and reviews', *SRV/ VRS: The International Social Role Valorization Journal/La Revue Internationale de la Valorisation des Rôles Sociaux,* 2(1), 42–6
(Also published in French in the same issue as: 'Annotations et nouvelles: la VRS en bref' (A. Dionne, trans.), 47–51.)

103   Wolfensberger, W., Thomas, S. and Caruso, G. (1996) 'Some of the universal "good things of life" which the implementation of Social Role Valorization can be expected to make more accessible to devalued people', *SRV/VRS: The International Social Role Valorization Journal/La Revue Internationale de la Valorisation des Rôles Sociaux*, 2(2), 12–14.

104   Wolfensberger, W. (1996) 'Social Role Valorization news and reviews', *SRV/ VRS: The International Social Role Valorization Journal/La Revue Internationale de la Valorisation des Rôles Sociaux*, 2(2), 45–51.
(Also published in French in the same issue as: 'Annotations et nouvelles: la VRS en bref' (A. Dionne, trans.), 51–8.)

105   Wolfensberger, W. (1998) 'Social Role Valorization news and reviews', *SRV/ VRS: The International Social Role Valorization Journal/La Revue Internationale de la Valorisation des Rôles Sociaux*, 3(1), 54–61.

(Also published in French in the same issue as: 'Annotations et nouvelles: la VRS en bref' (A. Dionne, trans.), 62–70.)

106   Flynn, R.J., Guirguis, M., Wolfensberger, W. and Cocks, E. (1999) 'Cross-validated factor structures and factor-based subscales for PASS and PASSING', *Mental Retardation*, 37(4), 281–96.

107   Wolfensberger, W. (1999) 'Social Role Valorization news and reviews', *SRV/VRS: The International Social Role Valorization Journal/La Revue Internationale de la Valorisation des Rôles Sociaux*, 3(2), 44–55.
(Also published in French in the same issue as: 'La VRS en bref: annotations et nouvelles' (A. Dionne, trans.), 56–69.)

108   Wolfensberger, W. (2000) 'A brief overview of Social Role Valorization', *Mental Retardation*, 38(2), 105–23.

109   Wolfensberger, W. (2000) 'Lessons from WWII martyrs, for the times ahead', *National Catholic Register*, March 5–11, 76(10), 9.

110   Wolfensberger, W. (2001) 'The normative lack of Christian communality in local congregations as the central obstacle to a proper relationship with needy members', *Journal of Religion, Disability & Health*, 4(2/3), 111–26. (Co-published simultaneously in Gaventa, W.C. and Coulter, D.L. (eds) *The Theological Voice of Wolf Wolfensberger* (pp. 111–26), Binghamton, NY: Haworth Pastoral Press.)

111   Wolfensberger, W. (2001) 'Response to the responders', *Journal of Religion, Disability & Health*, 4(2/3), 149–57. (Co-published simultaneously in Gaventa, V.C. and Coulter, D.L. (eds) *The Theological Voice of Wolf Wolfensberger* (pp. 149–57), Binghamton, NY: Haworth Pastoral Press.)

112   Wolfensberger, W. (2001) 'The story of the "Cruickshank chairs" at Syracuse University: a contribution to the history of the brain injury construct', *Mental Retardation*, 39, 472–81.

113   Wolfensberger, W. (2001) 'What advocates have said', *Citizen Advocacy Forum*, 11(2), 4–27.

114   Wolfensberger, W. (2001) 'The problematic nature of the victim role', *SRV/VRS: The International Social Role Valorization Journal/La Revue Internationale de la Valorisation des Rôles Sociaux*, 4(1&2), 10–16.

115   Wolfensberger, W. (2002) 'Needed or at least wanted: sanity in the language wars', *Mental Retardation*, 40, 75–80.

116   Wolfensberger, W. (2002) 'Social Role Valorization and, or versus, "empowerment"', *Mental Retardation*, 40, 252–8.

D) Minor articles, published letters, or articles in minor journals

1   Wolfensberger, W. (1957) 'Patients' chess club proves popular', *Mental Hospitals*, 8, 7.

2   Wolfensberger, W. (1961) 'The free-will controversy' [Letter], *American Psychologist*, 16, 36–7.

3   Wolfensberger, W. (1961) 'A note on "measurement of attitudes to institutionalization" by Jacobs, Butler, and Gorlow', *American Journal of Mental Deficiency*, 66, 290.

4   Wolfensberger, W. and Wilson, J.M. (1961) 'The employee screening program at Greene Valley Hospital and School', *Mind Over Matter* (Publication of Tennessee Dept. of Mental Health), 6, 11–14.

5   Wolfensberger, W. (1962) 'Employee selection at Greene Valley Hospital and School: a further note on local norms for the PTI Oral Directions Test', *Mind Over Matter* (Publication of Tennessee Dept. of Mental Health), 7, 28–9.

6   Wolfensberger, W. (1963) 'IQ scores and genetic trends' [Letter], *Science*, 142, 1620–1.

7   Wolfensberger, W. (1964) 'Reminiscences on a British Psychological Society convention' [Letter], *American Psychologist*, 19, 774–5.

8   Wolfensberger, W. (1964) 'Report on membership survey' *Michigan Civil Service Psychological Association Newsletter*, 4(1), 1–2.

9   Wolfensberger, W. (1964) 'What does the new Michigan community mental health act mean to a parent of a retarded child', *Plymouth Parents Link* (Publication of Plymouth State Home & Training School, MI), 2(1), 4.
     Reprinted in part in: (1964) *The Voice for Detroit Association for Retarded Children*, 4(4), 4.

10   Wolfensberger, W. (1966) 'Whom does AAMD represent?' *Channel 8* (Newsletter of North Central Region (Region 8), American Association on Mental Deficiency), 12(1), 8–9.

11   Wolfensberger, W. (1967) 'Experimentation: rights and risks' [Letter], *Science*, 155, 1618.

12   Wolfensberger, W. (1970) 'Large institutions set fifty year pattern' [Letter], *Focus* (Newsletter of Michigan Assoc. for Retarded Children), (February), 1.

13   Wolfensberger, W. (1970) 'Ideology power', *Nebraska Contributor*, (Publication of Nebraska Office of Mental Retardation), 1(1), 1–6.
     Reprinted in:
     a. Pennsylvania Association for Retarded Children (1970) *Residential Services: Gateway to Change*, Harrisburg, PA: Author.
     b. (1972) *Channel 8* (Newsletter of the North Central Region (Region 8), American Association on Mental Deficiency), (July).
     c. Region V Mental Retardation Services (1977) *Orientation Manual* (pp. 17–22), Lincoln, NE: Author.

14   Wolfensberger, W. (1970) 'Of human courage and dignity', *Mental Retardation News* (Publication of the National Association for Retarded Children, TX), 19(9), 6.
     Adapted and reprinted: Wolfensberger, W. (1970) 'Retarded youth died a hero', *Omaha World Herald*, 19 December.

15   Wolfensberger, W. (1972) 'New battles take shape in state', *Focus on Mental Retardation* (Publication of the Nebraska Assoc. for Retarded Citizens, Lincoln, NE), 4(4), 5.

16   Wolfensberger, W. (1972) 'Former Omahan, Wolf Wolfensberger, writes after hearing of the tragedy' [Letter], *GOARC Gazette* (Publication of the Greater Omaha Assn. for Retarded Citizens, Omaha, NE), August, 15.

17   Wolfensberger, W. (1973) 'A comment on "The sweeping generalization – 'right to read' " ', *Education & Training of the Mentally Retarded*, 8, 159.

18   Wolfensberger, W. (1976) 'Consumer participation in service planning and development', *Déficience Mentale/Mental Retardation*, 26(1), 14. (Appears in French in same issue as: 'La participation des bénéficiaires dans la planification et le developpement des services', 49.)

19   Wolfensberger, W. (1976) 'Comments of "discussion on involving mentally retarded persons to demonstrate teaching techniques before a live audience"', *Déficience Mentale/Mental Retardation*, 26(3), 38–42.

20   Wolfensberger, W. (1977) 'Crime and the elderly', *ADVOCATE! Newsletter* (Publication of Advocates Dedicated to Vigorous Ongoing Change in Attitudes Toward the Elderly, Syracuse, NY), April, 4.

21   Wolfensberger, W. (1978) 'Devaluation of our elderly', *ADVOCATE! Newsletter* (Publication of Advocates Dedicated to Vigorous Ongoing Change in Attitudes Toward the Elderly, Syracuse, NY), March, 3–5.

22   Wolfensberger, W. (1978) 'Prophetic messages', *Letters of L'Arche*, (17), 9–10.

23   Wolfensberger, W. (1978) 'Citizen advocacy is basically a one-to-one relationship', *Advocacy Exchange* (Publication of the Citizen Advocacy Division of the National Association for Retarded Citizens, TX), August, 4–5.

24   Wolfensberger, W. (1979) 'Letter on telethons' [Letter], *Education Unlimited* (Publication of Educational Resources Center, PA), 1(3), 2.

25   Wolfensberger, W. (1979) 'A case against New York State' [Letter], *Mental Retardation*, 17, 268.

26   Wolfensberger, W. (1979) 'Does Christianity imply a policy on integration of handicapped children?', *Special Education* (Newsletter of the Special Education Department, National Catholic Educational Association), 1(2), 1, 6–7.

27   Wolfensberger, W. (1980) 'To whose health?', *ADVOCATE! Newsletter* (Publication of Advocates Dedicated to Vigorous Ongoing Change in Attitudes Toward the Elderly, Syracuse, NY), February, 1–2.

28   Wolfensberger, W. (1980) 'The crucifixions of wounded people', *Unity Grapevine* (Newsletter of Unity Kitchen, Syracuse, NY), March, 4.

29   Wolfensberger, W. (1980) 'The hospice movement', *ADVOCATE Newsletter* (Publication of Advocates Dedicated to Vigorous Ongoing Change in Attitudes Toward the Elderly, Syracuse, NY), May, 5.

30   Wolfensberger, W. (1980) 'The extermination of handicapped people in Nazi Germany', *DD Polestar* (Newsletter of the Developmental Disabilities Training System & Technical Resource Center of Welfare Research, Inc., New York), 1(9), 2–3.

31 Wolfensberger, W. (1980) 'Extermination: disabled people in Nazi Germany', *Disabled USA*, 4(2), 23–4.

32 Wolfensberger, W. (1983) 'Prophecy and reading the signs of the times: a lesson from recent history', *The Unity Grapevine* (Newsletter of Unity Kitchen, Syracuse, NY), September, 3–4.

33 Wolfensberger, W. (1984) ' "Euthanasia" in our society today', *People With Special Needs/Down Syndrome Report*, 6(2), 12.
Reprinted in: (1997) *Inroads* (Newsletter of Person-to-Person Citizen Advocacy Eastern Suburbs, Perth, Western Australia), (5), April–July, 13–16

34 Wolfensberger, W. (1987) 'The peculiar paradox of violence in the language of peace', *The Unity Grapevine* (Newsletter of Unity Kitchen, Syracuse, NY), June, 2.

35 Wolfensberger, W. (1988) 'A painful new ethical dilemma?', *Augustus* (Publication of the National Center on Institutions and Alternatives), 11(2), 12–13

36 Wolfensberger, W. (1989) 'A note of caution about the composition of Citizen Advocacy assessment and consultation teams', *Citizen Advocacy Forum*, 1(1), 7.

37 Wolfensberger, W. (1989) 'Citizen advocates for the dead?' *Citizen Advocacy Formum*, 1(1), 8–10.

38 Wolfensberger, W. (1990) 'Was that the Catholic Church?' [Letter], *The Catholic Sun* (Publication of the Catholic Diocese, Syracuse, NY), 24 January, 5.

39 Wolfensberger, W. (1990) 'Questions Thea House' [Letter] *The Catholic Sun* (Publication of the Catholic Diocese, Syracuse, NY), 110(26), August 8, 5.

40 Wolfensberger, W. (1990) 'Service brokerage sanity and insanity', *The Safeguards Letter* (Publication of the Ohio Safeguards Project, Chillicothe, OH), (16), December, 2–5.

41 Wolfensberger, W. (1991) 'Warning: The U.S. is headed toward de facto military dictatorship', *The Unity Grapevine* (Newsletter of Unity Kitchen Community, Syracuse, NY), (9), 2.

42 Wolfensberger, W. (1991) 'Hype, lies, and mythology in drug promotion', *Biblical Reflections on Modern Medicine*, 2(4), 6–7.

43 Wolfensberger, W. (1991) 'The sad story of a mentally handicapped cannibal', *History and Analysis of Disabilities Newsletter*, (4) Fall, 2.

44 Wolfensberger, W. (1991) [Letter to the editor] *The Catholic Sun* (Publication of the Catholic Diocese, Syracuse, NY), 111(36), Nov 7–13, 2.

45 Wolfensberger, W. (1991) '20th anniversary celebration of Citizen Advocacy and First World Congress', *Citizen Advocacy Forum*, 2(1), 24.

46 Wolfensberger, W. (1991) ' "PC": the new censorship?' [Letter to the editor], *AAMR News & Notes* (Publication of the American Association on Mental Retardation), 4(6), 2, 3.

47   Wolfensberger, W. (1992) 'Effects', *This Brain Has a Mouth* (Rochester, NY), (12), 14–17.

48   Wolfensberger, W. (1992) 'One thing that is not true', *CMHERA (Community & Mental Handicap Educational & Research Association) Newsletter,* No. 1 New Series, April, 10–11.

49   Wolfensberger, W. (1992) 'The "if this, then that" formulation in SRV-related decision-making', *CMHERA (Community & Mental Handicap Educational & Research Association) Newsletter,* No. 1 New Series, April, 4–7.

50   Wolfensberger, W. (1992) 'Citizen Advocacy presentations: some thoughts', *Citizen Advocacy Forum,* 2(2), 10.

51   Wolfensberger, W. (1992) 'A guideline on protecting the health and lives of patients in hospitals, especially if the patient is a member of a societally devalued class', *Citizen Advocacy Forum,* 2(23), 26–7.

52   Wolfensberger, W. (1992) 'A call for Christians to withdraw from organizations that endorse deathmaking', *Biblical Reflections on Modern Medicine,* 3(5) September, 5–6.

53   Wolfensberger, W. (1992) 'More on birth control and Christians' [Letter to the editor], *Biblical Reflections on Modern Medicine,* 3(5) September, 4–5.

54   Wolfensberger, W. (1992) 'A caution against falsely interpreting Citizen Advocacy as having intrinsic ties to various ideologies', *Citizen Advocacy Forum,* 2(5), 11–13.

55   Wolfensberger, W. (1992) ' "Property" by default', *Citizen Advocacy Forum,* 2(5), 20.

56   Wolfensberger, W. (1993) 'A further comment on the 1990 formulation of Citizen Advocacy by the International Citizen Advocacy Safeguards Group', *Citizen Advocacy Forum,* 3(1), 21.

57   Wolfensberger, W. (1993) 'Acquaintanceship and friendship', *Citizen Advocacy Forum,* 3(1), 12.

58   Wolfensberger, W. (1993) 'Reconciling apparent discrepancies between different definitions of advocacy', *Citizen Advocacy Forum,* 3(1), 18.

59   Wolfensberger, W. (1993) 'More on mental retardation language' [Letter to the editor], *AAMR News & Notes* (Publication of the American Association on Mental Retardation), 6(1), 2.

60   Wolfensberger, W. (1993) 'Hidden agenda on feminine priest dolls?' [Letter], *The Catholic Sun* (Publication of the Catholic Diocese, Syracuse, NY), 113(28) August 19–September 1, 2.

61   Wolfensberger, W. (1993) [Letter] *Biblical Reflections on Modern Medicine,* 4(5) September, 5.

62   Wolfensberger, W. (1993) 'Strategies which I employ in order to maintain writing productivity', *CMHERA Newsletter,* (12) September, 19–21. (Earlier and briefer version of item 90 under 'Articles of significant scope and/or in major journals'.)

63   Wolfensberger, W. (1993) 'Questions about short-term Citizen Advocacy relationships as distinguished from crisis citizen advocacies', *Citizen Advocacy Forum,* 3(3), 17–18.

64 Wolfensberger, W. (1993) 'A core reading list on Citizen Advocacy and related topics', *Citizen Advocacy Forum*, 3(3), 25–8.

65 Wolfensberger, W. (1994) 'Courage and fidelity are required, even unto martyrdom', *The Unity Grapevine* (Newsletter of Unity Kitchen, Syracuse, NY), April–May, 6.

66 Wolfensberger, W. and Thomas, S. (1994) 'A few notes from the Training Institute', *Citizen Advocacy Forum*, 4(4), 7.

67 Wolfensberger, W. (1994) 'On advocating a fly to death during an ice storm in December', *Citizen Advocacy Forum*, 4(4), 9.
Reprinted as or in:
a. (1996) *Person to Person: Citizen Advocacy Newsletter* (Newsletter of the Person to Person: Citizen Advocacy Office, Syracuse, NY), September, 3.
b. (1997) 'When rights clash with the welfare of the person: a brief commentary from Wolf Wolfensberger', *Inroads: The Newsletter of Person-to-Person Citizen Advocacy Eastern Suburbs* (Perth, Australia), (6), 7.

68 Wolfensberger, W. (1994) 'What is grey integration, and is it good or bad?' *SRV/VRS: The International Social Role Valorization Journal/La Revue Internationale de la Valorisation des Rôles Sociaux*, 1(2), 35–6.
(Also published in French in the same issue as: 'Qu'est-ce que l'intégration grise, est-ce bon ou mauvais?', 36.)

69 Wolfensberger, W. (1995) 'History of a Swiss-German family: 1400 to 1995. The lineage of Dr. Wolf Wolfensberger's family', *Wolfensberger* (Newsletter of the Wolfensberger Family Association), 1(2) April, 8.

70 Wolfensberger, W. (1996) 'Wolfensberger tid-bits', *Citizen Advocacy Forum*, 6(2), 13.

71 Wolfensberger, W. (1997) 'AAMR professional conduct guidelines questioned', *AAMR News & Notes* (Publication of the American Association on Mental Retardation), 10(1), 2, 8.

72 Wolfensberger, W. (1997) 'A small thought about big Citizen Advocacy', *Citizen Advocacy Forum*, 7(2), 11.

73 Wolfensberger, W. (1997) 'A "Wolf note" ', *Citizen Advocacy Forum*, 7(2), 18.

74 Wolfensberger, W. (2000) 'Lessons from WWII martyrs, for the times ahead', *National Catholic Register*, 76(10) March 5–11, 9.

75 Wolfensberger, W. (2000) 'A note on spans across the seas', *Citizen Advocacy Forum*, 10(1), 16.

76 Wolfensberger, W. (2000) 'Time to think about establishing a Citizen Advocacy archive', *Citizen Advocacy Forum*, 10(1), 12.

77 Wolfensberger, W. (2000 and 2001) 'Yes, it's free: a tribute to Helen Zauha', *Citizen Advocacy Forum*, 10(2) and 11(1) , 29.

78 Wolfensberger, W. (2002) 'Some thoughts about the connection of the von Wolfsberg family to Rapperswil', *Wolfensberger Family Association Newsletter*, 8(1), 5–6.

E) Reviews

This section of the bibliography has the following order: title of the review, if any; item being reviewed and where it appears; where the review appeared; co-author, if any.

1 Reviews of (a) 'Understanding mental retardation', *Public Health News, 1957*, 38, Whole No. 10; (b) 'Proceedings of the Institute for Nurses on Mental Retardation', *Public Health News*, 1960, 41, Whole No. 9. In *American Journal of Mental Deficiency*, 1961, 66, 326–7.

2 Review of Thorne, G.D. (1965) *Understanding the Mentally Retarded*, New York: McGraw-Hill. In *American Journal of Mental Deficiency*, 1965, 70, 493–4.

3 Review of Robinson, H.G. and Robinson, N. (1965) *The Mentally Retarded: A Psychological Approach*, New York: McGraw-Hill. In *American Journal of Mental Deficiency*, 1965, 70, 623–5.

4 'Shortcomings and handicaps', reviews of (a) Adler, S. (1964) *The Nonverbal Child*, Springfield, IL: Charles C. Thomas; (b) Willey, R. DeV. and Waite, K.B. (1964) *The Mentally Retarded Child: Identification, Acceptance, and Curriculum*, Springfield, IL: Charles C. Thomas; (c) McNeice, W.C. and Benson, K.R. (1964) *Through Their Hands They Shall Learn: Crafts for Retarded*, Bloomington, IL: McKnight; (d) Abraham, W. (1964) *The Slow Learner*, New York: Center for Applied Research in Education. In *Contemporary Psychology*, 1966, 11, 70–8.

5 'Memories of childhood shared with an MR sister', review of Sowby, M. (1969) *Dorothea: The Story of a Retarded Child 50 Years Ago*, Toronto, Canada: United Church of Canada. In *Mental Retardation News*, 1970, 12(3), 5.

6 Review of Blatt, B. (1970) *Exodus from Pandemonium: Human Abuse and a Reformation of Public Policy*, Boston: Allyn & Bacon. In *Exceptional Children*, 1971, 37, 611–12.

7 Reviews of (a) Egg, M. (1969) *The Different Child Grows up*, New York: John Day; (b) Egg, M. (1964) *Educating The Child Who is Different*, New York: John Day; (c) Egg, M. (1964) *When a Child is Different*, New York: John Day. In *Déficience Mentale/Mental Retardation*, 1972, 22(3), 40.

8 Review of Clark, B. (1974) *Enough Room for Joy: Jean Vanier's L'Arche: A Message for Our Time*, Toronto: McClelland & Stewart. In *Canadian Welfare*, 1974, 50(6), 14–17.

9 Review of De Vries-Kruyt, T. (1971) *Small Ship, Great Sea: The Life Story of a Mongoloid Boy*, Toronto: William Collins & Sons (published in the USA as *A Special Gift: The Story of Jan*). In *American Journal of Mental Deficiency*, 1975, 79, 611–21.

10 Review of Murray, J.B. and Murray, E. (1975) *And Say What He Is: The Life of a Special Child*, Cambridge, MA: Massachusetts Institute of Technology. In *American Journal of Mental Deficiency*, 1976, 81, 207–8.

11   Review of Thompson, J.D. and Goldin, G. (1975) *The Hospital: A Social and Architectural Study,* New Haven, CT: Yale University Press. In *Canada's Mental Health,* 1977, 25, (3), 20–2.

12   Review of Rude, C.D. and Baucom, L.D. (eds) (1978) *Implementing Protection and Advocacy Systems: Proceedings of a National Developmental Disabilities Conference,* Lubbock, TX: Research & Training Center in Mental Retardation. In *American Journal of Mental Deficiency,* 1979, 84(2), 215–16.

13   'The History of Woodlands: 100 Years of Progress – A revision of a revisionist history of a provincial institution site', review of Adolph, V. (1978) *The History of Woodlands: 100 Years of Progress,* Victoria, British Columbia: Ministry of Human Resources. In *Canada's Mental Health,* 1980, 28(3), 21–2.

14   '*The Prophetic Imagination*: An interpretive review of Walter Brueggemann's book', review of Brueggeman, W. (1978) *The Prophetic Imagination,* Philadelphia: Fortress Press. In *The Unity Grapevine* (Newsletter of Unity Kitchen, Syracuse, NY), Jan/Feb 1983, 2–6.

15   Review of *The Client* (1979) 27 min., color, 16mm, New York: Focus International, Inc. In *Rehabfilm Newsletter,* 1983, 5(2), 12–13 (co-authored with S. Thomas).

16   'A history of one of the world's largest institutions for the mentally retarded', review of Cranford, P. (1981) *But for the Grace of God: The Inside Story of the World's Largest Insane Asylum. Milledgeville!,* Augusta, GA: Great Pyramid Press. In *Institutions, Etc.* (Publication of the National Center on Institutions and Alternatives), 1985, 8(8), 20–2.

17   'Racial Hygiene: Medicine Under the Nazis', review of Proctor, R. (1988) *Racial Hygiene: Medicine Under the Nazis,* Cambridge, MA: Harvard University Press. In *American Journal on Mental Retardation,* 1990, 95(3), 362–7; reprinted as 'Review of Proctor, R. (1988) *Racial Hygiene: Medicine under the Nazis*'. In: *CRTI Report* (Publication of the Center for the Rights of the Terminally Ill), 1991, 5(3), Supplement.

18   Review of Reiss, M. and Daley, K. (1989) *Building Bridges: Stories from the Springfield Citizen Advocacy Project,* Springfield, MA: Springfield Citizen Advocacy Project. In *Citizen Advocacy Forum,* 1991, 2(1), 14 (co-authored with S. Thomas).

19   Review of Emerson, E. (1992) 'What is normalisation?', in H. Brown and H. Smith (eds) *Normalisation: A Reader for the 1990s* (pp. 1–18), London: Routledge. In *CMHERA Newsletter* (Publication of the Community & Mental Handicap Education & Research Association, London), 1992, 3 (July), 3–6.

20   'Review of current service ideologies', review of Shaddock, A.J. and Zilber, D. (1991) 'Current service ideologies and responses to challenging behaviour: Social Role Valorization or vaporization?', *Australia & New Zealand Journal of Developmental Disabilities,* 17(2), 169–75. In *SRV/VRS: The International*

Social Role Valorization Journal/La Revue Internationale de la Valorisation des Rôles Sociaux, Spring 1994,1(1), 49–50.

21 'Review of "Impact of Federal Regulations" ', review of Holburn, C.S. and Jacobson, J.W. (1993) 'Impact of federal regulations on desired processes and outcomes in public residential facilities: national perspectives', *Journal of Developmental & Physical Disabilities*, 5(2), 109–20. In *SRV/VRS: The International Social Role Valorization Journal/La Revue Internationale de la Valorisation des Rôles Sociaux*, Fall 1994, 1(2), 53.

22 'Review of "Drugs: a case for normalization" ', review of Engelsman, E.L. (1989) 'Drugs: a case for normalization', paper presented at a conference of the Victorian Drug Rehabilitation & Research Fund, Melbourne, Australia, 10–12 November 1989. In *SRV/VRS: The International Social Role Valorization Journal/La Revue Internationale de la Valorisation des Rôles Sociaux*, Fall 1994, 1(2), 54–5.

23 'Review of "Normalization: theory and practice" ', review of Race, D.G. (1987) 'Normalization: theory and practice', in N. Malin (ed.) *Reassessing Community Care* (pp. 62–79), London: Croom Helm (paperback edition, 1988). In *SRV/VRS: The International Social Role Valorization Journal/La Revue Internationale de la Valorisation des Rôles Sociaux*, Fall 1994, 1(2), 55.

24 'Review of "Putting People First" ', review of Brandon, D. and Brandon, A. (1988) *Putting People First: A Handbook on the Practical Application of Ordinary Living Principles*, London: Good Impressions. In *SRV/VRS: The International Social Role Valorization Journal/La Revue Internationale de la Valorisation des Rôles Sociaux*, Fall 1994, 1(2), 55.

25 Review of Sobsey, D. (1994) *Violence and Abuse in the Lives of People with Disabilities: The End of Silent Acceptance?*, Baltimore: Paul H. Brookes. In *American Journal on Mental Retardation*, 1995, 100(2), 217–21.

26 'Normalization and deinstitutionalization of mentally retarded individuals: controversy and facts', review of Landesman, S. and Butterfield, E. G. (1987) 'Normalization and deinstitutionalization of mentally retarded individuals: controversy and facts', *American Psychologist*, 42(8), 809–17. In *SRV/VRS: The International Social Role Valorization Journal/La Revue Internationale de la Valorisation des Rôles Sociaux*, Spring 1996, 2(1), 38–9.

27 'Review of A.L. Chappell's (1992) "Towards a sociological critique of the normalisation principle"', review of Chappell, A.L. (1992) 'Towards a sociological critique of the normalisation principle', *Disability, Handicap & Society*, 7(1), 35–51. In *SRV/VRS: The International Social Role Valorization Journal/La Revue Internationale de la Valorisation des Rôles Sociaux*, 1998, 1(1), 37–47.

F) Poems

1   Wolfensberger, W. (1967) 'Geneticist's nightmare', *The Worm Runner's Digest* (Publication of the Mental Health Research Institute, University of Michigan), 9, 110.

2   Wolfensberger, W. (1971) 'Christmas carol for human management personnel', *GOARC Gazette* (Publication of the Greater Omaha Assoc. for Retarded Citizens, Omaha, NE), 3(2), 12.

3   Wolfensberger W. (1971) 'Farewell to Nebraska', *Focus on Mental Retardation* (Publication of the Nebraska Assoc. for Retarded Citizens, Lincoln, NE), 3(4), 3.

4   Wolfensberger, W. ('Sarah Binks') (1973) 'Hail, up and raise the ComServant', *ComServant* (Publication of Saskatchewan ComServ), (2) December, 1.

5   Wolfensberger, W. ('Sarah Binks') (1974) 'Study, study, study, study', *ComServant* (Publication of Saskatchewan ComServ), (4) October, 3.

6   Wolfensberger, W. ('E.A. Stern') (1975) 'Me thinks Binks stinks!', *ComServant* (Publication of Saskatchewan ComServ), (5) September, 3.

G) Interviews

1   Soeffing, M.Y. (1974) 'Normalization of services for the mentally retarded – a conversation with Dr. Wolf Wolfensberger' CEC ERIC's The Now Way to Know, *Education & Training of the Mentally Retarded*, 9(4), 202–8.

Index

CPSIA information can be obtained at www.ICGtesting.com
Printed in the USA
LVOW10s1826250913

353909LV00001B/1/P